Psychiatrists on Psychiatry

Psychiatrists on Psychiatry

Conversations with Leaders

Edited by
DINESH BHUGRA
CBE, MA, MSc, MBBS, DSc(Hon), PhD, FRCP, FRCPE, FRCPsych, FFPHM, FRCPsych(Hon), FHKCPsych (Hon), FACPsych (Hon), FAMS (Singapore), FKCL, MPhil, LMSSA, FAcadME, FRSA, DIFAPA
Professor Emeritus, Mental Health & Cultural Diversity, IoPPN, Kings College, London

Associate Editors
MARIANA PINTO DA COSTA, MD, PHD, MSC
Institute of Psychiatry, Psychology and Neurosciences, London

HUSSIEN EL-KHOLY, MBBCH, MSC, MD, MRCPSYCH
Associate Professor of Psychiatry, Neurology and Psychiatry Department, Faculty of Medicine, Ain Shams University, Egypt

ANTONIO VENTRIGLIO, MD, PHD
University of Foggia, Foggia, Italy

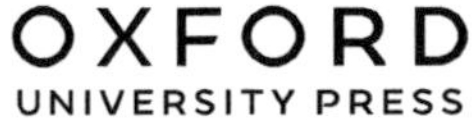
OXFORD
UNIVERSITY PRESS

OXFORD
UNIVERSITY PRESS

Great Clarendon Street, Oxford, OX2 6DP,
United Kingdom

Oxford University Press is a department of the University of Oxford. It furthers the University's objective of excellence in research, scholarship, and education by publishing worldwide. Oxford is a registered trade mark of Oxford University Press in the UK and in certain other countries

First Edition published in 2023

Published in the United States of America by Oxford University Press
198 Madison Avenue, New York, NY 10016, United States of America

British Library Cataloguing in Publication Data
Data available

Library of Congress Control Number: 2022943971

ISBN 978–0–19–885395–4

DOI: 10.1093/med/9780198853954.001.0001

Printed and bound by
CPI Group (UK) Ltd, Croydon, CR0 4YY

To Vera Sartorius and Norman Sartorius for their friendship and guidance with affection

Contents

Interviewees

1. **Professor Renee Binder**—Professor and Director of the Psychiatry and Law Program. Associate Dean for Academic Affairs, University of California, San Francisco School of Medicine and former President of the American Psychiatric Association.
2. **Dame Fiona Caldicott**—Former Master of Somerville College Oxford and former President of the Royal College of Psychiatrists. Dame Fiona Caldicott was the National Data Guardian for Health and Social Care for England.
3. **Professor Silvana Galderisi**—Professor of Psychiatry and Director of the training school in Psychiatry at the University of Campania Luigi Vanvitelli (SUN), Italy. Former President of the European Psychiatric Association (EPA).
4. **Sir David Goldberg**—Emeritus Professor Kings College, London and advisor to the World Health Organisation; he developed the General Health Questionnaire (GHQ) and established Primary Care Psychiatry. He chaired the Guideline for Depression in Physical Diseases for the National Institute for Health and Care Excellence (NICE).
5. **Dr Billy Jones**—Clinical Professor of Psychiatry at New York University and President/CEO of New York City Health and Hospitals Corporation. Commissioner of NYC Dept. of Mental Health; Medical Director at Lincoln Hospital and Senior Associate Dean at New York Medical College.
6. **Professor Shigenobu Kanba**—Former President of the Japanese Society of Psychiatry and Neurology. Programme Supervisor and Officer of the Japan Agency for Medical Research and Development and is involved with the Tokyo Metropolitan Institute of Medical Science, the Japanese Association of Medical Sciences, the Japanese Medical Science Federation and the Science Council of Japan.
7. **Dr Marianne Kastrup**—Consultant, Dignity—Danish Institute against Torture, Copenhagen. She headed the Competence Centre Transcultural Psychiatry, Copenhagen University Hospital, Denmark and has been on the executive boards of European Psychiatry Association and World Psychiatric Association.
8. **Professor Linda Lam**—Professor at the Chinese University of Hong Kong, former President of the Hong Kong College of psychiatrists and former Chief Editor of the East Asian Archives of Psychiatry. Dr Lam is also the founding President of the Chinese Dementia Research Association in 2009.
9. **Professor Saul Levin**—Professor at George Washington University, Washington DC, and CEO and Medical Director of the American Psychiatric Association.
10. **Professor Mario Maj**—Professor and Head of the Department of Psychiatry at the University of Naples. Former President of the European Psychiatric Association and World Psychiatric Association, and Editor of World Psychiatry.

11. **Professor Felice Lieh Mak**—Emeritus Professor of Hong Kong University and former President of the Hong Kong College of Psychiatrists and World Psychiatric Association. Chair of the Hong Kong Medical Council.
12. **Dr Sarada Menon**—Founder of the Schizophrenia Research Foundation (SCARF), an NGO in Chennai. Previously Superintendent of the state-run Madras Mental Hospital (now the Institute of Mental Health), and led on psychosocial rehabilitation by setting up industrial therapy centres and psychiatric facilities in district general hospitals in the state of Tamil Nādu.
13. **Professor Driss Moussaoui**—Emeritus Professor of the University of Casablanca, Morocco, and former President of the World Association of Social Psychiatry. Executive Committee member of the World Psychiatric Association, and President of the International Federation of Psychotherapy.
14. **Dr Carol Nadelson**—Professor of Psychiatry at Harvard Medical School, and former President of the Massachusetts Psychiatric Society, the American Psychiatric Association, the Association for Academic Psychiatry, the Group for the Advancement of Psychiatry, and the American College of Psychoanalysts.
15. **Professor Ahmed Okasha**—Professor of Psychiatry and Past-President of the World Psychiatric Association. Honorary President of the Arab Federation of Psychiatrists, and the Egyptian Psychiatric Association.
16. **Professor Tarek Okasha**—Professor of Psychiatry at Ain-Shams University, and Director of the World Psychiatric Association. President of the Egyptian Alzheimer Society, and the Arab Board of Psychiatry.
17. **Professor Maria Oquendo**—Ruth Meltzer Professor and Chairman of Psychiatry at the Perelman School of Medicine, University of Pennsylvania. President of the American Foundation for Suicide Prevention, and former President of the American Psychiatric Association.
18. **Sir Michael Rutter**—Emeritus Professor of Child Psychiatry at Kings College London. He was the first chair of child Psychiatry in the UK and directed the MRC Unit of Child Psychiatry. He subsequently became director of the Social Genetic and Development centre for its first five years.
19. **Professor Norman Sartorius**—Former President of the European Psychiatric Association and World Psychiatric Association. He is the President of the Association for the Improvement of Mental Health Programmes and a member of the Geneva Prize Foundation.
20. **Professor Alan Schatzberg**—Kenneth T Norris Professor of Psychiatry and Behavioural Sciences. Previously the Chair of the Department at Stanford University School of Medicine, and Director of the Mood Disorders Centre. Also a former President of the American Psychiatric Association.
21. **Dr Nada Stotland**—Consultant Psychiatrist, and former President of the American Psychiatric Association. Previous Director of Consultation/Liaison Psychiatry, Director of Psychiatric Education, Medical Coordinator for the State of Illinois

Department of Mental Health, and Chair of Psychiatry at the Illinois Masonic Medical Center.

22. **Professor Paul Summergrad**—Dr Frances S Arkin Professor of Medicine and Psychiatry at Tufts University, Boston. Former President of the American Psychiatric Association, Tufts Medical Center, and Secretary for Finances of the World Psychiatric Association.
23. **Dr Thara Rangaswamy**—Dr Rangaswamy set up the Schizophrenia Research Foundation in Chennai with Dr Menon, and remained involved as Director, setting up innovative services for rehabilitation and care of people with dementia using tele-mental health approaches.
24. **Professor Pichet Udomratn**—Emeritus Professor at the Songkla University in Thailand. Former President of the Psychiatric Association of Thailand, Pacific Asia Rim College of Psychiatrists, Asian Federation of Psychiatric Associations, and ASEAN Federation of Psychiatry and Mental Health.
25. **Professor Rutger Jan van der Gaag**—Emeritus Professor at the Department of Psychosomatic Medicine and Psychotherapy of the Riga Stradins University, Latvia, and former President of the Netherlands Psychiatric Association, and the Royal Dutch Medical Association.
26. **Dr Lakshmi Vijayakumar**—Founder of Sneha, Chennai, for the prevention of suicide. Head of the Department of Psychiatry, Voluntary Health Services, Chennai, and a member of the WHO's International Network for Suicide Research and Prevention. Vice President of the International Association of Suicide Prevention.

Introduction

What makes a good leader? Are leaders born or are they made? Can anyone be a leader? What are the differences between a good leader who can bring about sustained, real change and those who occupy leadership positions for the sake of personal glory? This book aims to explore some of these questions in depth by interviewing leaders in psychiatry.

The idea for the book came from Professor Norman Sartorius many years ago. A major reason for collecting the life stories of leaders in psychiatry emerged from discussions which took place during various leadership courses. For example, a good researcher or academic does not always translate into a good leader. Equally it is important for the younger generation of psychiatrists to remember not only the contributions various leaders have made in different areas, whether research, teaching, clinical developments, or policy, but more importantly they carry with them institutional memory. Being reminded of what it was like in earlier times, how things were then, and how leaders changed things or contributed to change in research, policy, teaching and clinical services is critical so that we do not keep repeating history.

What is leadership? It can be seen as an ability to convince people to follow and go with someone at the helm. There are different types of leadership styles and the purpose of leadership can change according to the situation, from leading from the front to shepherding people. We all know a lot about political leaders who tend to follow personal agendas, dogma, or political ideology which may or may not convert to the betterment of populations. Inevitably, leadership in various professional settings carries with it a number of roles and responsibilities. Key components of the definition of leadership include role, responsibilities, processes, and conceptual thinking. Each of these aspects carries with it notions of real and perceived power which can be used or misused by the leader. There are leadership roles which can be short or long term and each carry different concepts and actions with it. Leaders can also bring about transformation which can be transitional or permanent. It can be argued that some of the skills in leadership roles can be found in common across various roles and responsibilities and for other purposes specific skills may be required.

For leaders in transformative roles, their main function is to manage change in the short, medium or long term. They will need different skills with a clear focus on influencing individuals to deal with the leadership processes when decisions are made. In these circumstances, leaders have to be excellent communicators. In order to lead, the leader has to have followers; people who are willing to allow the individual to take charge for the betterment of the individual, community, or both. Leaders can lead from the front or from behind, be either directive or directional. Leaders are not above their followers but the power differential between the leaders and followers can play an important role in achieving and delivering the leader's vision. In some cultures, leaders are given an automatic higher status and followers may feel that their leader can do no wrong. It is important to recognize that the skills needed for leadership roles are conceptual, technical, emotional, communicative, and incorporate a broad understanding of issues that are facing the organization, institution, or the community. Often leaders can delegate tasks to the right people around them to help achieve their ambitions and aims. The individuals around the leader must have complementary skills so that a linked-up style can be formed. A good leader must be able to think creatively but also needs to be aware of their own personal strengths and weaknesses.

The interviews in this book highlight cultural similarities in leadership styles and also cultural differences which influence healthcare systems. As will become clear from these interviews, leadership is a process as well as a trait. Very often the skills that an individual has in adulthood are a result of development and lessons learned as a child which are very strongly influenced by the culture in which leaders have been born and brought up. Family influences and early life can have a major impact on individual's outlook and vision.

Virtually every leader who has been interviewed in this book illustrates the importance of childhood upbringing, support, a secure family environment, and expectations of their family. These traits encourage leaders to treat their followers in a confident way by challenging them and questioning in non-threatening ways. Skills needed in leadership roles must include a degree of technical competence. This means that leaders must understand their subject, be proficient and up-to-date with recent developments, and able to share their ideas and vision in cogent fashion. An understanding of complex technical nature of the subject is helpful but essential when trying to communicate these ideas not only to team members but also to policy-makers and other stakeholders in a simple, easy way for the purpose of advocacy for psychiatric patients who are very often ignored by healthcare providers. Several leaders in this volume have illustrated their role as advocates and innovators in developing and delivering services. Creating an environment of trust and sharing ideas ensures that leaders are sensitive to the needs of the team be that a large or a small one

Some of the leaders interviewed in this book are technical leaders in the field too. Their energy, enthusiasm, and commitment shine through these interviews. Through humour and communication, they illustrate emotional intelligence. The leader must also be aware of conceptual skills which comprise the ability to work with ideas; this is where thinking out of the box can help. Often having an idea is not enough and the leader must be able to share these; communication is vital. Equally importantly, leaders must be prepared to be challenged about the validity of their ideas and have the skills to change their mind in view of new evidence without feeling threatened. A good leader can turn their ideas into strategy and vision.

As is evident from the experience of the leaders interviewed for this volume, personal individual styles of leadership do matter but there are common features which are to do with vision, communication, the ability to stand up for their vision, finding ways to manage, deal with, or eliminate problems, and move the organization, unit, or institution forward. The leadership style can be both directive and supportive. Another point worth noting is that good leaders will change their leadership style according to the situation and the need. Organizations can also generate leaders. Individual personality traits also play a major role and are often inherited though certain traits can be overcome or managed in effective ways. Some skills such as communication can be learnt.

Often leadership and management are confused, especially in the context of healthcare systems. Leaders have vision, their role is to do the right thing whereas managers are supposed to do things right. Managers may have to manage complexity and leader will set out their vision and the direction of the organization.

In psychodynamic teams, leadership is about childhood development, attachment patterns, and the ability to use personality traits in a way to achieve their vision. Successful leaders, as exemplified in this volume, have shown time and again that they are good at coming up with an idea or a series of ideas, developing the vision to put this idea into practice, and then communicating their vision and strategy clearly. More often than not they have overcome various obstacles in their personal or professional lives and have had to managed conflict with others but also within themselves.

Problem-solving is an essential part of the role of leader in recognizing the nature of the problem, assessing of the potential impact, looking at various possible solutions, then choosing the right one, communicating it clearly, and taking responsibility for the actions and the outcomes. Problems can be managed using a number of approaches. Good leaders can delegate responsibilities but they are also keen to have succession planning and mentoring in place. The act of delegation is not about handing over difficult problems to the people leaders do not like but instead moulding skills and capabilities to ensure that not only the problems are solved but appropriate development at the personal level can be put in place for those that follow. Leadership is about leading the people and the organization; the focus is on the future developments and achievements.

The leaders interviewed for this volume have been researchers and teachers. They have developed services and non-governmental organizations. They have led departments and national and international organizations. All of the interviewees recorded here were asked same questions; their responses and follow up questions have varied. The interviews were recorded transcribed and then edited by DB and the interviewees. Professor Mario Maj preferred to offer his responses in writing. Regrettably, Dr Fiona Caldicott, Dr Sarada Menon and Sir Michael Rutter passed away but their families have been kind enough to give us permission to go ahead with the interview for which we are immensely grateful. The choice of interviewees is purely personal and regrettably we could not accommodate all who had expressed an interest to be included. The loss is entirely ours.

I would like to thank associate editors Doctors Mariana Pinto da Costa, Hussien El-Kholy, and Antonio Ventriglio for their diligence and hard work in interviewing, transcribing and editing some of the interviews.

Thanks are due to Ms Sagupta Ghosh and Ms Trisha Rudra who transcribed the interviews with great diligence. Dr Susham Gupta did a huge amount of work behind the scenes for which I am truly grateful.

Ms Sue Duncan coordinated the final stages for which thanks. Pete Stevenson, Adam Breivik and Rachel Goldsworthy of Oxford University Press were true believers in the project and their unstinting support has been truly valuable; thanks to them are inadequate.

Dinesh Bhugra

1

Renee Binder

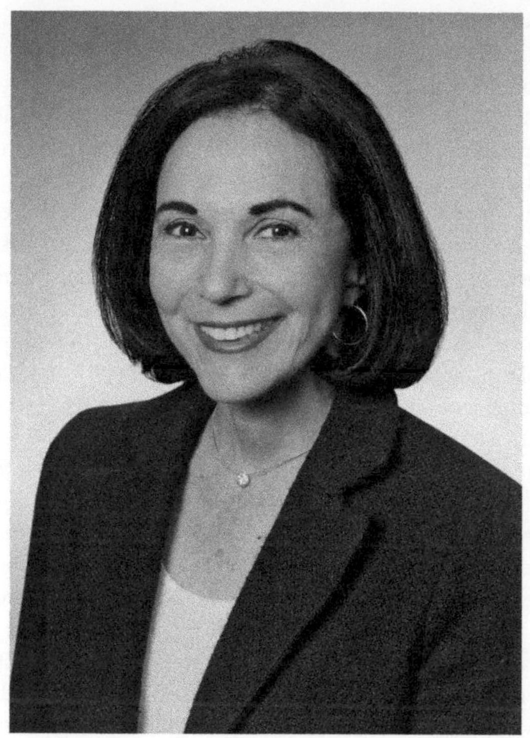

Biography

Dr Renee Binder is a Distinguished Professor of Psychiatry, the Founding Director of the Psychiatry and Law Program and Forensic Psychiatry Fellowship, and Associate Dean for Academic Affairs at the University of California, San Francisco, School of Medicine. She is also a past-President of the American Psychiatric Association (APA) and the American Academy of Psychiatry and the Law.

During her APA Presidential year, Dr Binder focused on advocacy for decriminalization of persons with mental illness. She has devoted her career to studying the clinical and legal aspects of the relationship between violence and mental illness. She has also conducted and published research related to diversion of individuals with mental illness from the criminal justice system to the mental health system as well as problem solving courts, homelessness, and Crisis Intervention Team training for law enforcement.

Dr Binder graduated from Barnard College and went to medical school at the University of California San Francisco. She did her internship and residency in San Francisco. She served as Interim Chair of the Department of Psychiatry and the Director of Langley Porter Psychiatric Hospital and Clinics for over three years. She also has served as Chair of the APA Council on Psychiatry and the Law and the Committee on Judicial Action.

Dr Binder has been an Associate Dean for Academic Affairs at the University of California San Francisco (UCSF) School of Medicine since 2004 and has been an active participant in making UCSF one of the most diverse, inclusive, and family-friendly medical schools and academic environments in the United States.

Dr Binder served as an APA Congressional Health Policy Fellow in the US Senate and worked on legislation related to healthcare reform and improving access to care. She also has a 2018 certificate from the Stanford University Graduate School of Business in 'Innovative Health Care Leadership'.

Dr Binder is the recipient of multiple awards including the Dr J. Elliott Royer Award for academic excellence and significant contributions to the field of academic psychiatry, the American Academy of Psychiatry and the Law's 'Seymour J. Pollack Distinguished Achievement Award' in recognition of distinguished contributions to the teaching and educational functions of forensic psychiatry, the American Academy of Psychiatry and the Law's 'Golden AAPL Award' in recognition of significant contributions to the field of forensic psychiatry, and the 2018 Isaac Ray Award for 'Outstanding Contributions to Forensic Psychiatry or the Psychiatric Aspects of Jurisprudence'.

Interview

I: Wonderful to have you involved here. Perhaps, we can start off by what was it like growing up and what was your childhood like?

RB: I grew up in New York. My father was a cantor and a teacher and my mother was a housewife who then became a guidance counsellor. I'm the middle child of three and all of us wound up going to professional school, because my parents put a high value on helping us get an education. My older sister became a paediatrician and my younger brother became a dentist.

I: What was that like? You have been a trailblazer in lots of ways, in terms of politics and research and clinical services. What drives you?

RB: My older sister was a significant influence on my career choice. She was always the smartest in the family. When I tell people that, they say that I am being modest and that I am really smart also. But honestly, my sister is a brilliant person. We did not have a lot of money and my sister received a scholarship to go to Barnard College, the all-women's college of Columbia University. Her idea was to become a high school biology teacher because that is what smart women from my neighbourhood who were good in science did. She took science courses at Barnard and a lot of the other students were pre-med. It had never occurred to her to be pre-med. We did not know many women physicians. She changed her career choice and went to medical school. Her choice really influenced me. I went to Barnard and also decided to become a physician. In college I was involved in political advocacy. There were all kinds of issues which may not seem very important now, but were seen as important then. My co-students and I tried to influence the administration about issues such as grades, the school bureaucracy, and changing the curriculum. Also at Barnard, they had a court that was run by the students. If someone was accused of cheating or other misconduct, they would come in front of the court, and I became very active in the student court. It was incredibly interesting and people told me that I seemed to be able to think about things in a complex manner and to see all viewpoints. It's very easy to decide that if a student cheated, she should be kicked out of school. I was always suggesting that we should first try and find out what was going on in her life and why she cheated and also to take into account whether this was a chronic issue or a one-time infraction. We would find out if she had significant life stressors, if she was severely depressed, or manic with poor judgement. I think people appreciated my contributions and I would sometimes argue for an unpopular position. These perspectives were probably early precursors to my becoming a psychiatrist and then a forensic psychiatrist.

I: I still remember coming to the meeting that you had organized in DC where you invited the sheriffs of about 300 counties to talk about changing the interaction of law enforcement with people with mental illness, so that was obviously taking a rather unpopular position.

RB: Right.

I: At what point did you decide that you wanted to go into medicine? Was it when you were at Barnard?

RB: I wasn't 100% sure that medicine would be the right career for me. I actually majored in art history but also took pre-med courses. I did my senior thesis on Salvador Dali and Freud's impact on Dali. As part of my thesis, I actually interviewed Salvador Dali. I knew that in the winter he stayed at the St Regis Hotel in Manhattan and so one night I called the St Regis on a whim and I said, 'Can I please talk to Salvador Dali?' The operator put me through and this man with his thickly accented English, said 'yes?' I was so shocked by actually being put through to him and I said, 'Well, I'm a student at Columbia University and I'm writing about you and I wonder if I could interview you?' He said 'Be here at three o'clock tomorrow' and so I went there with my brother as a chaperone. I interviewed him and used that as a part of my thesis about his relationship with Freud. I was interested in art and interested in psychology. Then I started to think about how medicine was a wonderful field and applied to medical schools. Most of my pre-med classmates went to medical school in the northeast area of the United States, I decided it might be interesting to go to San Francisco. At that time, I was not anticipating that I would wind up settling in San Francisco.

I: OK. And at what point did you decide that you wanted to do psychiatry?

RB: I always was interested in psychiatry but then I became fascinated with everything else in medicine. I remember that I really liked ophthalmology because I loved the idea that you could take someone who is blind because of severe cataracts, and could do surgery and help them see again. I liked internal medicine because it was so broad and intellectually stimulating. However, I realized that the most interesting thing for me was to try to figure out how people think and what can go right or wrong with their mental state. That was just the most fascinating thing to me. I found that when I was on other rotations, I would see a patient, take a history, complete my physical exam, write my notes, and then come back to the patient to discuss their emotional reactions and what else was going on in their lives. I just started to think that psychiatry was the most interesting part of medicine because I could learn about the mind and the brain and realized that psychiatry was the field for me.

I: Do you ever regret it?

RB: No. I mean psychiatry has been a fantastic field. It has never been boring, because there are so many different aspects of it. I have spent most of my professional life working with severely disturbed patients. I was the director of the inpatient unit for over 20 years, and I still enjoy working on the inpatient unit a few weeks each year when I cover the service for other attendings. It is rewarding to me to help people who are acutely ill with psychosis, depression, anxiety, or delirium. Together with a team of other professionals, we make interventions, and many of the patients substantially improve. I like working with a team and getting input from many people who may see different aspects of the patient. I also enjoy working within a system of care and with families. My heart goes out to family members who are trying to figure out how to help a beloved son or daughter who is currently psychotic. I work with them to be optimistic about prognosis, but also realistic. It is heart-warming to help these patients and their families.

I: A key part of the role of the psychiatrist, as I see, is giving the patients hope.

RB: Yes. I always try to be optimistic and convey to my patients and their loved ones that treatment really can help. It's rewarding to be able to do this kind of work. There are other aspects of psychiatry which I also enjoy. I work with the legal system and the courts. That work is very interesting and impactful on patients in a different way.

I: Do you run any court diversion programmes?

RB: I am the director of a Forensic Psychiatry Programme and we have contracts with jails, prisons, and the courts. We also work with diversion programmes. I work with medical students, psychiatry residents, and fellows who are advanced trainees. We do evaluations for the courts, and provide treatment in the jails and in the prisons. We work with court systems, judges, and attorneys.

I: Throughout your medical school and psychiatry training who were the people who influenced you, who would you see as your heroes and heroines?

RB: Well, my biggest heroine is my older sister and she is a prominent paediatrician and was Dean of a Medical School. She then got involved in the business world and earned an MBA from Wharton, a top US business school. She then worked on improving quality in healthcare organizations and ensuring equitable treatment of all members. She has been my role model for how to do things.

I: You have been looking after patients for a long time and you have done quite a lot of research. Are there any kind of memorable 'Eureka' moments which stick in your mind either patient-wise or in terms of research?

RB: I think the most exciting aspect of my research has been having the results impact policy and clinical care. For example, San Francisco set up a behavioural health court. When someone committed a crime and had severe mental illness, the person would be offered the opportunity to go to the behavioural health court and get treatment instead of being incarcerated. The court had been operating for a while and then there were proposed budget cuts that threatened the continuation of the court. I was asked to evaluate the court to show the San Francisco Board of Supervisors that the court actually made a difference in outcome. I gathered data, did the research, and was able to show that the courts decreased the number of days in the jails. Based on my research, the court was continued and this was very exciting. Another example is some of the research I have done about the risk factors for violence. We were able to improve risk assessment so that we were less likely to overpredict or underpredict violence.

I: Do you think psychiatry has changed during the period you have begun to practise and, if so, how?

RB: Well, I think the growth of neuroscience has clearly been a huge advance in psychiatry. We now know more about the underpinnings of mental illness. In addition, we have developed more specific and targeted types of psychotherapy that can be helpful to patients. It used to be that psychiatrists listened to patients and tried to understand the patient, but the techniques were not as specific as they are now. Depending on the type of problem, a patient can now be treated with cognitive behavioural therapy, dialectical behaviour therapy, and many other types of therapy.

I: What are your views on the current state of psychiatry? Are we in a good place?

RB: I think we are in a good place, but we have to make sure that we don't forget that we have to talk to patients. Recently, I was in a forum where psychiatrists pose questions to other psychiatrists. One psychiatrist related that she had a patient who was robbed and was very frightened of being severely hurt. She asked, 'What can I do to help her?' One of the consulting psychiatrists said you can give her a medication which will prevent her from storing the memory. I began thinking, 'Is this what psychiatry has come to?' The patient just had a very frightening experience and rather than advising her to block the memory chemically, someone needs to talk to the patient. How did she feel about it? Did it bring back other memories? What other areas of vulnerability does she have that made her feel even more vulnerable. You can't just give something to block a neurotransmitter. Her identity has changed. I hope that we are not moving too much in the direction where we just give medications and don't talk to the patient. We have to remember the complexity of psychiatry. When I was director of the acute inpatient unit, we administered the drug clozapine to patients. I still remember one patient that we treated with clozapine. Her husband walked on the unit and he said to me. 'I can't believe it', and I said, 'your wife is sitting right there, what can't you believe?' and he said, 'she's reading a newspaper. She has not read a newspaper for at least 10 years. She just wasn't interested.' The clozapine had had an incredibly powerful positive effect on her and the husband felt that it had worked magic on his wife. However, the patient would need much more that the clozapine to return to her normal life. She had missed 10 years of her life and would need therapy and other types of rehabilitation. So that's my concern about psychiatry. We need to incorporate all of the neuroscientific findings and not to forget that there is also a human being there. We need to continue to treat the psychological impact of mental illness and understand that when you have a psychiatric illness or a medical illness, it affects how you feel about yourself. A patient may have identity disturbances and other psychological stressors and they need to be able to talk to someone about that.

I: Do you think psychiatry is mindless or brainless?

RB: I don't think that psychiatry is mindless or brainless. Psychiatry a combination of the brain and the mind. We need to work with the whole person.

I: You are absolutely right to say that. What do you see as the problems of the current state of psychiatry?

RB: The problem is that we need to broaden our focus and not think that we will find a magic bullet, which will help us understand the aetiology and the treatment for psychiatric illness. Psychiatric illness is complex. Social and cultural factors have huge impacts on behaviour. We need to integrate therapeutic techniques, listen to patients, and be there in the moment when patients are talking to us. At the same time, we need to use our scientific and medical background, keep up with everything that's going on in the field, know that there could be other causes of the psychiatric illness such as thyroid disease, or infection. We need to use all our medical skills, but social factors are also important. One of the law schools in San Francisco recently set up a programme with geriatric medicine that includes a legal clinic that can deal with the social problems of the patient. For example, a patient may see their physician for hypertension and anxiety. A careful history might reveal that they are being evicted from their living situation and therefore they are anxious and have an elevated blood pressure. Medications alone will not fix their problem. The patients are referred to the law school clinic where law students are knowledgeable about the rights of tenants. The law students don't know anything about the medical aspects of the illness but they can help the patient stay in their apartment or get alternative housing. The medical problems are never going to get better until the social problems and the housing problems are also ameliorated.

I: I don't know what it's like in the States, in terms of recruitment into psychiatry and how would you improve that?

RB: Well, we do pretty well with recruitment.

I: Nationally or locally?

RB: Both locally and nationally. I think that the success of recruitment is related to exposing medical students to role models. When students see psychiatrists, who are doing interesting things and who are excited about their work, the students want to enter the field of psychiatry

I: You mentioned some of the characteristics of a good psychiatrist like being able to listen and doing innovative stuff. What else do you think a good psychiatrist has or should have?

RB: I think a good psychiatrist needs to have compassion and empathy and always be willing to learn about the particular individual that they are treating and what is going on with them. I think it is important to listen carefully to patients. I think a psychiatrist should also be willing to treat patients with serious mental illness and co-morbidities. These patients can be difficult to treat, but they need our services and help.

I: Do you think that's because of the gaps in training or gaps in demand or a mixture of the two?

RB: I think that one of the reasons that some psychiatrists don't want to treat patients with serious mental illness is that they feel that they need to spend too much uncompensated time coordinating the care with other members of the treatment team. In addition, there may not be available resources such as day programmes or hospital beds if the patient needs hospitalization. They don't treat these patients because there are not adequate community resources to help them with the treatment.

I: That takes us neatly into the (i) why don't they advocate for changes in the system and (ii) where does the psychiatry's social contract fit into that. It is a kind of three-way contract between psychiatrist, patients, and the funders, whether it's the government or insurance companies or whatever the system is, how can that be delivered?

RB: I feel very strongly that psychiatrists need to advocate for changes in our system of care. We need to establish relationships with legislators and try and improve health care delivery systems. Organizations such as the American Psychiatric Association can help psychiatrists learn how to do this.

I: And what would you tell your younger self?

RB: I would tell myself to be open to new opportunities about how to make a difference in people's lives. I would encourage myself to accept leadership opportunities even when I feel insecure about my ability to be effective. I would encourage myself to ask for help from mentors and senior leaders. I would encourage myself to continue to think about how psychiatric care can be improved. It is such a privilege to be a physician and be trusted by patients. Also, when we participate in advocacy, our opinions often have more weight than the average person.

I: As President of the American Psychiatric Association what were the challenges and what did you learn from that experience?

RB: I learned that as President of the APA, you actually can make a difference by choosing and trying to tackle several important issues. The issue I chose to highlight most was how people with mental illness wind up in our jails and prisons rather than in our mental health treatment system and the importance of trying to decriminalize mental illness. Under my leadership, the APA developed position statements, had Congressional hearings, convened meetings with stakeholders, and had a large conference to highlight the issues and raise money for the APA Foundation to continue its work on criminal justice initiatives. At that time, a popular American television show was 'Orange is the New Black' about incarcerated women. I invited members of the cast of the TV show to talk at the fundraising event. At the beginning of my Presidential year, at a meeting for the APA Board of Trustees in San Francisco, I arranged for members of the Board of Trustees to visit San Quentin State Prison and meet with some inmates as well as the staff. Another issue I highlighted during my presidency was the use of telepsychiatry as a means of increasing access to care. I convened a Presidential Task Force composed of psychiatrists who were national leaders in this field. They developed many tools and resources for psychiatrists to use to deliver psychiatric care to patients remotely. The results of this initiative have been especially helpful during the recent COVID-19 pandemic.

I: What would you like to be remembered for?

RB: That's an interesting question. I would like to be remembered for my accomplishments as President of the American Psychiatric Association. I also served as the Interim Chair of my Department of Psychiatry for three years. In addition, I started my forensic psychiatry programme. There had never been a programme in San Francisco and now the programme has national prominence. My program has trained outstanding forensic psychiatrists and they have provided high-quality services to the courts. Most importantly, I have two wonderful children. I mean, they are really good human beings who are wonderful parents and wonderful spouses. They have empathy for people and I'm very proud of that. I hope I'll be remembered for that.

I: Are they in medicine?

RB: My daughter is a physician. She is a neurologist who does sleep medicine specializing in behavioural interventions. My son is an attorney who is a partner in an entertainment law firm in Los Angeles.

I: They were there at your inauguration.

RB: They came to my inauguration and it was wonderful to have them there. I think they felt proud of me and wanted to support my presidency.

I: What are you most proud of? You have touched on the APA and your efforts to support the decriminalization of mental illness as things you are proud of. Are there other things that you would be proud of?

RB: I am proud of my efforts to work within the interface of psychiatry and the legal system. I have tried to bring about social change in how society and the legal system treat people who have mental illness and get in trouble with the legal system. I'm proud of my contributions in terms of trying to understand the motivations for people becoming violent and how to mitigate violence. I also have tremendous empathy for victims of violence and am proud of my work in helping victims of trauma and violence.

2

Dame Fiona Caldicott

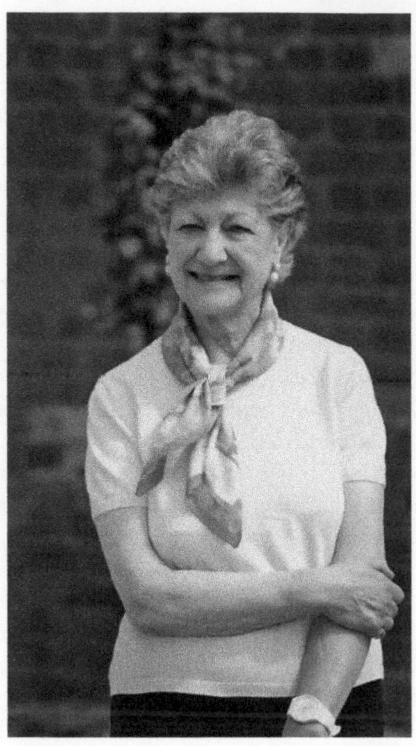

Biography

Dame Fiona Caldicott was the National Data Guardian for Health and Social Care for England. She passed away on 15 February 2021 at the age of 80.

In 2016 she published a review of health and care data security, consent, and opt-outs, which made recommendations to strengthen the security of health and care information and ensure that people can make informed choices about how their data is used. Her previous independent reviews in this area (in 1997 and 2013) had considerable influence on health and care services and led to the appointment of Caldicott Guardians in NHS provider and social care organizations.

Dame Fiona held a wide variety of roles in her illustrious career. She also worked at South Birmingham Mental Health NHS Trust from the mid-1970s to the mid-1990s, where she held several positions: Consultant and Senior Clinical Lecturer in

Psychotherapy, Unit General Manager, Clinical Director, and Medical Director. She retired from her 10-year-long position as Chair of the Oxford University Hospitals NHS Foundation Trust.

Having been Sub-Dean and Dean of the Royal College of Psychiatrists, she became its first Woman President (1993–1996), proudly noting that she was the first doctor to become a President of a Medical Royal College who had trained part time. She was also Chair of the Academy of Medical Royal Colleges (1995–1996).

She led the Royal College's work on Care in the Community, on staffing levels in the specialties of psychiatry, the overseas doctors' training scheme, and keenly supported the establishment of College offices in Belfast, Dublin, Edinburgh, and Cardiff.

She served as Principal of Somerville College at the University of Oxford from 1996 to 2010 and was Pro Vice-Chancellor in the University of Oxford, with responsibility for Personnel and Equality.

Interview

I: Thanks very much for taking the time for this interview.
The book is going to be aimed at trainees and other psychiatrists who are interested in what they need to learn from other people's experiences and learn about institutional memory. You have been really exceptional in UK psychiatry for all the things that you've done over the years and being the first woman President of the College and then going on to Somerville College as Master. What are the lessons for the next generations? So if we start off by hearing something about your childhood and what it was like growing up.

FC: I grew up in a suburb of London although I was born in Scotland during the war. My father was a chemist and he worked in a munitions factory, so I came to London when I was three and a half and I grew up there until I went to university at 19. I'm the older of two. My sister was born nearly six years after me, after the war. The important thing that I think about our childhood is that my grandfather was a greengrocer. His family had come from Continental Europe during the escape from repression. My father was a really firm believer in education but had to leave school at 16 to help his father at the shop. However, he got himself a bachelor's degree in Chemistry through evening classes and went on to get a law degree by correspondence. He was a great believer in education with two daughters, and didn't see any difference in how they would be educated if they were sons. I think that was an important thing during our childhood. I went to a direct grant school when I was 11, the City of London School for Girls, which was a school that set high aspirations for its students compared with some other girls' schools where their highest achievement would be, let's say, school teaching and nursing. Certainly the City of London saw that their girls could become members of all professions. And I decided quite early on that I was interested in medicine; very interestingly my favourite subject in school was history. My interest in medicine was stimulated by a book called *The Story of San Michele* by a Swedish doctor called Axel Munthe. It's a reminiscence about his career and I read it when I was like 10 or 11. It is a very inspiring book. In order to do medicine I had to give up subjects I liked, like history.

I tried to go to Cambridge in my second year of sixth form and failed. So I stayed at school to do an extra year thus improving my A levels and my CV. In the early part of that academic year I was offered an interview at Oxford and immediately that led to an offer of a place at Kings College Medical School. Quite interesting that London schools continued turning me down until I got an interview at Oxford. In those days, Somerville College attracted girls who wanted to do medicine and science because of its history, so like many of those girls I applied to Somerville and was sent to interviews, to other colleges, and was offered a place at St Hilda's which I accepted. I tell that story because it's relevant to later years when I was offered a different position at Somerville. I mean, my A-level results were really awful because I had been head girl in second year sixth, I think that probably is relevant to the rest of my career but it's difficult looking back to be sure. I think that the confidence of the teachers and the headmistress that I could fill such a role probably was quite good for me.

I: It's really fascinating to see the steps, particularly your interest in medicine because it obviously seems like a single book inspired you.

FC: As mentioned earlier, I think part of the story about Axel Munthe did inspire me. Also, my father became a patent lawyer and worked for Shell all his life after the war. He had a very prejudiced view that women shouldn't go into the law as they were much too emotional to become lawyers.

I: But they were emotionally OK to be doctors?

FC: Well, I'm not sure. (laughs). I did not really explore it (with him) but anyway it did not put me off. I suppose like most people wanting to do medicine, I do like other people like individual people and I like science, so it just seemed right. It was a very long-held aspiration, unlike some young doctors who think about it when they do their A levels or something. I was not to be deterred by getting really poor A levels. So getting into Oxford, the first member of the family to go to university, that was all very exciting. I thoroughly enjoyed the course. The course in Oxford and Cambridge is quite scientifically based as you know, and you end up with the science degree before you do your clinical studies and I think that was right for me. Well then again, I had some failures at university. I didn't do enough work, got distracted as many do. So part of my story is about some early failures that looked as if they might jeopardize what I really wanted to do and I think that's an important lesson actually.

I: Your clinical postings were in Oxford or were they in London?

FC: When I was deciding where to do clinical, I was engaged to someone who was on the medical course and we decided to stay in Oxford. Just before that there was a rather dramatic event when the relationship broke up and I decided to come to London. So I went to Westminster when it was a separate medical school which had great clinical training because there were a very small number of students to examine the patients. It had very, very good leading edge medicine going on such as early kidney transplants and so on. And in the middle of that course I got engaged to my now husband who's not a medic and that led to me applying to go to Birmingham to finish my medical training. And that led to the Professor of Psychiatry a few years later saying, when I applied for a more senior training job, 'Dr Caldicott you went to rather a lot of medical schools' or an unusual number of medical schools. The deans of the day took interest in women students' careers and they were probably more flexible when in practice. Anyway, I went to Birmingham and had the opportunity to work in local hospitals. I was the only student doing surgery and doing obstetrics in two postings, so had very good clinical training where I was given a lot of experience. After qualifying, I made the decision that I wouldn't go full-time into medicine because I was already pregnant. So the ambition that I gave up at that point was to go into academic medicine which didn't seem realistic for someone with a child. We are talking of a time when there were 10 women on the course in Oxford out of a 100 students. I think at that point, Guy's and Tommy's (St Thomas Hospital) and Kings used to take two women in a year, so it was a very different environment in which I qualified. I had the baby and immediately, really within weeks, I wanted to go back to work. I mean that. I had done a brief locum in emergency medicine and I went to a family friend who was a GP who gave me two afternoon surgeries a week. And my part-time work built up from there because during that period the local hospital was rebuilt with a small psychiatric unit. So I was working in general practice but had the opportunity to apply for a clinical assistant session in psychiatry, which I obtained, and I think that interest goes back to my tutor in Oxford, who was a married woman, a neurophysiologist, with three children and a very successful research career and was for me an inspiration. She was very much a woman who could succeed in medicine while fulfilling family responsibilities. I think that interest in the nervous system plus my enjoyment of general practice with the experience of lots of different patients from all sorts of backgrounds really led to my applying for the session in psychiatry and I've never regretted it. One of your questions is have I ever regretted that? No, absolutely not. I think it's a fantastic specialty, provided you have got that particular orientation of liking human beings with all their frailties but also the application of science to medicine.

I: For me one of thc interesting things about psychiatry is that it's very much person based but it is also about application of art and science along with a number of other fields which makes it really exciting and unique really. There are also quite a lot of parallels between general practice and psychiatry because quite often people who choose primary care or psychiatry are very similar minded, more art-based rather than craft, in that sense. At what point did you switch to full psychiatry training and then psychotherapy?

FC: While I was doing the one session at the local hospital and the general practice, the training schemes for doctors to work part-time in a specialty were put in place. I can't remember if the training scheme was actually named as if it was for women, I think it may have actually been but it was a circular of 1969. Up to that point, the only way you could do a proper training in medicine part time was in general practice and I actually did that. I worked in a practice where the partners were very willing for me to be pretty part-time with a small child. To get sufficient training to be seen to be trained as general practitioner; it wouldn't meet today's criteria but it was enough in those days. So the married women's training scheme gave me the opportunity to then train in psychiatry. The College (The Royal College of Psychiatrists) was founded formally in 1971, so at that point it was not clear that as a part-timer, you could become a member of the College.

I: The College was indeed founded in 1971.

FC: I know that people like Tony Clare were very active lobbying against the establishment of the College and also other things were going on. I wasn't at all political but I didn't think I could work in a specialty as a specialist, given I would only work part-time. So I did the Diploma in Psychological Medicine which was a three-part diploma, and I got that in 1975 during which time it did become possible for part-timers to get their membership. So I did Part 1 in 1973 and Part 2 in 1976. And the next hurdle was whether, as a part-time clinical assistant, I could actually get on to the formal training ladder. And of course once I got the membership, I could then apply for a senior registrar post; that was a bit of a hurdle. It was also unknown, really; you know what these strange doctors were trying to do. So I applied for a full-time registrar's post at the local asylum. I am quite a pragmatic person and I think the view I took was that if people were going to cast aspersions on my training, I would show them that I learnt everything that I could by treating the severely mentally ill in asylums. So I did about nine months as a full-time registrar and it gave me great pleasure when I was interviewed for my SR (senior registrar) post, one very senior consultant asked me if I learnt how to prescribe psychotropic medication during that placement. So I had to say that I had already been trained in how to prescribe competently before I went into that placement. I mean this idea that if you are part-time you are somehow second rate still bedevils some people and it is not fair because as you know, most part-timers do over and above what they are expected to do and their commitment is no different from full-timers. They are just choosing a different path, but anyway, that's another whole story.

I: When did you move to psychotherapy? Was it at the senior registrar level?

FC: Yes, as a senior registrar I got a placement at the local psychotherapy unit in Birmingham, the Uffculme Clinic, and pretty much did all my higher training there. Although I stayed pretty involved in general psychiatry because I could see that as my husband had a family business in the Midlands, geographically I couldn't really move about. By then I had two children and I wanted to keep my options open for promotion that I might not get offered a consultant psychotherapist post. I took up two sessions at the health centre for students at the University of Warwick as a consultant psychiatrist and eventually I think it was in 1979 or maybe 1978, I'm not sure about the exact year, I did get a consultant psychotherapist post at the clinic where I had done my training.

I: And how did you get interested and involved in the College?

FC: While I was a senior registrar, I had kept in touch with colleagues that I got to know and the man who had been a senior registrar when I did my Surgical House Officer post was on the Central Manpower Committee, which was a BMA (British Medical Association) committee which worked with the Department of Health on planning doctor numbers for specialities. He knew that the committee thought that they should have a part-time doctor on it, sort of token I think, I mean, maybe not (laughs). Anyway, he asked me if I was interested in going on to the Central Manpower Committee and I have to say that my motivation was very modest. You know, to commute from Coventry to London for a committee that was completely unknown to me and its function sounded like a very dry and uninteresting subject. But I think one of the points of my career is relevant which is that one should not turn down opportunities until you know that they are not for you, I mean I just think that is a mistake particularly when you are building your career, so I agreed to do it partly because I was an admirer of the work of the man concerned. And from there the College. Once the College realized that I was on this key committee they asked me to go on to the College Manpower Committee and as this often happened to me in my career, I was very quickly its secretary and very soon its chairman.

I: Then you became the Dean and the President and then you had a fairly big hand in establishing the Academy of Medical Royal Colleges and you were the first President of that.

FC: Yes.

I: How did that come about?

FC: I found the Conference to Medical Royal Colleges (precursor of the Academy) a very disappointing body. The first meeting I went to was with Andrew Sims (outgoing President of the Royal College of Psychiatrists). I was the incoming President so was introduced to the committee at the last meeting of the outgoing President. This group of highly distinguished doctors was divided across specialities, each pushing its own speciality without substantial collaboration which was affecting the substantial potential influence the medical profession could have had. Another feature of my career, I think you'll have observed is that I do tend to get involved in how things work, so if this is a committee to get something done, I'll tend to join it. So I could see that the future of the conference could be different and we began to look at what was required to put it on to a properly legal footing with a statutory basis and so on. I was a part of that thinking which led to our College asking for an interim chair of the nascent Academy. Before long, of course, it was agreed to have somebody as a full-time chair who had been a President (of a College) and would have had that experience and that they were not trying to do both jobs. I didn't have that opportunity because that developed as I was leaving but I'm sure that was right. I still think that the Academy as a body can speak up more than it actually does. It has been interesting during the pandemic that one of the remarks made recently was 'where are Medical Royal Colleges?' I know that the politics of the medical profession in the political arena are very complicated and I could talk a bit more about that in terms of psychiatry but I think that we are often pussyfooting. There is not enough worrying about speaking up for the profession and the patients.

I: In your experience how has psychiatry changed since you started in the late 1970s?

FC: I think it has become more evidence based. I think people have understood that we have to convince the policy-makers and the public that we know what we are talking about quite a lot of the time. We have allowed ourselves sometimes to be criticized because it hasn't been easy to have the same, if you like, standard of pure research in psychiatry given the many factors that affect why people become mentally ill, but we do know a lot. We tend to put up with people who all think they can be amateur psychiatrists, which I think is a pity. And we have gone on struggling with the issues of stigma particularly within the profession, which is powerful. I don't think we have done all that we might have done about that, but I think in the science we probably have done a lot in my lifetime compared with what we could offer in the 1970s and 1980s. Obviously we know much more about drugs and why they work for some people. We know much more about genetics which

I'm sure will lead us to improved care and support for patients and help them with life events that may have a particular effect because of their genetic predisposition. There is a long way to go, I know that, but I do think there are promising signs that we are more knowledgeable than we were 30 years ago.

I: Do you see psychiatry as mindless or brainless?

FC: I think that's a terrible question, I really do. I looked it up. I looked up both words: brainless means just very stupid, I don't know how you can call a medical field brainless. It doesn't seem a very good sort of choice to me. Mindless means not dealing well with the complexities of a thing, so if I have got to make a choice it would certainly not be brainless and I don't think it's mindless either, mostly.

I: It is interesting that almost everybody (I have interviewed) has said that psychiatry is neither brainless nor mindless. The question arose from a series of paper in the *British Journal of Psychiatry* and I think it might have been in Bob Kendell's time (as President of the Royal College of Psychiatrists); there were papers debating this issue of mindless versus brainless psychiatry particularly at that point of time as it was moving more from social psychiatry to biological psychiatry. Recently there has been a big push in the United States from NIMH (the National Institute for Mental Health) with R-Doc criteria, which means that structural brain changes are needed to diagnose although DSM-5 (the *Diagnostic and Statistical Manual 5*) is full of various diagnostic categories which appear very culturally bound.

FC: Yeah, well that's interesting. But no, I'm not a supporter of that question (laughs).

I: What do you see as the problems with psychiatry?

FC: Well, I have mentioned stigma. I do think that the negative attitudes ingrained in influential people are important. I'm not saying that we haven't done as much as we can but it's a very difficult area in which to counter prejudice, I think. So that's an important aspect for me. And well, we still have the problems of recruitment, which was another question, which I think partly relates to the stigma and I suppose it's partly the attitudes of the public as well. We have colluded with the idea that somehow, if you get severe depression, it's just like having a broken leg. I haven't spent a lot of my life thinking about the philosophy of these issues, but I do think it is a very fundamental questions for us where we may get a bit misled for good reasons into talking as if mental illness and all the things we try to help people which are straightforward and like having a physical illness. That is misleading in a rather fundamental way because the fear of mental illness is of a different order for most of us, the idea that your brain can stop functioning is terrifying, I think. So there are very big questions behind that and I don't know if we helped ourselves as much as we the so-called experts could do. Then one gets into the difficulties of persuading policy-makers that there should be investment when you are not always very good at explaining the treatments that would work for which group of people. I think we have some fundamental problems that our colleagues in physical medicine don't have.

I: One of the things that intrigues me in a way is that people are beginning to talk more about mental health as are the politicians and sports people and celebrities which is good in one way but talking about mental health concerns or mental health issues and also that you can't have simple depression you have to have bipolar disorder, which brings in another kind of stigma.

FC: Yes, I think that's right and I think we need to clear that up. I have just made a note to myself of the biopsychosocial model which I think is very helpful because the complexity of psychiatric disorders reflects that. For our patients, the proportion of each of the biological, psychological, or social factors contributing to the causation of their individual condition is very variable. We are having to explain that complexity in a world that really often is looking for relatively simple answers, it is something like that. I agree with you on the definitions or descriptions. I think that sometimes patients want a straight answer, so one can say to the patient that you have a psychiatric illness but it does not mean that you are a bad person. It may be the result of various factors such as maybe there is something wrong with your genes or what's happened in your life and these are the ways we can help you. So it is a much more complicated story that patients have so we need sufficient time for interaction with them (patients) and their families. So time is required with the patient, and the complex long-term nature of many psychiatric conditions increase costs which policymakers do not like, and so on and so forth.

I: It always amuses me when somebody stands up in a conference or a meeting and says so and so is *suffering* from mental health, why would you be *suffering* from mental health?

FC: (laughs) Exactly, isn't it that we are striving to have (good mental health)?

I: Absolutely. Earlier you touched upon recruitment and stigma. How do you think we can improve recruitment into psychiatry?

FC: I think we have to start young. We have to educate the kids at school. I think the psychiatrist should be willing to go out and talk to young people about their careers. Also, role models are a key part of this, a great psychiatrist who can go and make the work sound absolutely fascinating, and the compassion and the altruism of a specialty will inspire some young people in schools and universities. Having great role models in medical schools is important. Not enough women are heading up medical schools compared with men; women bring different perspectives inevitably to our specialties. I think giving young doctors the only experience of psychiatry in a relatively chaotic environment with failure to contain severe mental distress has been really harmful. So making sure those trainees, whatever their interests, have an opportunity to see different aspects of psychiatry is vital. One of the most telling phrases that was said to me when I was President was from President of another College who said' why would my trainees need to know any psychiatry?' You can guess which College. That says so much about what goes on in our profession, we all doctors need to know some psychiatry. You might not call it psychiatry, but you might call something like mental health or psychology because otherwise you'll fail the patients particularly the ones who got serious mental illnesses. We always have to think about the opportunities to show people what we can provide for those who have just as many needs as those with physical illness and great role models to illustrate what a rewarding career it is.

I: One of the things that intrigues me is that in Europe and the UK, it's the mind—body dichotomy and dualism that continues to persist as if somehow the two are very separate things and they don't talk to each other. This is where your recollection of the President's remark comes into play because for them it's burst appendix or broken hip or whatever. They don't care as far as they are concerned surgery went well and if the wounds get infected subsequently is the general practitioner's problem. Whether the patient can go back to work or not, is the patient's failure. They appear to think that they have nothing to do with that. Of course, not all doctors are like that. But there is a need to take it forward in a much more cohesive, coordinated way between mind and body. You touched upon some of the characteristics of a good psychiatrist, such as altruism and compassion. What do you see as the other characteristics you think that a good psychiatrist should have?

FC: I think a good psychiatrist should have quite a degree of personal insight (laughs). There are challenges in working with a those with mental illnesses. I guess we all have colleagues who for whatever reasons have not the insight to know when to separate from the emotional material of the patient and helping them remain well—functioning. I think compassion is hugely important. It is not just another patient with depression. It is this unique person, so the personal story I think is absolutely key, consistency and reliability. It is absolutely hopeless particularly for the seriously mentally ill or psychologically disturbed, to have someone who can't cope with the boundaries of care themselves, so for me punctuality, record keeping the basic housekeeping of the specialty are important. I have said over the years to trainees, 'you never know when your record of the patient's care will turn up in quite a different setting'. It may be different now, with the Electronic Patient Record (EPR), but lack of professionalism and patient information can catch up with them if it hasn't been of a high standard.

I: What do you see as the gaps in both practice and in training?

FC: I've always thought we don't do enough in the way that Continental Europeans do on neurology. One of the things that I spent a lot of energy on while I was involved with the College was the European Section for Psychiatry (UEMS). We went to all the other countries for our meetings so we knew each other's services. People couldn't believe that in the United Kingdom, you do not have to study any neurology except as a student to become a psychiatrist. And their observation is right. I had a patient when I was a trainee who had a very unusual presentation of depression, just not typical. I wasn't a very good neurologist but I just had a sense that there was more to this than appeared. We got a neurological opinion. That day I actually went to the theatre and her brain tumour was removed and the surgeon said to me 'it's very good to see a psychiatrist in my theatre'. It was actually a very good experience for me. It taught me that we can't leave behind the fact that we are doctors first. We can argue with psychologists as much we like but the professional platform from which we see our patients, as psychiatrists, is absolutely essential to some of them, so I would vote for students to study some neurology. Some more basic medicine is key for both training and probably Continuing Professional Development (CPD) because you never know when you will see an atypical patient and if you can make a diagnosis, so much the better. Now I know that the time for this is probably passed but that's something that I take from my training. Neuropsychiatry has changed in many ways I think because of radiology and all the imaging work that's now being done. Relating changes in the brain to how the person is functioning psychologically and mentally which may actually bring back some of what I am seeing as a gap. I have been very interested to read some of the things on the College website about that. I think that's an area where we could give more thought in the College. Maybe

I'm not as much in touch with the College as I was and maybe there's a lot going on which I don't know about but it seems to me that this is where our unique contribution is to patient care.

I: The College did get some money from the Wellcome Trust when Wendy Burns was the Dean to develop and deliver neurosciences training. The College has set up various meetings which have been well-attended. Shall we talk about psychiatry's social contract? What do we expect from our patients and what do we expect from government, what does government expect from patients and the public, so it's kind of a tripartite contract. How do you think that can be delivered, if it all?

FC: Because of the work I've done on data I would actually quite like to see a formal version of the social contract. I think that one of the problems for the NHS, and I'm not going off the subject, is that because it's a free good in many respects it's not valued as much as it would be if people knew what it cost either to them or to the taxpayer. One of the things I did raise from time to time when I was the Chairman (of the Hospital Trust Board) in Oxford was 'why don't we display the cost of 10 common interventions on our website?' Now as you know, that immediately raises all sorts of questions about trying to deter the poor from having care and that gets into very difficult areas. On social contract, my thought is that we have this almost universal service that is free at the point of contact. I know people pay for some things, that's all political, but if through consultation and lots of work the public would agree to some sort of contract that would be good; if you're given an appointment then you will keep it or you'll cancel it, you'll not throw all your new prescriptions into the bin, you'll take them back to the pharmacy; I mean, there's a lot of examples. So that people could see that actually healthcare is highly costly. I mean, they see these big numbers but the big numbers don't mean anything. If my hip (replacement) costs my Clinical Commissioning Group (CCG), say, £10,000, and I don't follow up with the aftercare that I should do; this is a problem. I'm a great believer in the social contract but haven't managed to get very far speaking up for it. So within psychiatry it's back to the obligations, you know. I'm always shocked when I go to my GP to see how many people didn't keep their appointments and I wouldn't be surprised if it is the same thing that happens with our patients, clinics, and psychiatrists. It would be a good idea if people signed up when they first entered the healthcare service, committing to keeping appointments, promising to let the service know when they can't attend so that the appointment can be offered to someone else. I wonder if we could lobby for more resources given that we see patients in a holistic way, which we and the GPs do. Could we lobby the policy-makers more to seriously consider this? The NHS is a political football with changes every four to five years. You know in all these things, like education, the public doesn't get what it deserves in my view, it deserves better.

I: I agree with you. There are two things that I have always been pushing the politicians that all they do need to say is if you give a pound to the NHS here is a pie chart which says 25% goes to staff, 15% goes for medication, 10% goes for surgery, etc., so at least people have an idea as to for every pound they pay what is it that they are getting. At the moment it is all very bizarre. I have been working with the BMA to talk about medicine's social contract, what it is, and what people expect from doctors, and what we expect from public and patients and the government.

My slight concern about a formal contract would be that it may become incredibly bureaucratic.

FC: Yes, that's true. I think it would have to be a very general statement that if I'm a patient of the NHS, these are the things that I would agree to try to do.

I: These are my rights, these are my responsibilities and obligations.

FC: Exactly. I think it would take us a long way, actually.

I: Looking back at your career, what would you tell your younger self?

FC: I do wonder if I gave up the ambition to be an academic doctor too easily? I look at what some people have achieved in their working lives and you could argue that given my career. paradoxically, I think I could have been more ambitious.

I: I am talking to a psychotherapist so obviously I'm making connections in my brain. Like you, I feel maybe bit more ambition would have been good but then where does it stop?

FC: Yes, and then immediately I say to myself, well look at the context, look at the time when I qualified. In my social group none of the wives went to work after they had children, so I have always been a social oddity and here I'm in my late 70s, still working. What a fantastic career from my own point of view and hopefully in terms of contributions! You ask the questions and I'm being very honest in this interview. It just struck me having had that original ambition to be an academic doctor which I would have loved, hence I guess my attachment to things in Oxford and the work I did at university. But you can't do everything all the time and my son died when he was 19 and if I look back, at the time I had two children if I had given up more of my career, I would have probably felt even worse. We make decisions at such a point in time, don't we? And it's no good now saying I should have been more ambitious. Too late (laughs).

I: It is never too late; people have different kinds of ambition. You moved from clinical work to policy to running an educational institution, running a hospital, etc. It is the skills set that you learnt in one field that are equally applicable to another, so yes, you would have been a stunning academic psychiatrist.

FC: I was not shortlisted for a lecturer post in Oxford. I mean the irony of that! That was my story at Somerville. They asked me at the interview why this and not any other college and I told them because you turned me down when I was 19 and sent me to St Hilda's (laughs).

I: What would you advise the trainees of today?

FC: I think I would encourage them to make their own choices. When I used to go to a lot of speech days, I would say to the kids it's what you want to do, it's which A-levels you want to do, it's not what your teachers say, not what your parents say. I have seen faces around the room and I just think that it's hard to make your own choices but, in the end, if you make choices you think other people want you to have or make, that doesn't lead to reward or even success usually. I think you need to be very careful about the choice of your partner. We had our 50th (wedding) anniversary at the beginning of the month. That has made a huge difference to my career, of course. I talked about women giving up work. I mean if I didn't have a husband who supported me in my career, I wouldn't have been able to do the things we did in terms of the childcare or cooking or all those shared responsibilities. I do say to young doctors that it is great if your partner is another doctor but it is going to make it harder for you to plan your career and in the end one of you probably has to plan rather than the other because somebody will get their first training and adjustments will be needed. I think medicine has particular ramifications. If you don't like what you're doing then, I say to them, find a way of getting out. That's one of the things that worries me about a number of young doctors who have chosen to leave the profession. Was it so awful for them or was it that they just didn't find the support they needed to go on with it?

I: From the BMA I led on a survey of mental health and well-being of doctors and medical students which we subsequently extended to 12 countries and the rates of burnout vary between 65% and 95%. These are bright, young, energetic, enthusiastic people; I don't know what we are doing to them. I can understand the highest figure was in Hong Kong with the political situation there. You can understand the uncertainty there but Wales, England, Italy, Canada, India, there are different kinds of pressures but still very, very high rates of burnout.

FC: Was burnout higher in the home-trained doctors or in those who came here from overseas?

I: Interestingly, the lowest number of burnout amongst doctors was in those from the Indian subcontinent. Doctors from Continental Europe showed fairly high rates and local doctors too were quite high. Trainees and junior doctors and Specialist Associate (SAS) doctors plus those who were coming up to retirement showed very high rates.

FC: I just wonder, what it reflects is the lack of support in a situation where people's expectations were dashed. The NHS should offer something better, particularly for the younger doctors (who have their lifetime ahead of them working in the field).

I: Very much so because lots of them were complaining that they didn't feel part of a team, they were doing their shifts and heading off. Often, they had no idea about the continuity of care that you were mentioning earlier. But also, they felt that medicine in particular has become far too technical and that they did not come into medicine to be a technician. That raises yet another issue. We are down to the last two questions: what would you like to be remembered for?

FC: I would like to be remembered for compassion, both towards patients but also for colleagues, so in the more senior positions I've had I have tried to understand what it's like for more junior staff, so that aspect of management or leadership is important: don't forget the people who worked for you. I think that applies both to colleagues and to patients. I suppose I would like to be remembered for the degree of efficiency; did I get things done according to whatever the role was, a degree of wisdom? Perhaps.

I: I think one of the major aspects of leadership is wisdom and yet humility.

FC: Yes, I certainly wouldn't like to be remembered as someone who has done the things I have done for my own gratification. I think I have tried to always put the patient first. That's one of the things that has kept me going with the data work, but you know the public out there is not well served by our legal and other systems, so I guess to be remembered for that and not seen as someone who wanted only to advance themselves in the things I've done.

I: Which of your many achievements are you most proud of?

FC: Well, I've got a very soft spot for being the first trainee who worked part-time to become a President of the Royal College. I don't know if there's been any since. I was and I'm still very proud of that because it said such a lot about what can be overcome and how a system can recognize how something different may be. I was the first President who was not a General Psychiatrist, a woman, etc., so there was something about that position that has many sorts of degrees of resonance for me. I'm really proud of what I have done for the data world.

I: Is there anything that you would like to add that we haven't talked about?

FC: We haven't talked much about role models. One of the people I made a note about when we were talking earlier was that. I talked about rather distinguished doctors at Westminster who were completely intimidating as far as I was concerned. When I went to do house job in Coventry there were doctors I wanted to be like. One such person was the surgeon I worked for who was compassionate, kindly, wonderful with his patients. We were talking about that mind/body split and he did not believe in it. Another doctor was rude; not what one would expect from a doctor. I've found it important going through my working life to identify people who I really admire and want to be more like. I didn't want to be like the chair who would always tell the committee at the beginning of a meeting what decisions were going to be made before any discussion of specific items occurred. Anyway, there are lots and lots of things really. It's been an interesting conversation.

I: It has been absolutely fascinating because what you talked about resonates very well with my own experience and worldview. In the last 40 years or so that you have been in psychiatry there has been a remarkable shift from the very social to very biological perspective within the field. I feel that the pendulum is coming to settle somewhere in the middle and we are beginning to understand that attachment patterns in childhood affect brain structures. So that's a big step forward and long may it continue.

FC: Absolutely, I mean there is a great deal to discover but meanwhile, and we need to build on that.

I: Thanks very much for your time and I hopefully see you before too long.

FC: Absolutely.

3
Silvana Galderisi

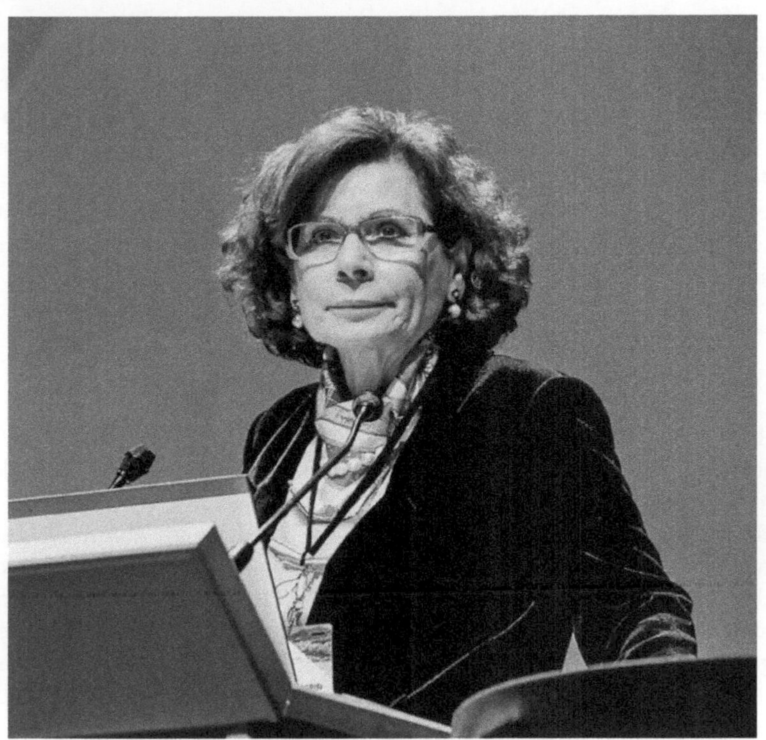

Biography

Silvana Galderisi, MD, PhD, is full professor of Psychiatry and Chair of the Department of Mental and Physical Health and Preventive Medicine of the University of Campania Luigi Vanvitelli. She is the Director of the Emergency Unit of the Department of Mental Health of the same university; Coordinator of the Outpatient Unit for Anxiety and Psychotic Disorders and of the Rehabilitation Program for severe mental disorders of the same Department.

She is President of the Italian Society for Psychopathology (SOPSI), Chairperson and Charter Member of the European Group for Research in Schizophrenia, past-President of the European Psychiatric Association (EPA); Co-chair of the Taskforce 'Minimising coercion in mental health care' and Chair of the Standing Committee on Ethics and Review of the World Psychiatric Association (WPA); past Chairperson of the Communications Committee of the Schizophrenia International Research Society (SIRS); board member of the European Scientific Association on Schizophrenia (ESAS) and of the Italian Society for Psychopathology and Italian Society of Biological Psychiatry. She is Honorary Member and Honorary Fellow of the World Psychiatric Association (WPA), Honorary Member of the Hungarian Psychiatric Association (HPA) and of the Polish Psychiatric Association, International Distinguished Fellow of the American Psychiatric Association-APA, International Advisor of the Japanese Society of Psychiatry and Neurology (JSPN), and Honorary Fellow of the European Society of Social Psychiatry (ESSP).

Her research activity focuses on schizophrenia pathophysiology, treatment, and outcome, with particular reference to the domains of negative symptoms and cognition and their impact on psychosocial outcomes. She is author/co-author of more than 400 publications, in national and international journals and books, a member of the editorial boards of several international psychiatric journals, Editor-in-Chief of *Schizophrenia Bulletin Open*, and handling editor of the British Journal of Psychiatry Open.

Interview

I: Welcome Professor Galderisi. Many thanks for agreeing to be interviewed for this book on leadership in psychiatry. I will start by asking you about your childhood and growing up.

SG: Thank you, well … I grew up in Naples, south of Italy. My family was from the lower middle class; my mother was a tailor, my father an employee; we were not rich but certainly not poor, and so my family could afford to send me to school. I had a nice life because although the house where I lived was very simple there was a garden, a beautiful garden. So, I had the pleasure of growing up among several animals, including cats, dogs, a sheep, chickens, and things like that. Overall it was quite a nice childhood; I went to school, had many friends, so it was a good childhood in spite of the fact that mine was not certainly a wealthy family, but overall, in the family, there was a good atmosphere.

I: What attracted you to medicine?

SG: Challenge. That's the only possible answer. I went to the grammar school, and all my teachers were convinced that my best future was in the humanistic field, i.e. literature, history, philosophy, or journalism, but I thought that it was too easy for me, and that's why I wanted to take up the challenge of studying something in the scientific field, not purely scientific (such as mathematics or physics), but sort of a bridge between natural and humanistic sciences, and the idea was since the beginning to become a psychiatrist, though I was not self-confident enough for that. In the beginning I thought that medicine was challenging but psychiatry probably even more so.

I: Why did you choose psychiatry? Have you any regrets?

SG: No, certainly not, I have no regrets about that. If I had a chance to go back and choose again, I would choose psychiatry all over again. Why did I choose psychiatry? Because, as I said, for me something that was really a bridge between natural and humanistic sciences was what really interested me, but I was also very curious about human beings in general, the way in which they think, they feel, they behave, they relate to each other, and I was also very curious about the mind in general: what is the mind? How does it relate to the brain? These were the questions I already had in mind when I chose medicine and then psychiatry. So, no regrets.

I: Who were your role models, heroes, heroines?

SG: Well, frankly in my experience I do not recognize heroes and heroines. This was not my style even when I was an adolescent. I do remember that my friends and classmates were in love with heroes and heroines, such as singers, actors, actresses. That was not the case for me, never. But what I can say is that yes, I had role models, especially people that gave me something in terms of teaching me something, and this has been the case on several occasions, especially in the field of neuroscience, psychiatry, electrophysiology, and psychotherapy. From people who were my mentors and teachers, I really learned a lot and I'm very grateful because there were many people that were really very generous in this respect. And I have very good memories and part of what I have achieved is certainly their merit besides mine.

I: Your impression of patients?

SG: Well, patients are other persons that gave me a lot, a lot in terms of experience, but also in terms of knowledge and personal growth. I was fascinated by psychotic patients since I took my first steps into psychiatric practice. I was very interested in all psychotic phenomena including delusions and hallucinations, and so whenever patients spoke about these I was extremely interested. In the beginning, these were my main interests. Then I became more interested in negative symptoms and cognitive dysfunctions because I learnt quite soon that while patients improve a lot with regard to their delusions and hallucinations, very often they do not improve in their negative symptoms and cognitive dysfunctions. I could see that even when we were able to get rid of the psychotic symptoms there was quite a lot left there that stopped people to go back to their meaningful life, to being satisfied with life. That's why I became very interested in those who had these kind of dysfunctions. In terms of psychotic experiences, what sometimes really struck me was that for people who were very psychotic, psychotic experiences were their reality, their world. I still remember a patient, a young lady, who once told me, 'Doctor, tell me the truth, everyone hears voices, and this is a little bit like sex: everybody does it but no-one speaks about it, everyone listens to voices but no-one says that they do.' Unfortunately I had to reject her statement because this is not certainly the case, though I said that yes, many people hear voices, probably more people than the ones we take care of, but it is not true that everyone hears voices. She was a bit disappointed.

I: So, what are the memorable occasions in practice or research in psychiatry you can share with us?

SG: I have many. I mean in more than 40 years of experience there are many memorable experiences in both practice and research. In practice, I always remember when I decided to go through a psychotherapy training. At that time, I was involved in research and treatment of people with panic disorder and we treated many women with this disorder; at those times we used tricyclic antidepressants for treating women with panic disorder and their improvement was impressive.

They went back to their lives and they were very happy with the treatment; all symptoms disappeared, but for many women the time came when they had to face the prospect of becoming pregnant and therefore the need to stop pharmacological treatments. That was very difficult for me as a young doctor because I thought that I had very little to offer. Although I told my patients that in several papers the authors reported that during pregnancy women experienced an improvement of panic, they were still scared about having to stop the treatment and were afraid of relapsing. I understood then that people cannot be treated only with drugs; they need something more and that's why I decided to undertake a training in psychotherapy even though I was in the very beginning of my career, I already had my specialization in psychiatry, and was working as a staff psychiatrist, with quite a lot of responsibilities. So it was not very easy to undertake the training, but I considered it as an essential part of my professional development. I think I improved a lot in my practice and that's the reason why now I suggest that all young trainees should be skilled in one psychotherapy approach at least.

I: How has psychiatry changed in your time?

SG: Somehow psychiatry has changed for the better, but somehow also for the worse. What do I mean? I mean certainly compared to the time I started to be interested in psychiatry, when I decided to become a psychiatrist, psychiatric hospitals were still open in Italy and we still had a system based on psychiatric hospitals. When I started to work as a psychiatrist, probably during the second or third year of my training, the psychiatric hospitals in Italy were closed and no patient could be admitted to a psychiatric hospital and so there was a sort of revolution, let's say, and that was a very difficult time when people really did not have any place to go because there were few services for psychiatric emergencies.

I: What are your views on the current state of psychiatry?

SG: Well, as I said before, certainly at the moment we are in a phase of transition because we really need to rethink the models treatment is based on. In several European countries at the moment there is a shift from a hospital-based to community-based treatment, but I'm not sure that this system is really sustainable because what we have seen, up to now, is that this is a type of system that needs resources and also there are many gaps in the pathway of a patient that undergoes diagnosis and treatment in psychiatry. We still have to solve the problem of early recognition and early intervention not only for psychotic disorders but also for many other disorders. We still have to close the gap between child adolescent psychiatry and adult psychiatry because in many countries there is a distinction between these two age-related services and there is a huge gap, meaning that many people get lost in this transition, and in many systems this gap is not being addressed properly and still is not a priority in the political agenda. Even among psychiatrists it is not seen as a priority among many colleagues. So I believe that this is a time of transition in which we need to address all these gaps and we know that the resources made available are not enough to address all these gaps properly. I think that besides identifying problems, we need also to identify potential solutions, and I can see potential partial solutions to all these issues. The implementation of Internet-based treatments, for instance, could be part of the solution. Of course, this is a new challenge. This is a new world to be discovered and developed with all its problems and issues, but as a complementary aspect of our practice, it could be very useful. It could save money and could help in terms of resources and also in terms of solving the lack of skilled personnel. So let's see whether we'll be able to develop the future through these pathways.

I: Professor Galderisi, is psychiatry brainless or mindless?

SG: Both statements are wrong. I mean, I would never support the premise that psychiatry is mindless and would never support the premise that psychiatry is brainless. Psychiatry deals with human beings, human beings have brains and have minds, and therefore neither should be excluded. We need to consider human beings as a unit, as one entire entity. Mind is not only brain. Mind is embodied and mind is something related also to the environment and especially to the interpersonal environment. So we cannot reduce mind to brain or brain to mind, but we need to take a larger perspective than this.

I: How would you improve recruitment in psychiatry?

SG: Well, first of all I think we should modify the curriculum of medical training in which there is very little room for psychiatry in most universities across the world. I think that this is an important gap to be filled, not only for recruitment in psychiatry but also for being a good medical doctor because, in my opinion, the fact that there is not enough training in psychiatry throughout the medical curriculum is something that prevents medical doctors from being very good doctors: they do not recognize many psychiatric disorders and do not feel confident enough in diagnosing and treating psychiatric disorders, but at the same time the fact that the training in psychiatry is very limited throughout the medical curriculum also determines, amongst students, the idea that psychiatry is not important; it's something like a discipline, as we say, in the B category. The other very serious issue is that in many countries, psychiatrists are viewed as inferior to other medical doctors and this, of course, creates stigma towards psychiatry, psychiatrists, and psychiatric patients, and at the same time discourages students from becoming a psychiatrist. So this should be addressed and improved. Then I think that we need very good role models in psychiatry, meaning that the idea that psychiatrists are always a little bit odd people, people who always behave in a quite strange way, is also something that should be counteracted. We should offer the message that psychiatry is a noble discipline, is challenging, extremely interesting, and complex, and is meant for people who are smart, want to study and work in a very serious and scientifically sound manner, while promoting a patient-centred approach.

I: What do you see as characteristics of a good psychiatrist?

SG: In 2018, together with Peter Falkai, I published an editorial in *European Psychiatry* entitled 'Psychiatry and Psychiatrists: Fourteen core Statements'. The idea behind this paper was that we wanted to provide two innovative definitions for mental health and mental health disorders, but we also wanted to highlight the core aspects of this discipline and of a good psychiatrist. I think it is worth reading the paper but would like to highlight the perspective proposed in the article that the psychiatrist should be regarded as an integrator *par excellence* of the biopsychosocial model. I mean that psychiatry is and should always be at the intersection between natural science, psychology, and social sciences. Good psychiatrists need to be good medical doctors because no psychiatrist can ignore the physical health of her/his patient; a good psychiatrist needs to be knowledgeable about pharmacotherapies, psychotherapies, and psychosocial treatments. And a good psychiatrist should be able to apply these methods and work within a therapeutic alliance in order to design, personalize, and integrate treatment plans. Therefore, the competencies cannot be limited to one or the other aspect. Psychiatric competencies must cover all these aspects: pharmacological, psychological, psychosocial treatments. In addition, we need to be advocates for our patients because sometimes we forget the need for advocacy in our profession. It is true that sometimes we don't have the time, perhaps we don't have the skills, but we should develop those skills and remember that there are many contexts in which we can be advocates of the rights, needs, and expectations of our patients. Last but not least, we should never collude with political expectation or demands; we should not serve any kind of political purpose but only the interests of our patients.

I: What do you see as gaps in the practice of psychiatry?

SG: The main gaps are actually the gaps relevant to different epochs of life: there is a very important gap between child adolescent psychiatry and adult psychiatry. There is also very often a gap between the places in which our practice takes place; sometimes psychiatrists working in an emergency ward are not in contact enough with those working in the community services, the exchanges are not very well organized and are not part of standard procedure in everyday practice. Another gap, in my opinion, is due to ideology: we still have psychiatrists who consider themselves only psychotherapists, and are not knowledgeable enough about new treatment options in terms of pharmacological treatments, or psychiatrists who consider that psychosocial treatments are not needed.

I: What do you see as gaps in training in psychiatry?

SG: I would like to address this question from a European perspective. As a leader of the European Psychiatric Association, I have been in touch with many colleagues and organizations, and, in my experience, there are very important gaps. Nowadays, in different branches of medicine it is possible to move from one country to the other and practise in different countries. For psychiatrists, to be able to do this several gaps need to be addressed. First of all, the language barrier should be overcome because people are able to study the language of the country where they wish to practise. This problem can be solved. But when it comes to the training in psychiatry, we have huge heterogeneity across Europe; there are countries in which the training is six years, others in which it is five, four, three, down to one year of training in Belarus. This is really unacceptable today. In Europe we should define a standard and stick to that standard. There is no single European curriculum. It has not been designed yet. I mean, there are several purposes but there is not a shared curriculum that is applied homogeneously throughout Europe in our training schools and there is no European examination in psychiatry. In other medical disciplines this has already been established but not in psychiatry, at least not yet. This is another important gap to be addressed.

I: How do you think the psychiatry's social contract can be delivered?

SG: Well, I think that as I said before, psychiatrists should be advocates for their patients and have the interests of their patients as their mandate. This should be the social contract as to the expectations from society versus psychiatrists. It is a bit different because very often psychiatrists are considered the people who should guarantee that psychiatric patients do not bother society in general, do not create trouble for society. Sometimes we are also considered as, how can I say, gods, meaning that we can predict behaviour, outcomes, treatments and the like. We are expected to be better than meteorologists at predicting, we are expected to know whether a person will be dangerous from the time they leave treatment, maybe in the next decade or so; whether a person can be harmful to himself/herself or for others. This is of course not a sound request because for all complex systems the predictability is very low, especially in the long term. Over the short term our predictions might be reliable but in the long term there is no possible certainty about prediction for complex systems, as human beings are. So of course we can help in making predictions but the legal responsibility that we are sometimes given is unrealistic. Sometimes our mandate is seen as something of very low level, such as custodial aspects or social control, and these have nothing to do with our profession. So we should try to clarify what the social contract can be but we should accept the contract, the social contract in which we consider ourselves as part of an improvement of the society, as instigators of programmes aimed to improve people's lives and the society in general.

I: How would you advise your younger self?

SG: I would have taken it easier, meaning that I always took everything very seriously and sometimes I had to force myself to take the next challenge. If I had a chance to go back, I would probably take it easier but it is easy to say this now because when you grow up and acquire more experience you also become more self-confident. Of course, when I was younger it was much more difficult and challenging but, if possible, I would have liked to have taken it a bit easier.

I: What is your advice to trainees of today?

SG: Be proud of your profession, it is the best one—is the best. So always be proud. Spend a lot of time with your patients; this is always worthwhile, you can learn a lot from your patients. Being with them can be a very valuable experience. Never give up, never get discouraged, and always study a lot because learning is a process lasting all life. We should always study and this will keep our health in good shape, not only our brain health or mind health but also our physical health, together with physical exercise. We should always consider knowledge as important. We should never be trapped in our everyday practice without continuing to be curious, aiming at taking further steps, innovative practices, and exchanges with the rest of the world in terms of best practices and good knowledge.

I: What would you like to be remembered for?

SG: I would like to be remembered for the effort that I put in my professional life, for my honest approach to different experiences and to my profession, and for the respect I always showed towards other people and especially towards patients and their relatives.

I: Which of your achievements are you most proud of?

SG: Many of them. I am proud of being a psychiatrist; I'm proud of being a university professor; I'm very proud of having been the President of European Psychiatric Association; I'm very, very proud, in my capacity as President of the EPA, of the decision of including the two most important associations of patients and relatives on the Board of the European Psychiatric Association as official members of the Board with voting rights; and I'm proud of having initiated a prize for women who contributed to the profession and to research in psychiatry.

I: Many thanks again Professor Galderisi for your time and for being a leader in psychiatry.

SG: Thank you very much.

4
Sir David Goldberg

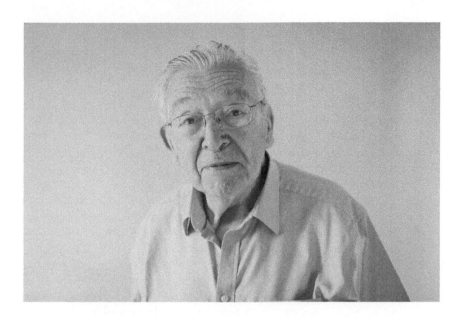

Biography

Sir David has devoted his professional life to improving the teaching of psychological skills to doctors of all kinds, and to improving the quality of services for those with severe mental illnesses. He has advised the Department of Health in the United Kingdom over many years about service developments, and has been extensively used by the World Health Organization as a mental health consultant.

His interests are in vulnerability factors which predispose people to develop depression and in teaching general practitioners (GPs) to offer a better service to psychologically distressed patients. His research over many years has been concentrated on the details of communication between GPs and their patients, and he has applied these principles to his teaching of mental health workers in developing countries. He was Chairman of the Guideline Development Group for Depression, and is currently Chairman of the Guideline for Depression in Physical Diseases for the National Institute for Health and Care Excellence (NICE).

His basic medical qualifications and his Doctorate are from the University of Oxford. After completing his psychiatric training at the Maudsley, he went to Manchester, where for over 20 years he was Head of the Department of Psychiatry and Behavioural Science. In 1993 he returned to the Maudsley as Professor of Psychiatry and Director of Research and Development. He is a Fellow of Hertford College, Oxford; King's College, London; and the Academy of Medical Sciences.

Interview

I: Can we start off by talking about your early childhood and where you were born and grew up in and what was it like?

DG: I was born in Hampstead Heath in London. From a little boy's point of view, I was not aware of the storm clouds gathering over Europe, I was a happy little lad, but I began to feel more seriously alive when my dad explained to me that if the Germans were to invade, he would kill us first.

I: Wow! That's an extreme step.

DG: Those were rough days. I was about six or seven at the time. He explained what various political parties stood for. Interestingly, he managed to sound as though he was reasonably objective about the Conservative Party but I knew already at the age of seven that he wasn't at all (laughs).

I: What was it like growing up with war on the horizon?

DG: It was very perplexing to think that people who never met me were determined to kill me. It seemed so irrational. I couldn't imagine why they would want to do that. But very clearly they did and that's what my dad had said. Those were eventful years and we were evacuated to Oxfordshire. The local people were not at all pleased to see us because we were outsiders and from London and thus dangerous people! Those were exciting years but we got so fed up with living there that we decided that we better be bombed in London than to go living with that.

I: How long were you in Oxfordshire?

DG: Three years. We went there in 1943

I: That must have had a major impact on your growing up and the fact that your dad said to you that 'before they kill you, I will'.

DG: I thought that was a good offer (laughs).

I: Why?

DG: I didn't have any confidence in the kindness of the Gestapo. I thought my dad would be more concerned with our welfare than they would.

I: So the whole family moved to Oxfordshire and then back? Or just the children?

DG: No, my mum was with us all the time.

I: Right.

DG: My dad was moved about by the government during the war and he was sent initially for just one year to the United States, and then a second year there.

I: And there wasn't any offer for the family to join him for that period?

DG: Oh no, it was very dangerous crossing the Atlantic at the time. My parents put us down for sort of British equivalent of *Kindertransport* to the United States. There were liners that took British children across the Atlantic. One that left, just before ours was due to leave, was torpedoed and every child was killed. My parents thought that suicide would be better or to take a chance on staying put, so we remained here for the duration and we never left.

I: How did this impact upon your education and schooling?

DG: Not much, I don't think it was disturbed. The schooling I received in Oxfordshire was not really special, you know it was pretty standard schooling. It didn't get much better when I started in primary school in London during the bombing. It started to get slightly better when I went to the North London Emergency Grammar School in Highbury which was for the people who still foolishly stayed put in London.

I: Why was it called the Emergency School?

DG: Because most schools were closed.

I: Closed or moved?

DG: Moved. The school that I was due to be sent to in St Albans wasn't open but my parents needed a school which was in London so we went to Highbury County which was now called the North London Emergency School.

I: What was it like after the war? What was the interpretation of the fact that the stress was over in some ways and that the strangers were not coming to kill you after all?

DG: Well, it was clear probably a year before the end of the war that we were going to win, so there wasn't really much anxiety about that. We may have been bombed but we were unlikely to fall into the hands of the Gestapo. A relative of my mother's (who was Jewish and was allowed to serve in the British army) was an official interpreter in the army. He wrote letters to us as they travelled through France, and later, through dispossessed, dismal hopeless parts of Germany telling us exactly what was going on. That was a great feeling as if I was in a tank with him. It felt almost certain that the tables would turn in the war and we might win; it did look as if there was light at the end of the tunnel.

I: In terms of history, did it affect your relationship with German colleagues in any way?

DG: I didn't have any relationships with German colleagues. You mean later? It did not affect my relationship with German colleagues.

I: So you went to Oxford in 1952?

DG: Yes.

I: And you were doing medicine there?

DG: No, because my dad insisted on me having to take exams in pure mathematics. Mathematics is not a part of requirement for going into medicine. Individuals who would study pure mathematics had a special subject called Advanced Mathematics for the previous two years. I hadn't done that subject and I found it extremely difficult. My dad started saying 'if you don't understand maths, you don't understand anything', which is more or less correct. But it was not helpful information about going to university because I was not really fit to go into any particular course. So I spent the first year, actually the first two terms of the first year, qualifying in botany which I hadn't read so that I could do the pure maths, which I enjoyed very much. I thought botany was a good subject and I had to be re-examined in Latin. I had to get a credit in Latin but that was fine too. I enjoyed it; it was no big deal. When I think of what kids go through now to get into medical school there is just no comparison, we had it easy.

I: You said you had to take your Latin exams twice, so in school had you studied Latin?

DG: Yes.

I: Was that compulsory or optional?

DG: No, it was not compulsory but it was very much something that I did. On the other hand, you could quit mathematics if you didn't like it.

I: Right, and so you did two terms of botany, took exams in Latin, and that's when you decided to go into medicine.

DG: No, I had to be examined in Latin before Oxford would look at me at all.

I: Oh I see. OK.

DG: So I did that when I was in London but when I got to Oxford, I had to do botany in order to make myself eligible for medicine. And this was again suggested by my dad. I didn't want to read medicine; that was the last thing I wanted to do. I thought doctors were boring and I disliked the way medical courses were really a set of factual texts that you had to memorize. I didn't like that. It didn't feel to me that this was the way to learn an academic subject. I liked psychology and the way I was taught the subject. My dad said that his condition for me reading psychology was that I read medicine as well. As he was paying, he had the whip hand.

I: At what point did you get interested in psychology?

DG: My dad helped me with that. The story becomes complicated because when I got to Oxford, I was already concerned about the rehabilitation of the mentally ill because of what my dad had been doing. The government training centres and industrial rehabilitation units which were across the whole country had been used to get injured soldiers and service personnel back to work. When they made the decision to empty the mental hospitals that was really exciting.

I: What was your father's job?

DG: He was a Civil Servant.

I: Right. He had the responsibility for these rehab units, so he came home and talked about it, is that right?

DG: He would tell me about the characters and the work that was being done. I was very interested in it. I met all the psychologists who worked with him as they often came and visited us at home and I liked the way they thought about problems.

I: So you wanted to do psychology; you said that your father's condition was that you read medicine first.

DG: Yes.

I: So you did medicine to please your dad, and psychology to please yourself?

DG: Exactly.

I: When you went to Oxford, did you go straight into medicine?

DG: No. I spent two terms qualifying for the medical course. Then I had to complete first Bachelor of Medicine and Bachelor of Surgery in four terms, which was really hard going. I had to dissect thorax in my long vacation in order to have done all the bits of the body by the end of my second year. As soon as I did that I went into psychology for two years.

I: How did it work?

DG: Well, you have to be a graduate at Oxford and most people take physiology. I took physiology and psychology for the next two years.

I: OK.

DG: I'm not the only person to do that.

I: In India, we had physiology and anatomy in the first MBBS which was 18 months, over three terms, and then we went into pharmacology and pathology and started with clinical placements. Obviously, the Oxford system was quite different from other medical schools, or was it fairly similar?

DG: I have never really compared it to any others so I don't think I can answer that question.

I: At what point did you move from psychology to psychiatry?

DG: Well, when I was working at St Thomas' and came back to London to do my clinical work, I went to all the psychiatry teaching. I won the Exhibition in Psychological Medicine there. I was reading very widely at that time and I came across Aubrey Lewis who wrote *Between Doubt and Certainty in Psychiatry* and I thought, that's the man who I could learn from. The way he thought, the way he formulated problems, was the way it needed to be and so I moved to the Maudsley, having failed the London membership a number of times. After I presented cases to him, life held no terrors for me. I took the membership examination again and passed (laughs).

I: Do you think the point that Lewis was making in terms of uncertainty and doubt that still holds true?

DG: Absolutely.

I: So why do people often pretend that psychiatry is a science?

DG: Well, I don't. It's a clinical subject. No more scientific than all other subjects.

I: But my own view has always been that both medicine and psychiatry are arts backed by science.

DG: Maybe the scientific methods are used to study particular problems but the idea that psychiatry is a science and it's just like medicine, that's nonsense.

I: After coming to the Maudsley, you did your Diploma in Psychological Medicine. At what point were you attracted to primary care psychiatry?

DG: During my time at the Maudsley, when I met Michael Shepherd. He had done a study of psychiatric illness in primary care, which is still the exemplar of systematic study, and I helped him. He wanted to have a screening test for screening clinical populations and that was where the General Health Questionnaire (GHQ) came in. Because we didn't really have a way of validating the screening test, I also had to produce an interview for making medical diagnoses, so I developed that. My first publication was the standardized interview, which was very different from the rigid official PSE (Present State Examination). The CIS (Clinical Interview Schedule) was my contribution to Michael Shepherd's work and we did various studies at St. Thomas's. I wrote a paper on the psychological aspects of the diseases of the small intestine. They were good days. It was very busy.

I: Looking back at the screening questionnaire and developing something, were you excited? Was it frightening? What was Shepherd like to work for?

DG: Oh, he was really fun, we got quite fond of him. He would spend Fridays in his research unit so we always knew Fridays were going to be Michael's. Sometimes he would not feel like doing any work and he would imitate his consultant colleagues hilariously. He would make them say such stupid things. He was a very malicious man. I liked him very much. He was a great friend, but not in a way Aubrey was, Aubrey was the only scholar that I ever met in psychiatry.

I: And at what point, did you go to America? Did you decide it or was it just an option?

DG: I decided to go. If you wait for people to offer you things, you can wait a long time (laughs). No, I decided that I would go and by that time I was married to Ilfra and we had two babies, Paul and Charlotte. One condition that they made in Philadelphia was that I had to go on an NP1 visa which will allow you to become an American citizen. They felt that everybody comes into the country when they are in need, then they have to go back home in order to apply for a visa from outside the country, but you are not allowed to do that when you have your NP1. That was a bit tricky because in the United States, the (army) draft was going on at the time and I didn't have any intention of going to Vietnam. I had already sussed out the quickest way of getting to Canada if I was drafted. I would have suppressed my NP1 and showed them my British passport and got on a British Airways flight.

I: By that time had you finished your DPM?

DG: Yes. I had done all that. I had passed my membership too. So, I went to the States in 1969.

I: Why Philadelphia?

DG: They offered me a job as an Assistant Professor.

I: Right.

DG: The head of department there had been trained at the Maudsley and he liked the British. The first year I was in the States, I was working only in Philadelphia. When I went back, I was working only in Charleston but that was the consecutive research money from the National Institute of Mental Health.

I: You mentioned in your paper about doing primary care work in Philadelphia and also the similarities between UK primary care and US primary care in terms of symptomatology.

DG: Yes, that's right. It was indistinguishable.

I: As a cultural psychiatrist I am always intrigued by cultural differences rather than similarities. I agree with you entirely that patients don't fit into neat diagnostic boxes, particularly in primary care.

DG: When I was validating the GHQ I realised that patients often would not fit into neat diagnostic categories.

I: And that is still the case.

DG: The world unfortunately had not agreed with me but it is what I think. The diagnostic model is totally unrealistic model for psychological disorder.

I: So where do you think psychiatry has gone wrong?

DG: I think it believes too much in the scientific basis and underpinnings and sees itself as wonderfully objective and amazing. It is not.

I: What do you think is the solution to overcome this? What should we be doing in terms of training medical students and postgraduates?

DG: I can't really say what we should be doing because I'm no longer in a university position, but I was interested in teaching communication techniques to students and that's what I did mostly both in Manchester and when I got back here.

I: I remember that.

DG: And I had certainly been teaching communication skills in Manchester for some time. I went on with that because it seems to be like it was the single most important thing that a psychiatrist has to be good at. It is communicating with people and finding out where they are at. As for the nature of mental disorders, most of the disordered people in the population don't receive a proper diagnosis because they don't fit with the diagnostic criteria. For example, what we now call bodily stress syndrome is multiple somatic symptoms that keep fluttering around. Now that's something that conventional psychiatry doesn't really make allowances for.

I: If you were starting with a clean slate with all your experience behind you, how would you set up the diagnostic system? I'm assuming that we do need a diagnostic system for a number of reasons.

DG: Yes, we do.

I: I'm interested in particular in both secondary care and primary care.

DG: So am I.

I: You have been absolutely spot on in terms of supporting primary care because those working in it deal with most of the psychiatric burden, as it were, and yet quite often they are abandoned; it's 'sink or swim' for them. Secondary care has another problem because we are creating more and more barriers within services. If you had the power to change things and with your experience, what would your advice be to the next generation about how things should be done?

DG: I'm not sure I can answer that question because I need to be much more in tune with what's happening at the moment. My understanding is that despite the confident statements of Mrs May (the Prime Minister at the time of the interview) and her Chancellor at HM Treasury, austerity has not gone away. At the moment, you have to do what clinical work you can and what research comes your way without trying to change the system. There is not enough money available. It's clear that the country's economy is going to have to get better before we can return to any interesting developmental model for what's going on now.

I: Do you believe that mental health is influenced by social determinants?

DG: Yes.

I: So should we as psychiatrists not act more as advocates than we currently are? We generally shy away from advocacy for our patients as well as for policy.

DG: I believe that social determinants are vitally important. We have to see what can be done to the patients who come to see us; we can't start changing that and saying, 'you are not to come'.

I: That's not what I meant. I did most of my training in asylums and the first consultant job that I did was run community mental health in Peckham, and then working in community rehabilitation and intensive care, etc. The changes in the practice of psychiatry have occurred but the training hasn't. This also raises issues about differences in primary care psychiatry and secondary care psychiatry. If I were redesigning courses, I would make sure that every trainee did six months of primary care; I tried to introduce that but surprisingly, the GPs won't play ball.

DG: I'm not sure how very good primary care physicians they would be if they are not prepared to study the problems of general medical illness and the psychological effect of medical illnesses. To me, that seems to be an important aspect of the problem.

I: When you were in Manchester and you were working with primary care physicians, what model did you think and find works best? Is it liaison between community teams and primary care or is it more about getting the psychiatry teams to sit in primary care settings and help?

DG: I think the important thing is the way you train primary care physicians. During my second year in the States, I learnt that there is a way of making primary care physicians more psychologically sensitive and better able to cope with the psychological disorders that they are faced with and patients present with. The method of teaching that I designed in Charleston was very labour intensive and impractical. You could not use that model for generalizing to what needed to be done here in the United Kingdom. When I got back to Manchester from Charleston I started to think about various ways that one could get that teaching to the whole generations of GPs. What we did was to have a weekly teaching session where GPs would bring videotapes of their interviews with patients and we would have special discussions. For these discussions, there would always be a GP teacher and a psychiatrist present who would be conducting the session. We would make sure that the GPs understood the way psychological disorder was affecting the patient being discussed and we would always look at an interview tape. We always concentrated on interview techniques. Thus we were helping doctors to understand the way they can influence the way you can revive an interview that's run into the sand and is no longer productive. I think that was quite important as there are various ways of working with GPs. Of course, it also depends very much on the GPs and how one can fit in usefully with them. I certainly added something to the service but I didn't think it was one of my better shots, really. It can be difficult to generalize this teaching model across countries and even within the same country. We were teaching trainee GPs in groups of 40, and every year we would have another 40 of them. I think we did a lot of good with those GPs who attended, but there is always more that can be done.

I: So these GPs will be with you for a year?

DG: No, not at all. They would have a day with us. And there is a lot of them to learn.

I: The fact that they came to your sessions must mean that they were keen and getting something out of the sessions which was going to make their life easier.

DG: I don't think that follows (laughs). I think that their teachers told them that's what they wanted them to do and they were just obedient. I had tremendous positive feedback from that teaching. The GPs liked it. It is a cause of great sadness to me that it was the only place in England that offered it and people in other places did not leap to follow it. One of the other things that I did in Manchester in addition to primary care was to look at manpower figures. We had fewer psychiatrists per thousand of population at risk in Manchester than anywhere in the United Kingdom but by the time I left Manchester we were at the top. We had more psychiatrists than anywhere. That was because I organized the teaching of psychiatrists and made sure that the most gifted psychiatrists were participating in that teaching; people wanted to come and work with us. I have always had tremendous concern for mental illness services. Another thing that I did was to adapt the Maudsley's rather fossilized view of a hostel ward to a very different concept of a ward. In these hostel wards, patients with chronic illnesses could take responsibility for their life and begin to see the world in a different way. It's a bit odd being asked what should be done now because I am no longer in a position to do things that would influence the system.

I: Looking at the problems with hindsight and in the context of your experience, highlighting what you see as problems and potential solutions is what we need to do, I think one of the other interesting things that you did in Manchester was develop a masters course for overseas trainees.

DG: Yes. I'm very proud of that. We sent trained people back to Africa and India and Pakistan. I wish I could say that every trainee returned to their home country, but some of them refused to go, Britain being a comfortable place. Often people didn't support me in encouraging them to go back to developing countries and the government did not want people to be obliged to go home. Many did not go home, which was a great fault of the system. It would have also been so much more efficient had we been able to bring people in for two years and send them home again with a completely different view of mental illness services in developing countries. The work I have done in low-income countries has been a very important part of my life and in that context, it was that teaching of doctors who wanted to come to Manchester was important. Unfortunately, the price we paid was that some of them wouldn't go home.

I: That raises a very interesting question about personal choice in the whole migration question. When you decided to set up that course, what were the primary aims from your perspective? What were you hoping to achieve?

DG: I was wanting trainees to learn that they have to turn the service upside down to be done differently, they must influence the Ministry of Health of the country that they worked in. This would allow them to innovate and help service development. This depressing mental hospital model that the developing world has, is expensive, inefficient, and doesn't achieve anything. To what extent did I succeed or not is really difficult to judge. Some of trainees went back and worked in the same service again and didn't try and contact the Ministry of Health and make suggestions about how to develop new services, as was my intention. I was hoping that they would be innovators who thought about and brought about change. I find some African countries really quite depressing and antediluvian in their views. So it's been a very mixed thing, but I have been proud to work with Professor Mubasshar in Pakistan who came nearest to revolutionizing mental illness services in that country. I was very pleased to help in that.

I: How did you select these trainees? Did the word spread and people put themselves forward, or were they sent by their respective governments?

DG: No, not respective governments. They don't do anything like that. We were paying. I was using National Health Service (NHS) money to train and I had arrangements from the banks so trainees could be given a bank loan as soon as they landed in this country because the trainees had a number of very costly things they had to do. Luckily, when we talked to the banks, they understood. It would be word of mouth; people would write to me and I said the same thing to all of them: just tell me what it is that you want to learn and how it would fit back into your service. They obliged me but they didn't always do what they said, but I do think it was worth it. The teachers and service providers were very interesting people in the north-west of England. They warmed to these doctors, it was something new for them.

I: Over the years your clinical practice shifted because you did liaison psychiatry and then you also did some gender identity work, did you not?

DG: Yes, that was just thrust upon me. It was John Hurley's interest; he was my predecessor in Manchester where he was the Reader in Psychiatry. I was appointed to the Chair in Manchester before I went to Philadelphia. I didn't do a day's work in Manchester before I left but I had a job to come back to.

I: Your clinical practice covered a range of patients and range of topics from liaison to primary care to gender.

DG: I realized that for the first 15 years I was in Manchester I was researching primary care and producing data. I was building the structure of my views of the problems facing mental health services and psychiatry. I am proud of that. I think I was the first person to relate rates of mental disorders in the community to rates in primary care, in psychiatric services as a whole but also in different arms of psychiatric services. These rates can give us a realistic model of what services need in terms of resources. You had asked me to say what needed to be done and I refused but now I have done so (laughs).

I: You have mentioned Sir Aubrey Lewis as one of your heroes; are there others?

DG: There was nothing to touch him; he was in a class by himself. There were other people whom I found quite impressive. In the United States, Paul McHugh and John Romano are both very well-known psychiatrists.

I: Anybody else in the United Kingdom you would see as your hero?

DG: No. Nobody else here.

I: Do you have any advice on how to improve recruitment to psychiatry?

DG: Well, I think we ought to give credit where it is due. I think that the (Royal) College has actually succeeded in improving recruitment in psychiatry and I don't know quite how the College did it. What we used to do was to have career fairs. One setup that I did when I was in Manchester was to encourage medical students who had passed the exams, especially those who were having to do sort of repeat courses to bring themselves up to scratch. We got them all to do research projects, not necessarily in psychiatry. My colleagues in psychiatry would always be pleased to have a medical student to do research projects. Many of the projects were psychiatric so that was excellent. You get these moments of freedom in your life when you are able to do things. I doubt whether you can do it now when the General Medical Council's dead hand is on the whole thing; you can't do it anymore.

I: I think that's a good point because I feel increasingly that clinical practice is being strangled by over-regulation.

DG: Yes, I agree

I: It seems to be becoming much more of a box-ticking exercise.

DG: People who don't really understand much about psychological disorders are in control and can make decisions which have a deleterious effect on both patients and clinicians.

I: One of the interesting things in recent times has become that often many managers are only interested in whether the regulations and regulators have been complied with by filling in forms. Looking back, the training approval visits that the College used to do were quite facilitatory. By looking at the training in a particular hospital or rotational scheme, you could advise what they needed to change. But reforms took that away from the College. What do you see as characteristics of a good psychiatrist?

DG: I judge a good psychiatrist mainly by their ability to interview patients and their families. I think what is good for me is having an open mind and being prepared to follow the patient where the patient takes you rather than imposing a strict model on what's going on.

I: You have made that point earlier about early days of GHQ and when you were working in St Thomas's about communication skills and the fact that the gastroenterologists were quite surprised with the information that you were coming up with.

DG: (laughs) I remember that. They were surprised.

: I don't know what we can do about that, nothing, I think. Organized medicine is such a focused business. Often doctors are not really prepared to hear what patients' lives are really like and it appears that nobody has the time to talk to the patients. I didn't have responsibility for looking after Crohn's disease or other conditions. I was there to discover how they functioned psychologically, which is what I did. The gastroenterologists were very surprised by the things I could tell them and it was a bit of a luxury being able to do that.

I: It links in with what you have done quite a lot in your career which is about training and communication.

DG: It's what I think is important.

I: Can you identify what you see as gaps in the practice of psychiatry?

DG: No, I don't think I can. I think I have been out of it too long.

I: You're still in touch with people, I'm sure. I mean, if you were writing to your younger self, what would you say?

DG: I think I'd advise him to do what I did. I think that I did the only thing that I'm likely to be able to do. I could see these huge problems between primary care and specialist care. I could also see the massive problems in low-income countries and I wanted to address both of them, which I did as far as I could. I think there are changes I made which are slight and not that impressive but on the whole, I think that we have succeeded in part in making the government realize that the huge mental hospital is a poor structure, really.

I: What would you have done differently if you were starting over again?

DG: You want me to suppose that I'm back there in an earlier stage with the knowledge that I have?

I: Yes.

DG: I don't know if I would have done anything differently, I'm quite happy with what I did, I mean I'm not complacent, it's just that . . . I don't know.

I: You have talked about your role both in terms of primary care psychiatry and psychiatry in low- and middle-income countries. These are the achievements that you said you are very proud of. Is there anything else?

DG: I'm not very proud, they were just achievements.

I: I think you are the first person to highlight those, weren't you?

DG: I think so, yes.

I: Michael (Shepherd)'s work was also largely in primary care research but yours was different.

DG: My contribution and his are quite different. He was taking all the things the GPs told him. I was interested in what they were missing, what was going on that they didn't seem to know about. But also what we should be doing about what they were missing and that was tremendously different from his work. That's why I said if I had my time again, I would still want to do what I have done. It takes a long time to do these things and did I succeed? No, I didn't. I didn't succeed in everything I tried but I was very impatient of the world order and wanted to see things done differently. I wanted to produce change, and at the time I was working I think I did just that. The thing that is sour for me is that the changes I produced have all been undone. Everything I did at the Maudsley has been undone. I think Manchester has had such a bad time since I left that there's probably very little left of all the things that I set up there. I see my life as having been a temporary phenomenon. I was reading George Orwell this morning and his thoughts and really, 60 to 70 years after he died people are still quoting what he said and what he did. They won't be doing that for me, I suspect. My children are my main products. I'm very proud of them. I produced four kids whom I like. I did what I could when I was at work and it hasn't had much of an effect on anything.

I: The fact that GHQ is probably one of the most commonly used screening tools is important, don't you think?

DG: The research I have done has been much imitated and I'm very pleased about that. It appears that in this area I have made the most impact. It has always excited me because of the information you can get from the screening questionnaire about the sort of symptoms that are common and what people have. The patients and their symptoms are often not seen in that way by the physicians looking after them. Yes, the rise of GHQ has been a huge success and it's the only thing that still pays me (laughs).

I: Is there anything else that you would like to add that we haven't talked about or covered?

DG: No, I was very glad that I had the opportunities that I did have to mould a big provincial university department, which I did, and made it innovative. We innovated, we brought in foreign medical graduates. We taught GPs what they had never been taught before. That was good. I think that the things that I did at the Institute were good but they haven't lasted and that's disappointing. Do you think I'm being unwisely pessimistic?

I: I think you are. If we look at your contributions, the GHQ and the Goldberg–Huxley model (which described the biopsychosocial model of mental illnesses and the pathways into care from being treated in the community, primary care, secondary care and tertiary care) will stand the test of time. Nothing that you said in that context has changed and very much the same model is still applicable. The work that you did for international medical graduates was truly impressive and ground breaking.

DG: The thing I haven't mentioned which I'm pleased about is that I have suggested a new way of thinking about comorbidity and I have done that for the WHO. Dr Devora Kastel is leading the mental health division. She hasn't got the option of not using my work. She's got to use it; it is what the WHO produced for the primary care diagnosis in ICD-11 (the International Classification of Diseases 11). We produced a lot of research based on the fieldwork we did. So I'm quite pleased about that. If you want me to start cheering up, I will (laughs).

I: Thank you.

5
Billy E. Jones

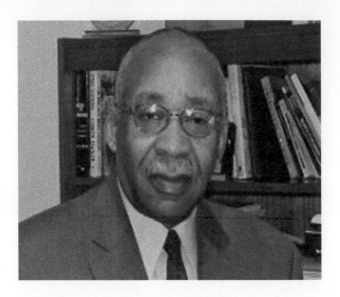

Biography

Billy Jones is a seasoned, board-certified psychiatrist. He has served as President/CEO, NYC Health and Hospitals Corporation; Commissioner, NYC Department of Mental Health; Medical Director Lincoln Hospital; and was Senior Associate Dean, NYMC, and Professor of Psychiatry. Dr Jones is the author of numerous articles, chapters, and books on treating African Americans and LGBTQ (lesbian, gay, bi-sexual, transsexual, queer) members. He is a co-editor of the recently published, 'Black Mental Health, Patients, Providers, and Systems'. Dr Jones is a Distinguished Life Fellow of the APA, the American College of Psychiatrists, the New York Academy of Medicine and is a past-President of the Black Psychiatrists of America. He is currently Clinical Professor of Psychiatry, NYU Grossman School of Medicine, and has a small private practice in New York City.

Interview

I: Thanks very much for making the time and taking part in this series of interviews. You have had an impressive career in different fields. Can we start off by looking at your childhood and growing up and what that was like?

EJ: My growing up/childhood and adolescence was most pleasant as I look back on it now. I grew up in the Midwest in Dayton, Ohio, where I was born. I am the second of three children from an intact family. My parents had been married several years before they had any children and were married for more than 50 years when my father passed away at the age of 77. The oldest child in my family was my sister and the youngest one was my brother. Hence, there were two boys and one girl. My sister was very bright and excelled in school. Neither one of my parents had finished high school, but they were very committed to seeing that their children were educated and did well. By the time I finished the eighth grade in elementary school, I absolutely refused to go to the high school where my sister had attended because the teachers sometimes forgot and called me by her name. This was obviously very embarrassing for a boy, so I said 'no more of this! I'm not going to any school where she went.' I attended a different high school than she did, which was really setting out on my own. From kindergarten to the fourth grade, I went to school with my sister. We would play along the way. We loved movies, so we would go to see the musicals, and we would dance and sing on our way to school. While my parents taught her to read before going to school, she taught me to read. I can remember learning to recite Abraham Lincoln's 'Gettysburg Address' as she was learning it in her fifth or sixth grade class. I was in the first or second grade. I was well prepared for elementary school, which gave me a good start. I did not go to the high school she had attended, which was mainly White in an all-White side of town. I did not want to go. I went to a different high school all the way on the west side of town. In order to attend that high school, I had to pretend I lived with my aunt who lived in the right district for that school. I had to get up earlier in the morning but it was worth it to be striking out on my own. I also had to make new friends because it was in a different neighbourhood. Hence my first two years of high school were different. I didn't study as much and I didn't apply myself as much as my sister. She was four years ahead of me so she had gone off to college. I very distinctly remember that on one occasion my parents and aunt looked at my report card and said, 'Billy, you'd better start applying yourself if you want to go to college'. So by the middle of my sophomore year, I settled down. Actually, I became a member of a group that was really very good for me in the sense of being young people who were much more focused on what they wanted to do and what they studied. I ended up doing very well in high school. At the same time, I needed to decide what I wanted to do career-wise. My aunt was a doctor. I had been more musically inclined. I had taken piano lessons for eight years or more. In high school, I took organ lessons and I just was drifting along, thinking that I would do something related to music. My aunt suggested that I should start thinking about what I wanted to do. My parents agreed with her. She pitched in saying that I would not be able to support a family as a piano teacher. I knew that I had little creative musical ability. I realized then that I did not want to struggle through life and not being able to at least try to excel in something. I decided that I would go to college as a pre-med student. I went to Howard University in Washington, DC, which was the first time I was that far away from home. I had a marvellous time. I enjoyed the college experience. I pledged to a fraternity and enjoyed being on my own even though I lived in the dorm. It was a very good time. I managed to major in pre-med which was a mixture of biology, zoology, and a little bit of chemistry, which I absolutely hated but managed to pass. Interestingly enough, physics was a subject I found one of the easiest and most enjoyable, so I did OK. Following that I was off to medical school at Meharry Medical College in Nashville, primarily because that College accepted me first. The first year I applied myself. I nailed myself to my seat and studied. I started out saying I was going to study six hours per night and once I got back the results from my first embryology test, I got a score of 100, the best grade in the class. I said, 'Oh wow! I don't have to study that much.' Medical school was enjoyable. I went from there to a residency in New York. My sister had married and was living in New York City and I went to a hospital out in Long Island for my internship. Following that, I came into the city to do my psychiatric residency.

How I decided to go into psychiatry is interesting. Throughout medical school I decided I wanted to be (like all the other medical students) everything. We would study a subject and I would like it and decide that that was my career path. We would then study and focus on something else as medical students and I would change and want to follow that direction. By the time I got to psychiatry, during my junior year, there was a new chairman of the department. He was a young guy, Lloyd Elam, who was outstanding and later became well known and the President of Meharry Medical College. I think he had an influence particularly on the students in my year because we were one of his first classes. At least six of us decided to go into psychiatry which was unheard of for Meharry. One of your questions asks: 'How was it that I picked psychiatry?' For me, it boiled down to being between psychiatry or paediatrics because I enjoyed working with the kids. I guess what turned me off paediatrics was when you end up treating or being with a really sick kid. It just would drain me emotionally. So I thought that I would never be able to spend my life doing this and I didn't just want to do well-baby clinics. Psychiatry was a new field and it was a challenge. It was more interesting to me being able to show my empathy. I liked the idea. I did my residency at New York Medical College and that was during the time the faculty was writing the *Comprehensive Textbook of Psychiatry* edited by Al Freedman and Harold Kaplan. Al Freedman was the chair of the department and Kaplan was the director of residency training. Kaplan was always off dealing with the book and was rarely at the College. Al Freedman became my mentor and a role model, as was the chairman at Meharry, Lloyd Elam. A few years later, when I was about to get out of the army, I had lunch with Al Freedman and he encouraged me to come back to the department and be on the faculty. He thought I might enjoy it, and indeed I did. Ben Saddock, who became one of the editors of the *Comprehensive Textbook* later, ran group therapy for the residents. I was in one of his early groups. As I look back at this picture of my training and early experiences, I see that I have been close to people who were successful role models.

Let me tell you about my time in the army. I had been in ROTC, the Reserve Officers Training Corps, for four years while in college. The deal was that you had to be in it for two years at that school. If you were in it for four years then you graduated not only with a degree but with a commission as second lieutenant in the military. I thought that joining for four years made sense because I did not want to be drafted out of college into the military nor to go into the army as a private. But mainly I joined because I wanted to be able to go from college directly to medical school and deal with the army once I had finished my medical training. Fortunately, that was the way it worked out for me. I graduated college and received a title as a second lieutenant and was deferred for four years to attend medical school. I then was deferred for four more years to complete my internship and residency training. Unfortunately, the deferment did not pay for medical school, residency training, nor did it provide a salary. When I got into the army, I was by that time actually a captain because I got a promotion doing my time as a reservist, when I was training. I still remember during the last year of my residency in my psychoanalysis lying on the couch, talking with my analyst about not wanting to go into the army. This was the time of the Vietnam War and I really did not want to go to Vietnam as I didn't believe in what we were doing there. I was spouting off about how I was going to run off to Canada. My analyst said to me that I needed to be a bit more realistic. 'The army has put all this time in you, and you will never be able to come back if you go to Canada,' he pointed out. I guess that reason won the day. I was assigned to Vietnam. I got off the plane in Vietnam and was met by an enlisted officer who was calling my name, had a jeep, and drove me to my assignment. I was assigned to run the mental health clinic in the stockade. The site looked like a stockade out of a Western. It was made of lumber, logs and all that stuff. The reason that they were so clear about where I was going was that they had their eye on me because there had been a race riot in this stockade the year before, and it had been nearly burned down. For the entire time I was there, more than 50 per cent of the prisoners in the stockade were Black. They were Black Americans and also from Puerto Rico. The stockade was for US soldiers (not for the Vietnamese). There was racial tension throughout almost the entire duration of the Vietnam War. This racial tension exploded within the stockade on one occasion and almost did so again at another time while I was there. For the military, here was this young, Black officer, who was a psychiatrist, coming on active duty that they felt they could use. Well, it made sense and it actually worked to some degree. There was an occasion when the Black soldiers/prisoners conducted a sit-in and refused to come out of their barracks. The commander of the stockade, who was a colonel, came and got me and we walked around the periphery. He was wringing his hands over what was he going to do. It was likely that his career would be over if there was another riot. I suggested to him that perhaps I should go in and talk with the prisoners on sit-in to find out what their complaints were. Along with a young Black lieutenant, I went in to talk with the soldiers who were saying that they were being mistreated. That was probably partially true but not quite to the extent that they saw it. We talked about what they wanted. In the end it boiled down to the fact that they wanted to be respected and that they did not like the way the guards were treating them. These were 18- to 22-year-old guys who were being guarded by the military police, who were also 18- to 22-year-old guys who were mostly White. Hence, there was always this adolescent push and pull of the one-upmanship kind of problem going on. I was able to explain some of that to the commander and got to the point of being able to negotiate a few changes that were sensible. This was very helpful to him.

A couple of months later, several different areas of the military in Vietnam were directed by the Pentagon to do an assessment and evaluation of racial tension in their areas, and of course they also asked the medical area. The Vietnam Medical Military command assigned me to do that assessment. I travelled around various areas and to different hospitals to assess racial tensions. I conducted focus groups in most of the areas with enlisted and with the non-commissioned officers, and also with the officers and local commanders who were in charge. The findings were as you would expect. The enlisted soldiers often did not like the sergeants and non-commissioned officers, and there were issues related to race. These were the ones with which they had the most problems. I wrote the report but never had any feedback.

The stockade was the only prison for US soldiers in the country. We saw marines, navy people, and air force personnel who might have done something wrong and were being detained. The marines guarded the US Embassy. One of the guys who guarded the embassy in Saigon had a psychotic episode. He was at the onset age of 21 or 22, when schizophrenia and other psychotic illnesses often start. He fired his weapon in the Embassy, killing a couple of people. He returned to his barracks, shaved his head, and wrapped himself in sheets. He was apprehended and like other marines he was brought to the stockade. As with others, it was my responsibility to evaluate and treat him. It was clear he had a psychotic episode requiring inpatient treatment, probably for a long time period. I told military command that he needed to be sent back home. I medicated him, of course, but none of the pilots were willing to fly him back without me being on the plane. As a result, I got a five-day trip to Tokyo accompanying the patient. This happened about a month or so after I just got there. There were experiences in the military that were interesting and these two I vividly remember.

When I returned to the United States, I spent my second year in the army working in Washington, DC in the Army Surgeon General's Office. Following that I joined the faculty at New York Medical College and ended up in the middle of a struggle between NYC mental health structure and the College over the community mental health centre. I ended up leaving because I did not want to be in the middle of that. I took a job in Brooklyn and then the Bronx, and became Director of Psychiatry, at Lincoln Hospital in the South Bronx.

I: That is really fascinating. How long were you in Vietnam?

EJ: Just a year. All that happened to me in one year.

I: Was there a point when your sexual orientation became important to you or an issue in the army?

EJ: Not really. I can remember dealing with that question before I went to Vietnam. I started my psychoanalysis while I was a resident in the second year of my training. I started seeing an analyst which was typical in the training programme that I was in. In many of the good training programmes in the States at that time it was the norm. Dealing with that whole question was one of the things that my analyst and I talked about. I said to him that I did not think it was going to be a problem due to several factors. At that point I had met the person that I have spent my life with and he wasn't going into the army. We communicated and made tape recordings we sent back and forth. Now if the army had intercepted them and listened to them, they probably would have thrown me out (laughs). I didn't feel it was necessary to come out in the army. I did not feel that I was going to fall in love with anybody that would cause me to come out, and none of that happened. What I felt was a bit of low-grade depression from being there throughout the whole year. No, that wasn't the problem.

I: And over the years, how do you think psychiatry has changed?

EJ: At the time when I went into psychiatry it was much less biochemical in focus and much more psychodynamic. This was the end of the time when the analyst ran things. They felt they were the cream of the crop, and some of them were. In New York Medical College I had an interesting experience. I haven't written about or figured out how to write about it so far. During residency training, my analyst was White and Jewish. When I came back and was thinking of finishing my analysis, he was the picture in my head of where I was going to go. After returning, I was talking with a very good friend of mine who was a psychiatrist and he suggested that I should see a Black analyst. He was Black and I figured 'well that's a thought' (laughs). I hadn't really consciously planned to talk with my analyst about it, but of course race was there as a subject and it came out and I said that I did not know any Black analysts. And my analyst said, 'if you can't find one, then nobody can find one'. My analyst thought it was a good idea to find one and encouraged me, so I did. I found somebody and with the blessings of my old analyst I started seeing him. Now the difference between seeing a Black and a White analyst is what I have really resisted trying to write about. I'm not really sure how much difference there was. I remember very distinctly being able to talk about some things more easily with a Black analyst. We would call my grandmother 'Big Momma', which is a typical term used in Black families for the grandmother. I felt a lot freer to talk about that with my Black analyst than with my White analyst. So that says to me that there certainly have to be other things that I haven't focused on, and that there are differences. And I think it would make a fascinating paper but I don't know quite how to get into it and overcome the resistance to this topic (laughs).

I: I would think that's partly about identity. One's identity is important in the way that one has been brought up and in the commonality of identity.

EJ: Yes, I think there were things that I could say to a Black analyst that I just couldn't otherwise. I just knew that he understood because he had a similar or common life experience to me and I didn't feel like I had to explain. I don't know how many of those things I kept from saying with the White analyst. There is certainly something in that.

I: Do you think that it might have also been helpful having had analysis for two years and then a break and then coming back to a Black analyst that might have opened up other possibilities?

EJ: I had not thought about the break because I would just have finished my analysis with the White analyst had not there been that break between seeing him and seeing a Black analyst.

I: Was Vietnam a traumatic time?

EJ: Yes. Being that far away and everything. I never was physically afraid because I was in the biggest US military post in the world. But it was like being in the middle of Kansas with absolutely nothing else around. It was six months of dust and six months of mud because it rained half the year and it was dry for the other half of the year.

I: What do you make of the current state of psychiatry?

EJ: I don't know if you are aware of some of the other things that I have done. It is different and it is like I have grown not only as a psychiatrist but as a physician. What I have done mostly has been community psychiatry and administrative psychiatry; that's what I had wanted to do. When I came back to New York Medical College, I came back as an assistant director of the community mental health centre. Then the city and the College had a fight about who was going to name the director. The College wanted to name me as the director and the city said no, because I was too young. So I left as I did not want to be in the middle of this fight. The difference now is that I have done everything in this city. I have run a department, grown the department, become the medical director of the hospital which is a general care hospital with psychiatry. I became the senior associate dean at the medical school and a tenured professor. I left when Mayor David Dinkin, the first Black mayor in New York City's history, asked me to be the commissioner of mental health for the city. I did that. There was a problem with the running of the city hospitals which I had trained in, not only Lincoln but all 11 city hospitals and with clinics and staff. So I moved from being the commissioner of mental health of the city to be the President and CEO of New York City Health and Hospital Corporation, which is the largest municipal hospital system in the country and I ran that. I have had a view from almost every perspective except the voluntary private hospital systems. I never particularly wanted to work there so I didn't. But I cannot imagine that they didn't have some of the same problems that the public hospital system had.

I: And when was that?

EJ: I was at Lincoln as the director of psychiatry from the mid-1970s to 1990. I went to work for the city in 1990 as commissioner. I was there for two years and then two years as the President of the Health and Hospital Corporation.

I: At the present time, what do you see as the problems psychiatry faces?

EJ: At the present time there are too few psychiatrists. Being a psychiatrist has never been sexy and well paid (laughs). So that is a problem and I think it takes a certain interest in people to want to be a psychiatrist because it involves taking on someone else's problems. One needs to have empathy even to consider the problems of somebody else.

I: You said that there are fewer psychiatrists than are needed. How would you improve recruitment into psychiatry?

EJ: That is interesting. I have obviously been on the faculty and done some teaching. I pictured in my own life that going into medicine was like a move into science. Then going into psychiatry is sort of like moving away from science because it requires not just science but art and human interest in humanness and in humanity, in human traits and the human condition which I don't see in surgeons and other medical professionals.

I: Do you not think medicine itself is an art backed by science?

EJ: I used to but it seems to me that it has moved almost the other way around

I: Talking about kind of science versus art and how you think we should improve recruitment, and in your role, what were the challenges that you faced?

EJ: When I was director of psychiatry at Lincoln, we restarted the residency training programme. Because of the particular needs of that community, we did a lot of recruiting in Puerto Rico because we needed residents from US-approved medical schools. We also wanted Spanish-speaking individuals. I don't speak Spanish but we went to Puerto Rico and recruited from the two or three US-approved medical schools there. It was difficult to find doctors who were interested in psychiatry. But once we found them, they were interested in coming to the United States. So that worked well, and we recruited some very good residents over a number of years. I always thought that we needed to get diverse residents. Diversity within the medical schools is important. Then one needs to move down the chain to interest medical students in psychiatry. Psychiatry can come across as being fairly esoteric. I am not sure if that's good for some medical students. For some, it needs to be a bit more concrete. If you think about surgery, cutting and moving bones and that sort of thing can be very attractive to some people. I have always thought that the teachers who were involved in teaching the medical students were really the key to getting more residents into psychiatry. I did teach residents. I had a little experience with teaching medical students at City University when I became commissioner. I was restricted by the Conflict Board from doing a lot of work in other arenas. I think students seeing teachers that are more like them, in the sense of what they were doing and having some connections to the community was encouraging for people who might look at psychiatry and wonder if it was for them. The type of questions are: 'what kind of patients am I going to see?' And 'what is the field going to be about?' Or, 'am I going to make any money' " All these sort of issues come up when you try to decide what you want to do after you graduate, particularly if you are from a minority population. Also, whether White patients are going to come to see you, and where one should set up practice. I thought these issues were important and needed to be addressed. Unfortunately, not a lot of non-Black, non-minority psychiatrists could actually respond to those kinds of questions in any meaningful way. A Black woman psychiatrist, June Christmas, was the commissioner for several terms before me and she ran a medical training programme for mental health at City University. I had been lecturing along with Phyllis Harrison Ross, at New York Medical College, who was a Black women psychiatrist. We were able to do a course on Ethnicity and Culture for the students. The particular students that we seemed to interest were interested not only based on their ethnicity but were interested in community psychiatry.

I: What do you see as gaps in training in psychiatry at the moment?

EJ: I think I had a little concern about it earlier concerning the direction in which training is going. There is no doubt that you need to teach the science of psychiatry because that needs to be understood. There appears to be a decrease of teaching about the art of it and other aspects of the mind as compared to the brain. Yes, you want to teach about the brain but you also want to teach about the mind. You also want to teach about the art of psychiatry.

I: One of the things that interests me personally very much is psychiatry's social contract. It is about how society expects us to take people's freedom away and lock them up. How do you feel that can be delivered? It is a three-way contract in the United Kingdom between the government, the patients, and the doctors, within the United States it would be the government and the insurance companies and psychiatrists and patients. What do you think we should be doing as psychiatrists to deliver that?

EJ: I have always felt that of the different aspects of medicine, psychiatry was the one that should be leading the way with regards to the social aspects and the social contract. That means psychiatrists need to be particularly careful in what image they present. They must be cautious and aware of patients' rights. When you started to talk about this, I recalled a patient I had as a resident who caused me to learn a lot. This was a woman who lived next door to the hospital and was an alcoholic prostitute. As it turned out, she had slept with most of the policemen in that vicinity. She developed a crush on me so we had to figure out how to deal with that (laughs). I went to my supervisor to find out how I could deal with this. I came up with this scheme and the supervisor agreed. I would turn her chair around when she came in, so that she didn't face me because when she was facing me, all of the other stuff would come up. After a few sessions of doing that, she was able to concentrate and talk about various things that were important to her. But I did think that I should be treating her. The answer was not to say that this was an inappropriate patient. She might have been that in a lot of ways, but it wasn't appropriate to close the door to treatment. I learned more from struggling with how to do this than I would have otherwise. It was an interesting task to figure out how to do that and also to engage with the community. I was still a resident when I was in the community working with community organizations and I was the one who had been sent out there rather than the supervisor. I was always concerned as a resident that I would overly identify with what the community was pushing for or asking for. I don't know if I'm answering the question.

I: In the end it is all about patient care and you are giving a very fascinating example being on the frontline and trying to do your best and everything else is secondary to that. So, moving on, what would you tell your younger self?

EJ: About going into psychiatry (laughs)? Actually, now looking back I would jump at the chance of going into psychiatry. As mentioned earlier, my two favourite rotations among all were paediatrics and psychiatry. As I said, I didn't pick paediatrics because well babies are fine but sick babies were too much for me. Neither paediatrics nor psychiatry paid much, so it wasn't because of that. I think there are still new opportunities for psychiatrists that exist. It is still a relatively new, fresh area. Back then, when I started, the establishment of the community mental health centres encouraged me and I went into it. Now that's not the case. However, I have just finished participating with some other psychiatrists in applying for a SAMHSA (Substance Abuse and Mental Services Administration) grant related to the establishment for a Center of Excellence for Black Psychiatry. Along with colleagues, we established an Institute of Black Psychiatry named after Chester Pierce. Did you ever meet Chester Pierce?

I: I don't think so. I know the name but I don't think I actually met him.

EJ: He has passed away now. He was a very distinguished Black psychiatrist at Harvard. The other person we named it after is Carl Bell. Did you meet Carl?

I: Yes, I did. I met Carl on several occasions.

EJ: Yes, so it's the Pierce Bell Institute of Black Psychiatry and that entity is one of groups applying for a SAMHSA grant to establish a centre of excellence for Black psychiatrists. The SAMHSA funding is over five years. SAMHSA is also funding a similar grant for a centre for excellence in LGBTQ matters. It is a way of acknowledging that there's still more to be done in these areas and still more things to be learned. I like being part of that because I recognize and feel that it's needed. I don't know if I have moved away from your question.

I: I'll come back to that later on because I think that's quite important but do you want to talk about your journey as a gay psychiatrist?

EJ: I struggled with that when I laid on the couch in my analysis and clearly accepted the fact that I was gay. During that time I met the person who has been my life partner. I was in my second year of residency when we met and we have been together now for 53, going on 54 years. It is clearly a part of me and my various interests. We have a son that we adopted when he was three weeks old, so we are a family. We do things as a family and we have been a family for a very long time. I think even though analysis in those days was saying that this was an illness and I was training at probably one of the worst places that taught that. There were people like Irving Bieber on the faculty. There were also faculty that did not believe it was an illness.

I: How did analysts respond to you being in analysis and you moving on from a Jewish analyst to a Black psychoanalyst. How did they deal with it?

EJ: How did they deal with me? Well, they knew it. I mean clearly, they knew it. It wasn't a hidden fact because Ben Saddock had established an analytically oriented group for my year of residents. There were 13 or 14 in that year and I came out in the group. Though I was in analysis I never wanted to be an analyst nor go to an analytic school. My analysts certainly knew it. When it became time for me to go into the army, that was talked about. People thought it might be a problem though I never did because I was not publicly out. Of course, people knew. When I look back now, I could have stood up and said I did not want to be in the army but that never crossed my mind at that time. After I got there, I felt that it was unfair for me to have refused to go because of my being gay when there were 18- to 20-year-old guys who went wherever they were sent. They needed me as a physician and they needed treatment. That would have been a little bit too selfish of me to refuse to go because I was gay.

I: You didn't have spurs in your heels, did you?

EJ: No (laughs), but it didn't sit right for me morally. So, I went. Since then, there have been times when I have been discriminated against because of my sexual orientation. I am sure there have been times when I didn't find out. There were certainly times that I was discriminated against because of my colour and race in ways that I probably never realized.

I: In a way you were facing double discrimination, so one doesn't know whether you were being discriminated against because of orientation or because of ethnicity or colour of your skin. The third discrimination often is that of being a psychiatrist.

EJ: I have been discriminated against for all those reasons. Let me tell you about being a psychiatrist. I became the President of the medical staff at Lincoln Hospital, but when they were looking for a medical director for the hospital, the director of the hospital wanted to appoint me. He talked to the President of the Health and Hospital Corporation about it. He was told that I was a psychiatrist I could not be the medical director for the hospital. In that case it happened anyway. There was a time also that I was discriminated against because of my age and I was told I was too young. The time I was discriminated against for being gay I was at Lincoln Hospital at the time as the Director of Psychiatry and the position of Director of Psychiatry for Harlem Hospital became available. The Chair of Psychiatry at Columbia University called and asked me to meet with him and he talked to me about it. Now I wasn't sure I wanted to move but by the time we finished talking he offered me the position. Well, a day or two later, two friends in two different conversations called me to tell me that some of the other staff in the department of psychiatry at Harlem had heard this and had called a meeting and talked about not wanting to have a director who was gay. As a result, I never heard from the chair of the department at Columbia.

I: So the letter never arrived?

EJ: The letter never arrived. I never heard from him. The second time was while I was in New York City Government as commissioner. I was interviewed to be the President of Downstate Medical School in Brooklyn. It comes under the NY State University system. The deputy of the state university system arranged to have dinner with me to talk with me about whether or not I would be interested, and he encouraged me to go for it. They then sent the recommended finalists to the public elected officials in the Brooklyn area where the school is located and someone else got picked. My thoughts were, 'well, you win some and you lose some'. A month or two later, one of the elected officials in Brooklyn told me that I had not got the job because I was gay. There has been discrimination I knew about at the time, some I knew about later, and I'm sure some I didn't know about at all.

I: What would your advice be to the trainees of today?

EJ: That they pick the right field. That is the first thing I want to tell them. They should endeavour to do whatever role they want to take because psychiatry is open enough as a field. I tell them that they can be successful in almost anything they want to do if they work hard at it.

I: What would you like to be remembered for?

EJ: I guess most importantly as a good father and as a good spouse. I think also as a good physician and good with my patients.

I: Do you still see patients?

EJ: I have a day of patients a week. I don't want to not do anything.

I: Which of your achievements are you most proud of?

EJ: I guess some of the things that I ended up doing at Lincoln. We did some research, we did some writing, we published. Recently I edited a book with Altha Stewart and Ezra Griffith about Black mental health. I guess some of the contributions that I have attempted to make, both academically like writing and for what I have done in patient care, are things I am proud of.

I: I'm a great fan of Ezra's. He has been doing some fantastic stuff. Is there anything that I haven't covered that you would like to talk about?

EJ: Well, there will be when I finish, I'll think of something (laughs).

I: That's been absolutely fabulous, Billy, Thank you so much for your time.

6
Shigenobu Kanba

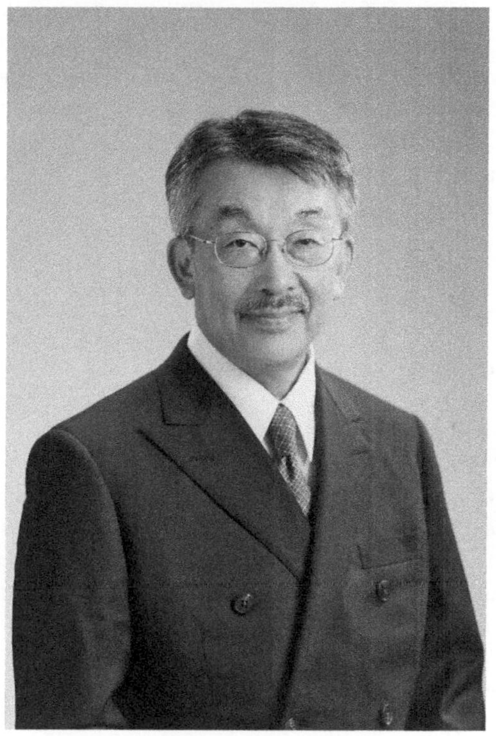

Biography

Professor Kanba trained at Keio University Medical School in Tokyo and then trained at the Mayo Clinic in Rochester, Minnesota, United States before returning to Japan. He has been Professor and Chair of Psychiatry at Yamanashi University School of Medicine and then Professor and Chair at Kyushu University Graduate School of Medicine where he is Professor Emeritus. His research interests have been mood disorders, psychoneuroimmunology, and psychopharmacology and his work has been published widely. He is the immediate past President of the Japanese Society of Psychiatry and Neurology (JSPN) and an honorary member of the World Association of Psychiatry (WPA). He was President of the Asian Federation of Psychiatric Associations, Vice-President of the International Society of Bipolar Disorders, and associate secretary of the World Federation of Societies of Biological Psychiatry. He is currently programme supervisor and programme officer of the Japan Agency for Medical Research and Development (AMED). He is a member of Directors of the Tokyo Metropolitan Institute of Medical Science, the Japanese Association of Medical Sciences, and is executive secretary of the Japanese Medical Science Federation. He serves in Science Council of Japan, the Committee of Health and Medicine of the Japanese Cabinet Secretariat, Social Security Committee of the Japanese Ministry of Health, Labour and Welfare, Pharmaceutical and Medical Devices Agency, and served in Brain Science Committee of the Japanese Ministry of Education, Culture, Sports, Science and Technology and in the Japan Society for the Promotion of Science. He is Editor-in-Chief Emeritus of *Psychiatry and Clinical Neurosciences* and a member of the Editorial Board of several international journals. He has received numerous honours and awards. Currently, he is President of the Japan Depression Centre (Tokyo), advisor to the Iida Hospital (Nagano), and director of the Fukuoka Institute of Behavioural Medicine (Fukuoka).

Interview

I: Thanks very much for agreeing to be interviewed.

SK: I am happy to see you Dinesh and thank you very much for your inviting me to this interview. I feel very honoured.

I: How are things? What's COVID like in Japan?

SK: I think we are experiencing the second wave now, but I think we are controlling it pretty well. (The interview was conducted on 30 August 2020.)

I: Right.

SK: There are about 1,000 positive cases each day now, but fortunately we don't have many seriously ill people.

I: That's good.

SK: How about the situation in the UK?

I: The numbers have gone down but the schools are opening next week and restaurants opened about two weeks ago so I think there will be a second spike, but nobody knows and I think part of the problem with the current government has been that it's given out very mixed messages.

SK: It's the same here.

I: One day you hear something and the next day the government changes its mind and you hear something completely different. It's really quite irritating. So, thank you very much for agreeing to do the interview, Nobu. I am delighted. You have written to me earlier and answered questions about your childhood and growing up. Do you want to say a bit more?

SK: You mean in addition to my written response? So, what do you want to know more about?

I: Normally what I do is interview people and then as you are conversing, other questions come to mind and one can explore bits about you, your childhood, interest in psychiatry, and so on and so forth. There are, of course, no right or wrong answers, just your story. Some other interviewees too have given written responses some of which have been in addition to interviews. The interviews focus on what people see as important milestones and about their leadership roles and achievements. The aim of the book is to introduce younger psychiatrists to a range of leaders in psychiatry and their views and their experiences from different cultures and different parts of the world, their different ways of doing it. The main purpose here is much more biographical. It is a collection bringing together institutional memories.

SK: Ummm, it is simple. When I got older, I began to realize I didn't have any physical ability for sports (laughs).

I: Neither do I.

SK: I used to play baseball and soccer a lot. However, I remember giving up on it because I had friends that I just couldn't compete with. On the other hand, I was a good student. I loved arithmetic, mathematics, and science, and aspired to become a scientist. I used to read biographies of mathematicians and scientists. I even created a simple laboratory space at home to conduct chemistry experiments that I read about in my textbooks, and to attempt to perform new chemical reactions. I also liked reading novels a lot. A children's book series by Erich Kästner was translated into Japanese, and I used to read them as my father bought them for me.

I: And were you the first one in your family to go into medicine?

SK: Yes.

I: Why did you choose medicine?

SK: It is simple. I watched doctors and lawyers in popular TV dramas, and both of these professions seemed very attractive. I wanted to pursue an intellectual profession. I was not particularly adept at public speaking. Since I liked science and mathematics, I had a vague notion that the field of medicine would suit me. I admired the image of doctors saving people's lives. Also, in Japan, it's very hard to get into medicine, and it was common for high-performing students to advance to medical school.

I: Which medical school did you go to?

SK: I went to the Medical School of Keio University in Tokyo. It is a competitive private medical school in Japan.

I: At what point did you decide that you wanted to become a psychiatrist?

SK: During high school, I was very inspired by an introductory book on psychoanalysis. Since then, the mysteries of the human mind have fascinated me. Medical school focused on biomedical subjects such as anatomy and physiology, so I was not introduced to psychiatric medicine until I was in my fifth year. I visited a psychiatric hospital as part of my psychiatric practical training. It was then that I learned about patients who spent many years hospitalized in closed wards. It was shocking to find out that these patients had been suffering with unimaginable symptoms for decades, in some instances all their lives, and were spending their lives in a cloistered hospital environment. Then I became obsessed with finding out why those incomprehensible symptoms emerged; how I could help in making them better and help those patients leave the hospital.

I was also fascinated with the brain, which is a complex organ. I was fascinated with the mechanism by which some drugs improve psychiatric symptoms through their action on the brain, while other substances, in contrast, cause hallucinations and delusions.

I: And do you regret doing psychiatry?

SK: I have experienced many instances where patients showed no improvement, got worse or committed suicide. On numerous occasions, I experienced the powerlessness of psychiatric medicine and my own inexperience. I am not sure how good a psychiatrist I have become compared to 40 years ago. However, I have never regretted becoming a psychiatrist. I think I was meant to be one. I must admit that there are times that I feel that I am not a 'real' doctor, like surgeons or emergency physicians. At this moment in time, it is a pity that I cannot be on the frontline against COVID-19 saving people's lives.

I: Who were your role models?

SK: In my youth, my role model of a doctor was Hideyo Noguchi of the Rockefeller University who identified causes of neurosyphilis, and who was researching yellow fever and died from it in Africa. I was also impressed with Albert Schweitzer's biography. I like his organ playing too. There is also an unforgettable image in my mind of my residency days at the Mayo Clinic where I saw, almost every single day, a famous child psychiatrist walking side by side inside the courtyard with a short and emaciated female patient with anorexia nervosa. He wasn't trying to force her to eat. I thought that the image of the doctor walking along with the patient was the epitome of what a psychiatrist should be.

I: What were your other memorable occasions when dealing with patients?

SK: I am mostly interested in mood disorders such as depression and bipolar disorder. I once received a letter, after an interval of a few years, from a patient whom I used to treat at a hospital where I worked. This was a patient who had suffered from depression for nearly a decade. I was ineffective and could not help the patient get better. However, the letter said that the patient was getting married. This was a marriage where the partner knew about and accepted all that the patient had gone through. The letter said that the patient felt as if they had hit a home run with two outs in the bottom of the ninth innings.

I also got a New Year's greeting card this year from a patient who was a housewife who switched frequently between manic and depressive episodes, and she mentioned that her mood swings had finally subsided after 16 years.

Another patient that I oversaw for six years wrote me a letter and gave it to me after hearing about my job transfer. The letter had a few lines of gratitude and it said: 'Thanks to you I have been able to stay alive until now.' That sentence left me speechless, and it made me realize how much the patient was relying on me.

In some cases, I regret the limits of my ability in psychiatry. One depressed lawyer, in what was to be his last interview as we were coming to the end of his treatment, stood still silently, as if he wanted to say something. I made an appointment for the next treatment and ended the interview without questioning the meaning of it. A few days later I received a call from his wife saying that he had killed himself. I remembered his silence and that it was something out of the ordinary. If I had listened to him more or asked about his silence, maybe he would have let go of his suicidal thoughts.

I: But I think psychiatry has changed dramatically in the last 40 years. Are there specific challenges for Japanese psychiatry? Because from here it is still very much seen as inpatient psychiatry. And the duration of admission is quite long; the median is about 400 days.

SK: Forty years ago, patients with severe mental illnesses were locked up in psychiatric hospitals. It was probably a time when patients who were once admitted to psychiatric hospitals could not rehabilitate into society and find a place to live safely. The world was full of prejudice. Some families did not want the patients to come home. In an extreme sense, once a patient was diagnosed with a severe mental illness, he or she was probably not considered a member of society.

In recent years, the average duration of hospitalization has been shortened, and there are various systems, institutions, and highly competent allied health professionals that support patients' social rehabilitation. Social prejudice against people with illnesses such as depression has lessened substantially, making it easier for patients to visit psychiatric departments. But, prejudice against patients with schizophrenia is still strong.

There are laws in place that mandate companies to hire a certain number of people with disabilities including mental illness. However, there are many patients with severe mental illnesses that psychiatry is not able to bring back to their original state of health. Their own and their family's desires are to 'want to return to how they were before they developed the illness'. I sometimes wonder how my patients from the first hospital I worked at 40 years ago are doing now.

Last year, the government spent a year developing a community mental healthcare plan to ensure that people with serious mental illnesses can live safely, and in their own way, in their communities. I was the chairman of the committee. There are many obstacles to overcome in order to make this project a reality.

I: In Japan you have changed the term 'schizophrenia'. Has that made any difference at all on stigma?

SK: Yes, I think so. Japanese is an ideographic language. You can tell what it means by looking at the letters. The previous name of the disease meant 'a split mind'. The new name '*togo-shicchou-shou*' means 'a disorder of mental integration'.

I think the change in the Japanese word for 'schizophrenia' has made a big difference in terms of how people understand the disease and how people see people with schizophrenia. In the past, I hesitated to say the diagnosis, using the old name, to patients or families but now it is easier to communicate with them using the new name.

I: How did that come about? I mean it's relatively recent, isn't it?

SK: I think it was in 2002. The World Psychiatric Association (WPA) made a very strong impact on Japanese psychiatry when we hosted the World Congress in Yokohama. We decided to change the Japanese name of schizophrenia during the meeting. It was 1993 when the request was first made by the family association to change the name.

Before the WPA World Congress in Yokohama, the psychiatric community in Japan was kind of 'closed off' to the rest of the world. The Yokohama meeting was a major moment in the change of designation.

I: Right. Is there a good relationship between the Japanese Society of Psychiatry and Neurology and associations of people with severe mental illness and family looking after them?

SK: There are patient and family associations, but they are not yet strongly organized or united. Their power is not strong enough to change the government's mental health policy. There is also a lack of cooperation between them and professional societies. As President of the Japanese Society of Psychiatry and Neurology, I would like to change this situation and established a task force to accomplish this objective.

I: That can be a problem because there can be too many organizations, and each has its own agenda.

SK: Exactly.

I: Some would say psychiatry is bad and others would say psychiatry is all good and that's a tension in itself. In your notes, you talked about lasting impressions about patients and memorable occasions. But I want to focus a bit more on talking about how psychiatry has changed in your lifetime. You said that you were planning to reduce the number of beds. Has there been any movement towards community mental health?

SK: Yes, the government has a policy of reducing psychiatric beds. As I mentioned earlier, we need to create better community psychiatric care where patients can live in the community in safety and peace. We cannot be so cruel as to force a patient to leave the hospital and put them on the street.

I: Is psychiatry mindless or brainless?

SK: The interesting part of psychiatric medicine is that one can learn subjects such as brain science, neurology, psychology, and philosophy, and broad knowledge is required to optimize understanding psychiatric problems and treatments.

I am also careful not to become brainless or mindless, and it is something I am mindful of when educating young people. In research, brain science, psychology, and psychopathology are separate fields of research; however, in the future, unless they are integrated it will not be possible to understand mental health phenomena.

I am a psychiatrist who has devoted my time to researching the brain. Tremendous progress has been made in neuroscience, and I hope that one day the pathological conditions of severe mental illnesses will be revealed. However, I believe that emotional wounds can only be healed by the affection of others. That is why I believe that psychopathology and psychotherapy are very important, and this is what I tell young psychiatrists.

I: What do you see as problems in psychiatry?

SK: Compared to cancer and heart disease, research investments by government in mental health are low in Japan. The government understands that mental health is an important issue; however, a medical care system that addresses these issues is not yet fully available. The same can be said about the cost of research of mental illnesses.

I: One of the things that I was really impressed with is that in Japan, you have had no problem in recruiting trainees in psychiatry. Is that true?

SK: I think the number of residents who want to be psychiatrists is increasing slightly. When I graduated from medical school in 1980, there was a strong prejudice against mental illness and a culture that made it difficult for patients to visit a psychiatrist.

However, the number of patients has increased and society has come to understand the importance of mental health and the role psychiatry plays in this. The prejudice has faded a little bit, and the resistance to visiting a psychiatrist has decreased.

I: Somebody showed me data that for every resident vacancy in Japan there are about seven applications. Is that correct?

SK: I don't think this is an accurate number. Psychiatry programmes in big cities such as Tokyo, Osaka, Fukuoka, etc., are very popular, while programmes in small cities in local areas are not. There is a huge difference in the number of psychiatrists between big cities and small towns. Also, the quality of psychiatric services varies.

I: I think that's true everywhere. One of the things that I was looking at in the United Kingdom was that for a very long time for every training vacancy we had 1.1 or 1.2 applications. So the numbers were really quite small, but there was also a tension between primary care and psychiatry. When primary care becomes popular, psychiatry becomes unpopular, and vice versa. There appears to be a cycle that changes every seven years. I was told that two countries that have no difficulties recruiting were Japan and Armenia. One of the reasons this appears to be the case for Japan was that a lot of it is inpatient psychiatry, so people feel safe, there are no risks such as those you face in community psychiatry. What's your thinking on this?

SK: I believe that medical students understand the need for psychiatry, and with the development of neuroscience and psychopharmacology, modern psychiatry may be attractive to talented young students. I don't know much about community psychiatry in the United Kingdom so I can't make comparisons, but in Japan, patients with serious mental illnesses are mainly treated in psychiatric hospitals, and treating them in the community is a challenge for the future.

I: In your opinion, what do you see as the problems in the current state of psychiatry?

SK: In Japan, there seems to be a gap between psychopathology/psychotherapy and neuroscience/psychopharmacology. Each group claims its own superiority. We should integrate these disciplines to improve our understanding and treatment of our patients.

There is also a gap between the medical care that patients are getting and the medical care that medical professionals are able to provide.

I: Let's talk a bit about recruitment. You went into psychiatry because you read about psychoanalysis. The question I suppose for me is how applicable is a talent in psychoanalysis to Japanese patients? And how would you encourage residents to go into psychiatry?

SK: I was attracted by psychoanalysis theory when I first read an introductory book. But as I gain more experience in psychiatry, I have realized that psychoanalysis is useful for mild neurotic patients but not for the severely mentally ill. But a small number of psychiatrists are still very interested in psychoanalysis.

I: Yes, I know.

SK: But now, young psychiatrists are more interested in neurosciences, psychopharmacology and also AI/IoT [Artificial Intelligence/Internet of Things], big data analysis, or computational psychiatry.

I: Yes. This indicates that it is possible to combine modern technological changes with patient care because Japan has been at the forefront of using AI and robots for companionship, particularly for older people.

SK: Exactly. National research projects are underway to predict the onset and recurrence of psychiatric symptoms of mental illness and dementia. In addition, an AI/IoT-based system is being developed to provide cognitive therapy via the Internet.

I: I was hearing that there was a trial going on between a university in England and one in Japan about robots who are culturally sensitive. This raises very interesting questions about the role future psychiatrists may have.

SK: I believe that COVID-19 has accelerated tele-psychiatry and the application of new technologies such as AI and IoT in psychiatric research. This was a major change in our field. Some of us are still very traditional and conservative, but the COVID-19 pandemic has forced us to change our attitudes. I think we are going to see a change and a rapid integration of new technologies into medicine and psychiatry.

I: How would you improve recruitment into psychiatry?

SK: It may not be a high-paying profession; however, I emphasize the interesting and in-depth aspects of psychiatry that explore the mysteries of the brain and mind. If the starting point of medical care is to help those who are vulnerable then it is the psychiatrist's job to stay close to the most vulnerable. It may not be as glamorous as being a heart surgeon but it is actually a highly impactful profession, as shown by the Disability-Adjusted Life Years (DALYs) of patients and the number of patients who visit.

Also, life is not only about success and happiness and one cannot avoid failure and setbacks. All these life experiences help in understanding patients. In other words, the more experiences one gains, the more one can grow as a psychiatrist.

I: And what do you see as the characteristics of a good psychiatrist? What makes a good psychiatrist?

SK: First of all, one would need adequate diagnostic skills, especially the ability not to misdiagnose neurological and physical diseases. Also, the ability to empathize with the experiences of the patients, to choose words that reach the heart of the other person, to maximize the effects of drugs while carefully avoiding side effects, and to utilize welfare fully and social support resources are all important.

Good psychiatrists need to be aware that sometimes we can't cure a patient as a surgeon can. We need to have strong tolerance of negativity, so-called negative capability. I mean that we shouldn't give up our efforts to be with our patients even when they are at their most challenging.

I: So, a good psychiatrist needs to hold out hope for the patients?

SK: Yes, exactly.

I: We talked a bit about the role the government plays. With regard to the question about psychiatry's contract with the society, it's an implicit contract, it's not straightforward. There is no signed commitment that doctors and psychiatrists will look after patients with problems, that the patient's liberty might be taken away from them, that they may be, forced to take treatment which they do not want. At the same time, the third partner in the contract is the government because it has to allocate money for the services and the hospitals. How do you think we can build a better contract and how can we deliver that?

SK: This is a very difficult question. The importance of mental health is more widely acknowledged than in the past and there is also less stigma towards psychiatric care. In Japan, more than 4 million patients undergo psychiatric consultations every year. Mental illness ranks as one of the five major diseases in our society. Society perceives psychiatry as a valuable profession.

However, in severe mental illness, the patient's behaviours may sometimes be restricted and coercive treatment has to be provided. This kind of treatment can be very traumatic for the patient. Even in these cases, thoughtful treatment is necessary to minimize psychological damage. In order to achieve this, healthcare expenditures must also be raised. Psychiatric associations and patient or family associations need to work together to change the health policy of the government.

I: I agree that we as professionals have to educate the policy-makers and we also have to educate the families. In addition, we have to be advocates for them and they have to advocate for us to the government. So this is the kind of three-way relationship that can work well and has to do so in order to deliver the social contract. What would you tell your younger self?

SK: My younger self? I wanted to be a researcher in neuroscience and psychopharmacology, so the disciplines I devoted myself to may have been biased towards those fields. Even if it was the long way around, I should have studied neurology and psychotherapy more in depth. But I don't think it is too late to start now.

I should have kept a record of all the cases that I experienced. If I had recorded each case, I would have learnt whether my initial diagnosis was correct or not and how I could have structured my treatment to achieve better results. I could have written my own textbook. However, I was too busy to make the effort.

I: What do you see as gaps in psychiatry?

SK: As I said, there is a gap among those in the fields of psychotherapy, neurobiology, and psychopharmacology. They blame each other for their own shortcomings, but they should acknowledge each other's advantages and work together to create better integrated medicine.

There is a heavy burden imposed on hospital doctors who look after patients with severe mental illness.

The remuneration for medical services at psychiatric departments is kept low compared to other departments, and the community mental healthcare and welfare systems are inadequate, compared to other fields such as cancer or cardiac medicine.

While the public's interest in mental health is rising, there is still strong prejudice against severe mental illness.

I: What are the gaps in training in psychiatry?

SK: Due to the introduction of the medical specialist system, one is able to learn from a broad spectrum of subjects, from psychotherapy to biology, child psychiatry to geriatric psychiatry, and psychotherapy to drug therapy. However, there is an urban–rural disparity in medical resources and the quality of available instruction.

I: What would you advise residents?

SK: I would advise them to observe each patient carefully, case by case, each time reading relevant articles and textbooks. Familiarize yourself with each case to the level of being able to write a case report. Try to understand patients from different angles using the biopsychosocial model. Have discussions with your supervisors.

Study a wide range of fields of psychiatric medicine to the extent possible during medical training. Find good role models and aim to follow in their footsteps.

In retrospect, I've learned that the more cases I've struggled with, the more I've learned. In other words, patients are teachers. As for the cases I could treat easily, I don't remember many of them.

I: What would you like to be remembered for?

SK: That's a really difficult question (laughs). As a professor of psychiatry or the President of the Japanese Society of Psychiatry and Neurology, I may have accomplished some things. However, while what I have accomplished is important, I believe that what is more important is how I have lived my life, and most importantly, how I have contributed to the next generation of psychiatrists. We will not be able to evaluate them until much later.

I also have regrets for what I didn't accomplish.

I: What do you think that is?

SK: I have not been able to make a significant contribution to improving the quality and equalization of the psychiatric care system in this country even though I was President of the Japanese Society for four years and Vice-President for five years.

I: Right. Which of your achievements are you most proud of?

SK: (laughs) I do not have anything in particular that I am proud of. However, I would venture to say that I have trained many talented apprentices and trainees. I may have made a small contribution in getting the government to acknowledge the importance of research in psychiatric disorders, by having paved the way for neuroscience and psychopharmacology in Japan. To a small degree, I may have also promoted the globalization of our society, the JSPN. To some degree, I may have been able to pave a small section of the way for the younger generation.

I: Thank you so much Nobu really appreciate you taking time this late on a Sunday evening.

SK: No, not at all, I'm so glad that you invited me to this interview.

I: Thank you so much for your time.

SK: Thank you very much.

7
Marianne C. Kastrup

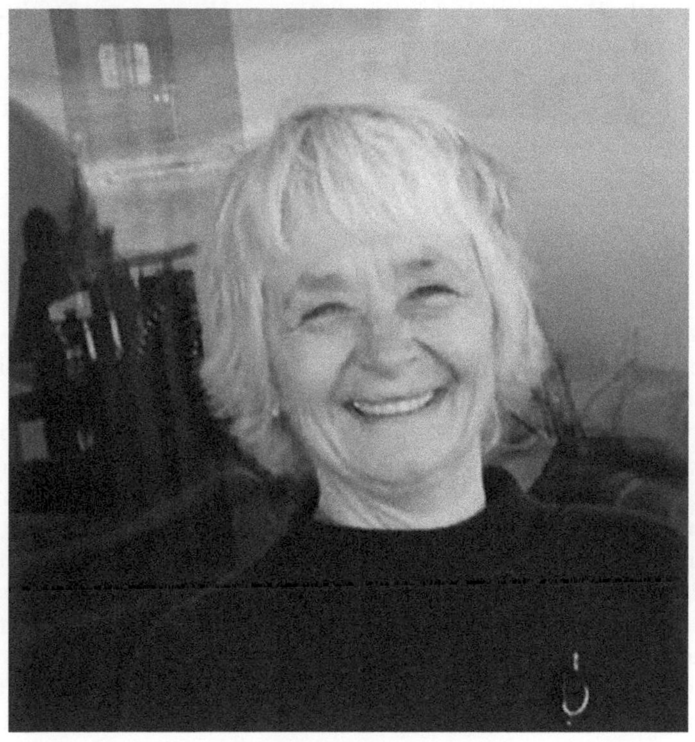

Biography

Dr Marianne Kastrup was born and trained in medicine and psychiatry in Denmark. She has always been interested in working with under-privileged populations. In this role she was the Consultant to Dignity—Danish Institute against Torture, Copenhagen. She led the Centre for Transcultural Psychiatry at the Copenhagen University Hospital, Denmark for several years and was the Medical Director of the International Research and Rehabilitation Centre for Torture Victims, Copenhagen as well as the Consultant and head of the department of psychiatry, Copenhagen University Hospital, Hvidovre. She advised the Norwegian Research Council for Mental Health, the United Nations Optional Protocol to the Convention Against Torture (OPCAT) function under the Danish ombudsman, the GESEMI Charité Hospital, Berlin, and the Eppendorfer Hospital, Hamburg, the Expert Advisory Panel on Mental Health,

World Health Organization (WHO), and has been an expert advisor for the European Council Committee for the Prevention of Torture, Inhuman or Degrading Treatment and Punishment. She was a member of the World Psychiatric Association (WPA) Executive committee and has been involved in various activities within the organization. For a number of years, she was Secretary General of the European Psychiatric Association (EPA) and chaired its Ethics Committee. She has been a member of the Executive Committee of the World Association of Social Psychiatry, chaired the Ethics Committee of the Danish Psychiatric Association, and has been the Danish editor of *Nordic Psychiatrist*. She was also a member of the Nordic Joint Committee as Treasurer and later Secretary and a member of the Board of Mental Health Europe. She has been on the Scientific Board of the *Danish Medical Journal* and a member of its Ethics Committee. She has received various accolades and honours both nationally and internationally, and has published widely in books, chapters, and papers.

Interview

I: Thanks very much for agreeing to take part in the series of interviews with eminent leaders in psychiatry. Perhaps we could start by you telling us a bit about your childhood and your growing up?

CK: I grew up in Denmark in a nice, middle-class background. I come from a family where, in particular, my mother felt it was important that I look ahead and not back towards the war. When I was a child, my mother would read the United Nations (UN) children's book to me. I still remember that very vividly; it made a great impression upon me. It was very important for my mother to emphasize that all children are born equal. I remember her telling me that no matter the ethnicity, we are all alike. I still have a vivid memory of the book; on the last page of the book you can see a globe and a small child sleeping; all children are alike and we all sleep in the same way. This was what I was brought up to believe. I don't come from a religious family and was brought up as a Protestant but we never went to church and religion did not have much bearing upon us. But I was brought up believing in the good in human beings, in justice, and that we should reach out to those who are different. I am very indebted to my mother because when I was young, she taught me to accept everyone, whether homosexual, Christian, Jew, etc., and she told me to read about them and understand that there are different religions, different ways to live, and in spite of all these differences, we are all equal. So this I learnt from my mother. To my father it was important that you were brought up as honest person and he believed that if you had the ability, you had a duty and should work for the common good. I was brought up to believe a girl is as good as a boy, and since I managed well in school, I was encouraged to believe that a girl can do anything she likes.

I: What attracted you to medicine?

CK: I was not attracted to medicine; frankly it didn't interest me at all. I would never study medicine again if I had the chance, but I was very good in mathematics. When I left school, I was the girl who was good in almost all topics, and so in university I could choose anything I wanted, and I wanted to choose mathematics.

Later I started studying mathematics but my teacher in high school told me to realize that there was a 99 per cent chance that I would end up as a high school teacher. And I started thinking, is that what I want? My grandfather was a lawyer and had enormous influence over my thinking. He told me, 'Marianne, you like to see the world; you need to do something useful, why don't you become a doctor? It's always better to be a doctor; don't be a lawyer, that's a lousy job.' My father, on the other hand, thought becoming a doctor was too easy; we had many friends who were doctors and he suggested that I become a nuclear physicist instead. In the end I decided to try and become a doctor. I am embarrassed to say that after a couple of years, I didn't like medicine at all. I told myself that I had started with mathematics, gave that up and chose to become a doctor, and now I can't skip that. So I finished medicine without, frankly, having the slightest interest in it. I have disliked hospitals my whole life; I didn't like the smell of one, I'm afraid of people who may die due to my ignorance. I have not been a very courageous doctor. I don't think I have done bad work but I have been afraid very often.

I: Why did you choose psychiatry?

CK: I chose psychiatry because when I finished medicine, I didn't want to become a doctor. I didn't want to go to work at a hospital, and by sheer chance I saw an ad in the university paper that they wanted someone to do—in Denmark it's called a 'Gold Medal Dissertation'—I felt this was interesting, because that was an epidemiological study, which happened to be on child psychological/psychiatric aspects. So I thought that is far away from a hospital and I took part in it, and I won a gold medal. This meant that I moved in circles within mental health. And when I had to decide, I didn't want to become a psychiatrist. I'm a socialist and I wanted to work where I could do something good for the poor. I wanted to do community medicine, but back then it was not a possibility in Denmark. I then looked at all the specialties and wondered about choosing the easiest field, and psychiatry was the easiest, so I decided to pursue it. That was one reason. The other is that I'm also a feminist. I was very active in the feminist movement and there was a lot of discussion about women's depressive disorder, women not being able to do a lot of things. I said to myself that I needed to meet female doctors and discuss all these issues about women's mental health. These were two of the reasons why I joined psychiatry.

I: And are there any things that you regret?

CK: I don't regret things in life, but on the other hand I would never choose medicine again and never become a psychiatrist again. I don't regret it, because I've had a very good career, but I would not do it again.

I: If not psychiatry, then what would you have done?

CK: There are two things that interest me; one is that I believe a lot in fighting for animal rights. I don't eat meat, and I think the way the Western world has industrialized meat production is a disgrace. I think animals and humans are very close so I might have become a vet, or I might have become a judge because I'm also very interested in human rights.

I: Who were your role models?

CK: I have been very lucky because I have not only had good role models but I've also had good mentors. When I was a junior doctor, by sheer chance, I met a famous professor, Johannes Ipsen, who was an epidemiologist at Harvard. He was a Dane, and when he retired he came back to Denmark and got an honorary professorship at the university where I was. When I finished, for some reason I met him, I don't remember how, and he had this very American style that was very open and informal. So when I was doing my dissertation, I could call him and he would say: 'Marianne jump on your bicycle and I'll tell Alice (his wife, who was American) and let's discuss it.' I never felt like he was so much more senior than me, that I was just a junior to him. I just felt like we were two equals discussing things. He meant an enormous amount to me.

My first boss, Annalise Dupont, was a woman and she was fantastic. She was also very keen on women's rights, and I was the only young doctor in my workplace who was working with the feminist movement. And so she and I became very close and I admired her a lot, even after I left the job. She was also a role model. Meeting Norman Sartorius has also made an enormous difference in my life. Only a few people have meant so much to me during my career and I feel extremely fortunate that I was on the Executive Committee of the WPA when he was President. I have learnt a lot from him; he was a fantastic President and a great human being. Also worth mentioning is (Juan J.) López-Ibor, who passed away; he was a fantastic President too. I have been very fortunate to be associated with people who have been unique in psychiatry.

I: And are there any lasting impressions about patients that you would like to share?

CK: Unfortunately, many psychiatrists (at least previously) talked to their patients as if they were not on the same level. When I was the head of a psychiatric department there was a tendency for psychiatrists not to share anything about patients with the patient's relatives, often looking at relatives as a nuisance. However, I have had good contact with relatives' organizations. Some of them called me for personal advice. I may seem too naive but I have always been keen on the rights that a patient and their relative have. This has meant a lot to me to be able to talk about the right of a patient and that they are treated with respect.

I: Do you have any memorable episodes that you would like to share either in terms of practice, leadership, or research?

CK: When I was a junior doctor, Professor Strömgren, a famous Danish professor who worked on International Classification of Diseases (ICD) and International Pilot Study of Schizophrenia (IPSS) and was in charge of a WHO collaborating centre. so often there were visitors to the centre. It was not a Danish tradition to interact socially with foreign guests but I had a boyfriend who was from India and I was used to a more cosmopolitan approach. So I frequently had social contact with them. The professor found out that I shared this interest so he once asked me if I wanted to go along with him to a WHO meeting in Geneva. I was at a meeting chaired by Norman Sartorius, I was just an observer and had no say whatsoever. This was a very decisive moment in my career because I didn't believe how kindly they treated me, as if I was one of them, which I wasn't because I had only just graduated.

Another moment that I can share is from when I started surgery, when I had already begun research. Back then there were not a lot of women who were doctors. This was at a big university department where there were 18 male doctors and me. I was the youngest and I had told them that I would probably become a psychiatrist. So they looked at me rather weirdly, but I didn't have low self-esteem and was quite confident. But I was absolute nil when it came to surgery. It was a very interesting moment in my life because I was standing there at the operating theatre and the doctors were working in shifts because it was an extremely complicated operation. Me, I was only allowed to go out to the bathroom and get some juice and come back and then had to stand there. Around 6 in the evening, the whole team went home and the professor was called from his house; he had to finish the operation because it had gone completely wrong. He came and changed and stood on the other side of the operating table and then he looked and called out to me. No-one had replaced me. I had been standing there all day. And he looked at me and told me that I was strong as a bear. I said, 'yes, no matter what you do, I'm not going to give up, And then everybody started laughing and he told me to go home. I shall never forget that moment in my life because for the first time I was visible in that department. Then after the surgery he came up to me and told me that they were going to have a staff meeting and he had heard that I was doing epidemiological research. He asked me if I wanted to give a presentation on the epidemiology of that disease. I was surprised but said I would be delighted. This was to me frankly more decisive than many things I experienced in psychiatry. You see, this was in Copenhagen and I was not from there, and when you go to Copenhagen from the provinces, you're expected to speak their language. So you have to fight doubly hard because you're not from Copenhagen. At the end of the day I managed this by sheer hard work and nothing else, in spite of being a woman from the provinces. So that was a very important moment for me.

I: How has psychiatry changed in your time?

CK: Some things have changed for the better but there is still quite a lot to be done. When I started, one of the first papers I wrote was with a mentor of mine. He was a psychiatrist but also a politician. We wrote a paper, 'Patients without a Corner'; in those days if you were in the more chronic wards, there were about eight patients in one room. We said, 'they don't even have a corner or a cupboard with their own belongings', so we wrote this article out of social indignation. This has of course changed for the better and the condition of the wards overall has improved drastically. When I was the head of the department there was more money and so we created community psychiatry where there was drama and events with patients being taught arts, music, cooking, and therapy, making the patients feel more empowered. Now little by little these things are closing down and many community psychiatric settings are turning into outpatient clinics. I think some of the ideals we had have been lost. Some things are getting worse, maybe due to the shortage of money, but what is better is there is much more emphasis on patient consent and collaboration with relatives. So some things are definitely better and some are not. Another sad thing is that in my country there is a huge recruitment problem because not many people want to become psychiatrists.

I: What are your views on the current state of psychiatry?

CK: There are several aspects to this. If you look at it from the medical aspect, I have always been involved in medical work and I'm very much a clinical doctor that way. I think it's sad that so few doctors want to join psychiatry. I think it's also sad that very often politicians take decisions about health reforms without consulting medical professionals. To me this is a very sad development. I have deep respect for psychiatry and I think it's sad if you think that you can replace doctors with other professionals. But on the other hand, maybe we have not been very good at showing what we are good at. I once came across someone who believed in doctors but he said that psychologists will say that they're better than doctors at talking to patients, but psychologists see patients only in nice settings, or in larger groups, while as a doctor he had seen human beings being born or dying. Sitting in an emergency clinic I had seen patients who were suicidal, homicidal, seen their happy moments, sad moments, basically all aspects of human life. There are not many professionals who have not only seen these but have had to decide what to do in such situations and stick to it. In many situations, the staff call the doctor only in very serious cases. When I was a junior doctor, the nursing staff on duty would call me and ask if they could let a patient go home, or if the patient was suicidal, and I would ask them what they thought, having been with the patient for hours. They'd reply that I had to decide, since they weren't the doctor. Now I had never seen the patient before so how could I decide?

This medical responsibility is something we haven't been good enough in showing, because we have a unique profession in many ways. And even though I wouldn't become a doctor again, I'm proud of it because I think we have the courage to get involved deeply and do things.

I: And do you think that psychiatry is 'brainless' or 'mindless'?

CK: It's neither. Psychiatry is a scientific profession and we should use the same standards in psychiatry as in other medical disciplines. It's not a profession where you just sit and talk. The impression given by some politicians is different. I remember that some time back there was a discussion in Denmark where some politicians said psychiatry is only a matter of speaking with love and empathy towards a patient and that's all that is needed. If you have the notion that psychiatry is just about speaking nicely to a patient then you don't understand what a mental disorder is. On the other hand, I fully agree that if you don't know how to speak nicely to another human being, especially one who is severely disturbed, or depressed, then you are mindless. But you need both a sound mind and a working brain, and both are equally important.

I: What do you see as problems with psychiatry?

CK: I think in most countries the amount of resources allocated to mental health is very limited. If you check WHO and see the percentage of gross domestic product allocated to health services and compare it with that allocated to mental health, it is quite poor. I don't think the balance is properly maintained in any country. I also think that it is sad that there is so much animosity against pharmaceutical industries, and many big pharma companies are no longer making drugs for psychiatry because they are constantly being accused of destroying people's mental health, that they're in the pockets of big psychiatrists, etc. I have never been involved in the pharma industry but I think we can't do without good pharma companies and we do need to develop more drugs. So to me, this is quite sad seeing that there is decreased development of new drugs. Having said that, I have seen many of my colleagues being too positive when the second generation of antipsychotics were launched. I think many of them either overlooked or were not aware of metabolic syndrome, and kept saying that there were no extra side effects. I don't know if putting on extra kilos or becoming diabetic is any better. It's also sad to see research on psychiatric patients dying having a life span several years shorter than normal.

I: You mentioned that recruitment in psychiatry in Denmark is poor. How would you improve it?

CK: I don't think it's easy but in Denmark child psychiatry is a different discipline from adult psychiatry. Child psychiatry wanted to recruit more doctors so they started emphasizing research aspects. They made it obvious that it is extremely important to carry out research as part of your training. I think this could be play a part in better recruitment. After seeing how much time young doctors spend in cardiology and internal medicine I can understand that they are attracted to such disciplines because there are so many new things going on and you perhaps feel more like a real doctor than you might in psychiatry. I don't know how we can recruit more doctors into psychiatry, but perhaps if we could show that psychiatry is also a medical discipline there could be some change. In my opinion, psychiatry has moved away from regular medical disciplines. At least here we have all somatic medicines in one health authority and then psychiatry is situated in a completely different health authority. So, in university hospitals, as a psychiatrist you're no longer a part of the medical council, which is seen as a different world.

I: What do you see as a characteristic of a good psychiatrist?

CK: A good psychiatrist should be humble. The Danish philosopher Søren Kierkegaard said when you want to help somebody you have to find him where he is and start from there. I think a good psychiatrist needs to be humble and should listen to the patient's story. I have been running a Centre for Transcultural Psychiatry and there it has been extremely important to hear the patient's version of their experience, especially if they come from different parts of the world. Thus, they may have a very different explanation about why they think they feel sick. And to listen and understand what they're telling you, I think you need to be a good psychiatrist. You shouldn't immediately try to ask them questions from a structured interview; yes, you have criteria that you must follow, but don't tell them: 'yes, you're suffering from depression, I can help you', and so on. That is not the sign of a good psychiatrist. That doesn't mean a good psychiatrist shouldn't know pharmacology and not know which treatment is appropriate, but I think they should first try to get the overall picture of the patient. They must understand their patient and ask what they are looking for. It takes time, but it can be done. I know it is easy to say but sometimes there is no time to go through these questions. At the same time, I think you need to allow the patient to express themselves through their own language. And I also think that neglecting traumatic events in life can contribute to psychopathology, and so a psychiatrist must understand the patient's life history in detail.

I: What do you see as gaps in the practice of psychiatry?

CK: I think there are many gaps. There is a treatment gap in the sense that there are many disorders that are not properly diagnosed. I think we also have a gap in gender issues; even though we see more and more women in psychiatry, it is men who still have the decisive power in many cases. Gender issues also exist with relation to the treatment of patients. There is also a power issue in the sense that mental health professionals may not have power politically and so many major decisions are being taken by people who know very little about mental health. I think the treatment gap is the worst. Also in certain parts of the world, it is only people who are well-off that manage to get treatment while many who cannot afford it get none. In my country we're seeing many doctors migrating from former Eastern European countries, and there is a huge shortage of psychiatrists because they've moved to Scandinavia where perhaps the salary is better, but I'm not sure if life is better, but they go there anyway, to get a better paid job.

I: And what do you see as gaps in training in psychiatry?

CK: I think it depends on which country you are looking at. Bedside training in many places may be problematic if senior doctors are not very welcoming to young doctors so that they can go and talk to the patient. I remember when I was a junior doctor myself, I had a very famous professor in whose hospital I did my residency. I asked him if I could join him for interviews and he looked at me and said, 'No way'. He wouldn't allow anyone to accompany him, a matron maybe, but no junior doctors, and that to me was very strange. Many doctors are very reluctant to let others accompany them on their rounds, so this I think is a gap. I also think it could be very useful if doctors are encouraged to go to other countries during their training, to see how things function differently there, especially with regards to training. I was recently speaking to a colleague who mentioned how many famous psychiatrists felt it was only natural to move to different countries during their training; this was even common in Denmark. Now you can see how junior doctors are trained only in a single setting. I don't think that's wise at all and it's extremely important to see as many settings as possible. It's also better to go out and see what working in hospitals can be like. We do give too much importance to hospitals, but most psychiatric work is done in primary healthcare settings.

I: How do you think psychiatry's social contract can be delivered?

CK: I have worked a lot on the topic of human rights and there you may see that psychiatrists are taking care of those patients whom the society refuses to accept; drug addicts, alcoholics, etc. We are just an arm of government and doing the right thing because society does not accept deviant personalities. So you can say we have an obligation, a negative one, because these people are not 'mental patients'. When I was a young doctor, abortion was not freely allowed in Denmark. You could have one if you were suicidal, depressed, or had other severe mental health issues. But when I was a student, I remember during my psychiatric training, a young woman was referred to the psychiatric ward and she was pregnant and wanted an abortion and there was nothing wrong with her. But how do you get an abortion? By saying how depressed you are? I believe in free abortion, so I wrote down how the woman was depressed, etc., and she managed to get an abortion. She was not mentally ill, but the system used a psychiatric diagnosis to help a young woman to have an abortion, or she would have had to travel to Poland, or perhaps an illegal clinic to get one. I also remember once I was in Romania many years ago and someone had been admitted in the hospital, possibly to protect him from being sent to a camp, but he was not mentally ill. I think there are both good and bad aspects of this. But as doctors, most of us are doing what the system has asked us to do. And it was not only in Germany, this was in Denmark as well; bad examples of doctors around the 1930s.

I: What would you tell your younger self?

CK: Work hard, take a chance, life is full of chances. Sometimes you may not win them all, but take them. I have friends who are scared to take chances, who ask me, 'what if someone takes advantage of you?' I said that this has never happened to me. We should try to see the good in all the tasks we've been given and always look for the social relationships available in any work you do. I remember Norman Sartorius had told me once that at the end of the day it is the human relationships that lasts and I think that I'm here, not only because of my profession but also because of my relationship with human beings whom I like very much. So I always say collaborate with others, either through research, training, or organizational work. And I always go out of my comfort zone and meet people of different cultures, learn from them, etc., and you will gain much more than you give. To me this is the nicest thing about my whole career: where I have collaborated and become friends with people across countries.

I: What advice would you give to trainees nowadays?

CK: My advice is that they should not be afraid of working hard. I think there is a tendency, at least in my own country, to become very protective of the time spent with our own family. I was recently involved in a reception celebrating 50th anniversary of an institute. This reception took place on a Friday afternoon and many individuals would not participate because they were going shopping, or Fridays are family afternoons, etc. They made excuses, which I think 30 years ago would not have been offered; people did not prioritize this way. Back then, we would prioritize broader human contact and responsibility. I think people are becoming alienated from one another and concentrate on the narrow family circle

I: What would you like to be remembered for?

CK: I would like to be remembered as being a no-nonsense person, one you couldn't corrupt, one with a sense of integrity. I want to be known as someone who worked hard and did not have to use sneaky tactics to grow in life and that I progressed due to sheer hard work. I was someone you could trust and someone who didn't change their but always followed a set path.

I: And who would you want to remember you?

CK: I don't know, as I've never given this much thought really.

I: Which of your achievements are you most proud of?

CK: I'm not proud of anything really but I'd like to see myself as someone who's managed to be a part of many things. I have not harmed anyone on my journey, haven't used illegal ways, and can look back and remember everyone I have collaborated with. This is important to me as this is what all my values have always been.

I: Thanks very much for your time, it has been great chatting with you.

8
Linda Lam

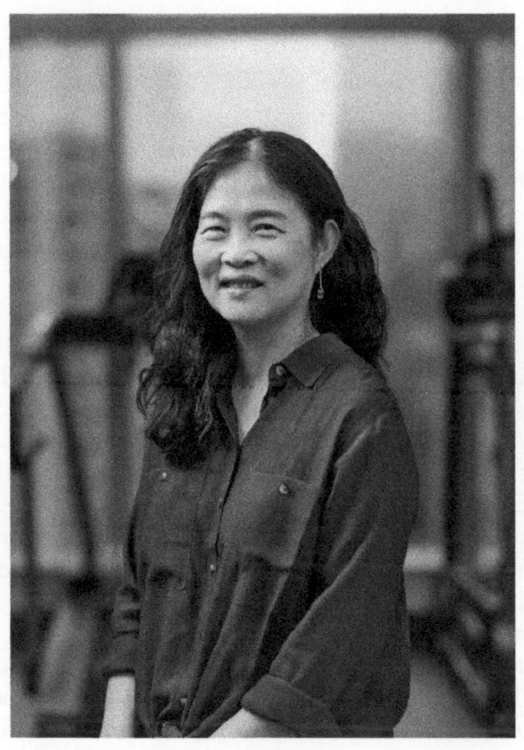

Biography

Professor Linda Lam is Clinical Professor and Director of the Chen Wai Vivien Foundation Therapeutic Physical Mental Exercise Centre, Dementia Research Unit at the Department of Psychiatry, the Chinese University of Hong Kong (CUHK). She received her undergraduate medical and doctoral degree at the CUHK.

Dr Lam was trained as a psychiatrist specializing in old age mental health. She is a Fellow of the Hong Kong College of Psychiatrists and the Royal College of Psychiatrists (United Kingdom). She is past-President of the Hong Kong College of Psychiatrists, and past-Chief Editor of the *East Asian Archives of Psychiatry*. Dr Lam is also the founding President of the Chinese Dementia Research Association in 2009. Since 2017, she has served as a member at the Advisory Committee on Mental Health in Hong Kong.

Her research interests include early detection and intervention for mild cognitive impairment and dementia. She conducted the first territory-wide epidemiological surveys on mental disorders and dementia in Hong Kong, and pioneered lifestyle cognitive and physical exercise, and non-invasive brain stimulation interventions for older Chinese adults with neurocognitive disorders.

Dr Lam serves on the Editorial Boards of a number of psychiatric journals and is grant reviewer for the grant review boards in Hong Kong, the Alzheimer's Association in the United States and the Alzheimer's Society in United Kingdom. She is now the Secretary General off the Asian Society Against Dementia. In 2017, in recognition of her contribution to the promotion of mental health in the community, Dr Lam was awarded Honorary Fellowship of the Royal College of Psychiatrists of the United Kingdom and Honorary Membership of the World Psychiatric Association.

Interview

I: Thanks very much Linda for agreeing to be interviewed. Not only have you been incredibly effective as a leader but you are also an immensely popular one. You have achieved a lot. Being a woman and being a leader brings their own challenges so perhaps we will start off with your development as a leader.

LL: Thank you, I didn't have any distinct plans, including a plan to study medicine. I'll start with my early days. I was born in Hong Kong into a family which was not a wealthy family. In fact, I was educated in an underprivileged secondary school that was run by nuns. Not many graduates from that school became doctors. This school had been in existence for 40 years but had produced very few doctors in all that time. It was an all-girls' school and very few students went on to become professionals. When I was a teenager, a teacher from the Bible and Religious studies class mentioned something that impressed me. At that time teenage girls often would go to factories to work, to earn money to give back to their families because they were very poor. That teacher said to us: 'You girls have to think for yourselves. Don't think of your family. You're still young and if you have a chance to study do so and don't quit, otherwise your life is not your own.' I didn't think too much about that at the time. After I passed my O levels, I went to work in a factory during my summer vacation in order to save some money for my school fees for the next year when I would take my A levels. I did quite well in the factory; the factory supervisor asked me to stay on and said: 'If you stay, I'll groom you for a supervisor's position.' I was 16 at that time. It was very tempting because I would have made money immediately for my family. I was the eldest of four siblings and the money would have helped them enormously. When O level results were out, I thought maybe I should give the factory a second chance and asked my mother what she thought. My mother said, 'Why not just carry on and study?' I had been earning my own school fees from when I was very young and I was a very well-organized person. After finishing my day at school I would come home for two hours, then go out and tutor young students to make some money. Then I would return home and cook for the family. Everything had to be done to a very tight schedule so that I could make room for myself and what

I wanted to do. I did my A levels from a secondary school which was very underprivileged, and almost none of my fellow classmates felt that they had any chance of getting into a university. We expected to just finish the two years of A levels and then become secretaries. I studied quite hard and had two teachers who told me that I shouldn't give up, that I had a real chance of getting into university. I didn't take much notice of this and just carried on and thought nothing. Actually, my primary wish was to become a pharmacist. Don't ask me why (laughs)! I just thought that I should be a pharmacist but in Hong Kong at the time, there was no school of pharmacy so it was impossible for me to pursue this dream. I didn't have any money so I just thought perhaps I could go study biology in the university. My A level results turned out to be surprisingly good so my teachers at the secondary school forced me to apply for medicine. They said: 'Don't waste this chance; try for medicine. It is a once-in-a-lifetime opportunity and it will make history for our school.' I was scared because I did not have that kind of confidence and I refused to apply for medicine at the University of Hong Kong (HKU). I told myself that I'd apply for biology because it was an easy way for me to get into a university. Studying biology felt like a dream come true, an impossible dream. I didn't plan it. It was sheer coincidence that at precisely that time, the Medical School of the Chinese University of Hong Kong (CUHK) took its first intake of students. I could use my A level results to apply for CU Medicine. I had a forceful teacher who trapped me in his room one day and demanded that I apply for medicine. I said to him: 'OK. I will apply for CUHK. I'm not going to apply for anything else because this is a real chance and I want to take it.' So I applied to study medicine. Do you know who was the professor who interviewed me? It was Professor Chen, the founding Professor of Psychiatry at CUHK.

I: Was he the person who was awarded the honorary Fellowship of the Hong Kong College of Psychiatrists a couple of years ago?

LL: Yes. Maybe it was all foretold! When you ask me why I am organized, I have had to be, from my earliest days as a child. At CUHK, I didn't feel under much pressure because I didn't feel I was setting any precedent for anyone other than myself. Luckily, I got scholarships every year, and that allowed me to keep studying without the burden of financial problems. I just carried on and really enjoyed my studies. I did quite well, especially in psychiatry. I became a psychiatrist! This is something else I didn't plan. Initially I wanted to do psychiatry for just one year. I really wanted to do internal medicine.

I: At what point did you decide you wanted to do psychiatry?

LL: In my internship. I realized that psychiatry was important when I was a medical student.

I: But it did not interest you at that time?

LL: I knew psychiatry was important. I thought it was interesting, but I thought medicine was more interesting. After I finished my internship, I asked myself whether I wanted to go on to psychiatry or medicine, and decided that I should spend one year in psychiatry before I went back to medicine. I asked Professor Chen if I could take a trainee's role and he agreed. The first year of my psychiatric training was a mess, a total mess. I had a number of patients who committed suicide and I wanted to know why they did. I couldn't figure it out and became intensely frustrated, so much so that my supervisor was not able to give me any support. I applied to leave psychiatry and go back to medicine, but somehow, I was given a rotation in medicine which I didn't like, so I stayed in psychiatry. That's when I met another supervisor who was a psychotherapist. He was a psychodynamic psychotherapist who really helped me to understand patients from different perspectives. Then I took College membership (MRCPsych) in the United Kingdom. At the time I took my Part II examination, Hong Kong had a shortage of senior doctors, so immediately after gaining membership, a qualified doctor would get promoted. I got my Part II of the membership and finished my training in Cambridge with Professor German Berrios, a real gentleman. I spent nine months with him. He was and is very inspiring. I'm not sure I follow everything he says because his writings are truly philosophical and take into account history of psychiatry but I still find him very inspiring. I returned to work in Kwai Chung Hospital as one of the youngest, possibly *the* youngest, senior medical officer. Being young, people had different expectations of me. I was under Patrick Sham at that time. He was the medical superintendent and was very busy so I had to take care of other junior doctors. It was here that I learned how to supervise others and learned administrative skills. It was one of my formative years. Thus, very early on, in my fourth year of training, I became a supervisor. Assisting the medical superintendent at that time, I learned how to lead a small team. Dr Sham was very efficient, a very effective person in hospital administration. I developed an interest in psychogeriatrics because I felt the field held great potential for older people. At the time, nobody cared much about dementia; the patients would just sit around very often doing nothing and staring into space. I felt very strongly that was unacceptable. So I took up an academic position in psychogeriatrics.

I: Why academic psychiatry? The move from Kwai Chung to the university department was quite a big deal, a huge leap, wasn't it?

LL: Yes. At that time, a horizontal transfer from Senior Medical Officer to lecturer was easy and transferring back from lecturer to consultant position was also very simple. I felt that perhaps an academic position would give me a better chance to learn about old age psychiatry outside Hong Kong.

I: Right, so you went back to Chinese University of Hong Kong, is that correct? Is that because it was your old medical school and it was easy to go there? Or did you want to work with Professor Chen again?

LL: My mentor in CUHK at that time was Professor Helen Chiu. She wanted somebody to help her build up old age psychiatry. She was the senior lecturer. I returned as a lecturer in old age psychiatry.

I: OK. Have you had any regrets in doing psychiatry? In ending up in psychiatry rather than in medicine?

LL: No, I don't have any regrets. I have done a lot of research in neurological conditions and dementia. I have no regrets being a psychiatrist but if I had done the same thing as a neurologist my influence would probably have been very different.

I: You mentioned Professor Chen; are there any other role models or heroes or heroines that you had dealings with?

LL: The first role model was Professor Chen, who got me into the medical school. The second was German Berrios. For nine months I studied with him. I learned how to construct concepts and frameworks and I learned about interesting aspects about academic psychiatry.

I: Was Eugene Paykel the professor at Cambridge at that time?

LL: Yes. I mainly studied under German Barrios because he organized courses for people from outside the United Kingdom. For nine months it was just straight course work. Professor Paykel was there at that time, I knew him but I didn't work closely with him.

I: What attracted you to psychiatry? Is it clinical work, academic work, or policy development?

LL: Initially the attraction was clinical. Clinical expertise in psychiatry is wonderful. I always tell my trainees that clinical skills are like the scalpel of a surgeon. A good surgeon needs to have good hand skills and hand-eye coordination, but for us psychiatrists, our clinical skills are all in our minds. To do well, we need very good clinical skills in order to look after our patients. You need to start by asking basic questions of your patients, then move on to deeper and complex questions. That's something that stimulated my interest in research. I have learnt a lot from my patients. I feel that if I want to do more and contribute more to the field, I have to start off as an advocate for them because often they don't or can't speak up for themselves. That's why I started doing more policy work, so that I can speak for them.

I: Over the years that you have been in psychiatry, how has the field changed?

LL: I can only talk about my experience in Hong Kong. When I started, the field was pretty much only general adult psychiatry, no other specialty existed in psychiatry. Everybody was treated in the same way with a cocktail of drugs. You had 10 drugs available to you and could prescribe only those 10 drugs for the patient. There wasn't a great deal of consideration of what the individual's exact problem might be. Psychiatry has gradually evolved into different areas that help with specific problems. Some areas are built on increased knowledge in psychiatry, others on psychological theories, some on patients' needs, and some on developmental aspects and special areas. This has been a tremendous evolution. Another thing worth mentioning is that medical students in Hong Kong are now keen to go into psychiatry. There is still the dominant interest in getting into medicine or surgery, but we constantly see medical students who are really interested in psychiatry from very early in their studies where something has really inspired them. That's why I think psychiatry education at undergraduate level is very important, for inspiring the potential psychiatrist but also making other specialties aware. The other thing is society. I'm not sure whether the stigma of mental illness in society has changed a lot but at least society knows much more about mental illness than it has known in the past. Eliminating prejudice has a long way to go but at least people have started feeling free to talk about mental health. In the last couple of years, I feel that the government here has begun to be much more committed to mental health.

I: Has something changed in government?

LL: Somethings have changed, yes, but there is still a long way to go.

I: How did you end up running the Hong Kong College (of Psychiatrists)?

LL: Ah! Another coincidence rather than a definitive plan! I'm a very low-profile person. I still remember when I was a lecturer at CUHK 20 years ago there was only one reserved position for a Council member who was nominated by each of the university departments.

I: OK.

LL: It must be over 20 years ago when it was my turn, by rotation, to represent the University on the College Council. It was not a competition. I become very familiar with how the College worked during my six years there, after which my term there finished. I was not on the Council for a few years. Then the Council needed a chairman for the publications committee for the College journal. There were not many people around who were willing to take up this job because at that time the journal was not indexed and was often behind schedule due to lack of submissions. Anyway, I became part of the publications committee. After a few years as Chief Editor, I managed to get the journal indexed in the *Index Medicus* and got the journal back on track with regular publication. So, I think it was Dr Hung, the person who was running for the Presidency, asked me if I would consider becoming the Vice-President. Dr Hung is one of my very good friends and a senior colleague with immense passion for his work. I didn't want to say no to him, so I agreed to take this on even though I wasn't entirely sure I could do the job. So it is because of Dr Hung I became the Vice-President for Censor and Education.

I: Often people think that you sat down and worked out a plan: this is what I'll do in three years, five years, seven years, 10 years. Life is never like that; it's always a series of coincidences and opportunities, and if you take the latter, then it is up to you. You could have easily said no, I don't want to be Vice-President. I want to focus on something else as a leader. Were you the second or third female President of the Hong Kong college?

LL: Third. Felice (Felice Lieh Mak), Helen Chiu, then me.

I: What was it like? Obviously, the time when Felice was President was very different than yours, they were different times. As you say the number of drugs available was rising along with newer therapies and investigations.

LL: They were three very different women. Felice was strong and powerful, assertive all the time. She was always very direct and everybody looked up to her because she was a senior Professor.

I: Was she the first President of the College?

LL: No, I think she was the second. She was already a well-known professor of psychiatry when she took up the presidency. Helen was a very good planner and used to plan everything well ahead of time. For me, being a Vice-President for Censor and Education was not very easy because I was the associate professor and comparatively young compared to the senior consultants on the committee. When I wanted to modify the existing guidelines I struggled. Few of my colleagues were interested in what I had to say. It took almost a full year for them to begin listening to my ideas, perhaps because I'm a woman or because I am not forceful. It was important for me to observe my role seriously. The issues at stake included education, accreditation issues, education guidelines, the curriculum, trainee manual, lots of things, and all had to be dealt in a very clear manner, so I persisted. I talked to my colleagues again and again about all these things. Eventually, I think at the end of the fourth year, I gained their trust. The committee members started talking to and communicating with me and we began to work well together. Most of the guidelines were revised during those four years. Maybe because of this, I gained a lot of experience on how to lead a big team and how to convince a senior person that something needed to be done.

I: It seems to me that it must have been very difficult to take people along with you. What strategies would you advise the younger females and upcoming leaders to take? What ought they to do to achieve what they want?

LL: I remember your lecture about leading from the front as opposed to leading from behind. When I first listened to your lecture, I realized that I am a person who probably leads from behind. I have tried to clarify the roles of the leader and the team members in order to avoid any confusions. I am determined and patient, and I want to see change. To be a leader, you need these three things. Also, I think that one of the key pieces of advice for somebody who wants to be a leader, especially for women, is that family and work need to be balanced carefully, that's important. I also have passion and enthusiasm for my work. I would never make excuses about not working hard. I want to lead is because I want to serve my patients better. I am not a person who talks a lot or forces people to do things. My way of working is to tidy up any confusion so that many paths become a couple of paths. I try to remove obstructions for my colleagues so that they can see what it is we are trying to achieve. Leading from behind works for me very well and many of the junior, younger doctors feel more comfortable with this style of working than working in a more hierarchical way.

I: What do you see the problems in the current state of psychiatry.

LL: Psychiatry still has a lot of problems. We are still working in the most difficult areas of healthcare. Psychiatry works with the person's mind, but not actually the person's brain. There is a big difference between the mind and the brain. What we know about neuroscience and brain structure is only very elementary to understanding human behaviour. There is still a huge knowledge gap in why and how human beings behave in particular ways and sometimes in non-adaptive manners. This is the biggest problem and limitation in psychiatry. On the other hand, this limitation is also very attractive because it offers us a chance to explore behaviour and the mind. I don't know how we can fix it but my own research and my own practice seeks to help people become more adaptive in their lives. We may not be able to treat mental illnesses directly because we still do not know what leads to them. But we can help people to become more adaptive and feel happier, and more fulfilled in their lives. This needs to be put forward as one of the treatment goals.

I: You were saying earlier that there is a knowledge gap between brain and mind. There has always been a debate about whether psychiatry is brainless or mindless. What would you see as the way forward?

LL: Talking from my personal experience, as a psychiatrist, I'm very interested in symptomatology, psychopathology, disease pattern, the presentation of abnormal, non-adaptive human behaviour, which all constitute significant parts in psychiatry. I was trained as a doctor and thus I am interested in how the brain works, so the neuroscience aspects of brain structures and resulting behaviours are important, I believe. I strengthen my knowledge in this aspect of my work as much as possible. One thing I feel very important is that to be a good psychiatrist, one needs to be open-minded. We need to think about the other aspects that help explain how a particular person will behave in a particular way at a particular time, and that probably goes beyond neuroscience brain structure and symptoms; it even might have something to do with the philosophical.

I: When you talk about other aspects, what are you referring to? Spirituality? Anthropology? Sociology?

LL: Yes, I'm thinking about things like spirituality. Seeking spirituality is like finding a way to feel that there is a meaning in life and it is very helpful for all kinds of mental disorders. Finding meaning in life and asking how to stay at least calm and at ease during a crisis are very helpful in the management of patients. Spirituality as a philosophical aspect of life is something that I would like to add to symptoms, brain structures, activities, and the like, and it is probably the connection and the links between all these influence the relationship between the brain and the mind.

I: In addition to being open-minded, what are the characteristics you think a good psychiatrist should have?

LL: They should like people. They should be passionate about other people, not just themselves. If they don't have empathy and curiosity about other people, it will be very hard for them to be good psychiatrists.

I: Sometimes people go into psychiatry because they want to find themselves.

LL: Yes, and that is something I would not advise. I think most medical students can become good psychiatrists, except for people who want to seek their own self in the process of being a psychiatrist. This search for the self in the psychiatric context can be demanding and perhaps too much.

I: How would you improve recruitment into psychiatry?

LL: We have some strategies in Hong Kong from the medical student days. We take student feedbacks every year and we change whenever we think that the feedbacks arc constructive and modify our curriculum accordingly. Different times and different cohorts may have different needs. We modify our curriculum to what our students want, although we insist that some core values and proper ways to study stand the test of time. Whenever we identify a student who really has a passion for psychiatry, we offer them special personal coaching. For a few, we ask them to become volunteers for our seminars so that they get early exposure to the field. This is very effective because most of those, almost 90%, who have been volunteers in our seminars and conferences in the past go on to become psychiatrists.

I: So it's a kind of early engagement, mentoring, and coaching?

LL: Engagement and coaching, yes.

I: In training in psychiatry, what do you see as the gaps? You have mentioned gaps in Hong Kong clinical practice; are there any others? I heard that there is not a lot of intellectual disability training in Hong Kong. Is that correct?

LL: It is minimum in Hong Kong.

I: If you were redesigning the curriculum for post-graduate training, what shape would it take?

LL: We talked about this before. We have six years of psychiatric training. The first three years of training is a broad-spectrum training for different areas and this should persist because it's very important. For the senior training from fourth to sixth years, because the volume of knowledge has expanded dramatically, we should give more opportunities to people to choose different areas of their preferred specialization. Some people may be interested in psychotherapy, we give them special training in psychotherapy. Others may be more interested in things like psychopharmacology so you should give them special training in psychopharmacology. Others may be interested in legal aspects or different neuromodulation strategies and their training needs will differ. I think that with the senior training at the current time, the training blocks are insufficient. We should offer more flexible blocks of training; one block in psychotherapy, another in psychopharmacology, addictions or cognitive assessment. The current curriculum in Hong Kong is not like that. We need more psychiatrists with more special skills, not the generic psychiatrist, and six years is just the minimum training.

I: You have had a fascinating career. If you look back at your career and you were writing a letter to your younger self, when you were 16, what would you say?

LL: The message that I would like to give my younger self is trust your ability, be confident, and stick with whatever you feel that is right for you and also for people around you. What I don't like and I really regret is that I had missed a few years of my life due to a lack of self-confidence.

I: Surely one of the things is that confidence depends on our background, where we come from, and if there are no role models when you're growing up, then you may feel like an imposter, so it's not surprising to hear you saying this. Now, when you look at what you've achieved, how does it make you feel?

LL: I think I'm quite happy with what I have done. More than happy at what I've achieved. I am very happy that some of my younger doctors stay in touch with me. Sometimes they write to me and say that they like me, or admire me and feel that I have been a good role model for them, particularly for young women studying to be psychiatrists. This is something that makes me really happy and I appreciate it very much.

I: When people write to you and express their views about you being their role model, what would you advise them? What should they learn or do? One of the major things that you flagged up is about spirituality which connects brain and mind. If I were a newly qualified doctor deciding that I wanted to do psychiatry and then I came to see you, what would you tell me?

LL: I would tell young psychiatrist that if you want to become a good psychiatrist, you first have to learn the basics. You have to keep up with the knowledge. The academic base is expanding dramatically so you have to read your books but also you have to see your patients and listen to them, feel that you are with them all the time. The next is how to develop frameworks, frameworks of mapping the book knowledge on to patient presentations. Knowledge of how clinical decisions are made is important. It is important to know why a decision, big or small, is taken. The decision may be right, may be wrong, but knowing that it is your decision and yours alone is important, and knowing that if it is wrong and you know that it is wrong, then you should change it. So that's why a framework is important. You have to have a framework for clinical management. This is the academic part or the work part, the other part is the personal growth. I frequently talk to young psychiatrists about personal growth in different roles. For example, some women doctors feel that they cannot be a perfect mother and consequently they feel depressed and say they want to drop out of their career. I would tell them that nobody is perfect.

We just have to accept our roles realistically, our roles at that particular moment in time, which will change as our lives change and we grow. I always tell them that a healthy lifestyle and taking some time off work are important, otherwise you will burn out.

I: What would you like to be remembered for?

LL: I mentioned that Dr Yung, who made me stay on in psychiatry, is a psychotherapist. When I was going through the training with him, he mentioned to me that when the patient forgets you after the therapy and doesn't need to come back that means you are successful. If he forgets you, forgets that he has ever gone through a period of psychotherapy with you, and he is living his life free of you, that is real success. I think that this is a very important message: if a patient doesn't come back to you and doesn't relapse and has no problems at all and even forgets you, that's good. That's the same for my trainees.

I: I think one of the things that you said that was absolutely right was that we all need portfolio careers; I mean a mixture of research and teaching, politics and policy, and clinical work. Your journey from a clinician to an academician to a policymaker has always had the patient at its core. You went into policy because it was another way you could see to offer change and support to your patients.

LL: Yes.

I: Of all the areas you have worked in and all your achievements, what are you most proud of?

LL: I'm most proud of being a good psychiatrist who helps patients.

I: OK. Thanks very much for your time and sharing your life story.

LL: Thank you very much for your time.

9
Saul Levin

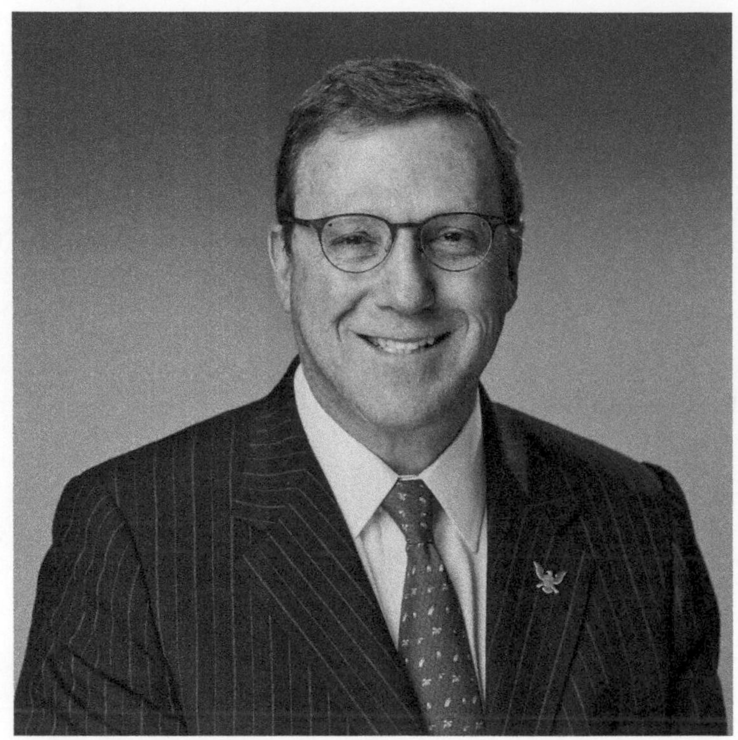

Biography

Professor Saul Levin, MD, FRCPE, MPA, is the Chief Executive Officer (CEO) and Medical Director of the American Psychiatric Association (APA) which is the largest psychiatric Association in the world, with over 38,500 members. He was previously the Head of the Department of Health of Washington DC, the American Medical Association Vice-President for Science, Medicine & Public Health, and the President and CEO of MESAB (Medical Education for South African Blacks), an educational trust started during Apartheid to provide medical and professional scholarships for Black South Africans to become doctors, dentists, and healthcare professionals. His career has focused on integrating primary care, mental health, and substance use disorders, for which he received the Royal College of Physicians fellowship and an Honorary Fellow of the Royal College of Psychiatrists.

He is a full professor at Department of Psychiatry, George Washington University, Washington, DC.

I: Thanks very much for making time. Shall we start off with what was it like growing up in South Africa?

SL: My parents immigrated to South Africa as young kids. I was born in the apartheid era as the only boy of four children. My father came from a large family and my mother had one sister. We were close to both sides of the family. My parents were very liberal. In fact, my mother was arrested one day for challenging a police officer who was trying to arrest a Black man. She was six months pregnant at that time and had to be bailed out of jail. My father was active politically in the opposition United Party, but the party could never muster enough votes to get many people elected to parliament.

One exception was the great icon Member of Parliament (Congress) Helen Suzman. While in parliament, she challenged the ruling apartheid government by asking questions that it did not want to hear. Years later we became close while I was President and CEO of the non-profit organization Medical Education for South African Blacks (MESAB), which served to provide scholarships to South African Black students entering the health field. One of my fondest memories of her was overhearing a phone conversation she had with Nelson Mandela. During that call, with her voice raised, she told him that he was not doing enough for the poor and downtrodden to help with housing, electricity, running water, and jobs. When the call ended, I said, 'Wow, that was honest!' She replied, 'Well, I think I am a little hard of hearing and he needed to hear it. He often doesn't hear things as he is surrounded by people who want to protect him.' Such was their relationship, close and honest, and they truly cared for one another. I believe it serves as a model for how people should work together.

On a personal note, I knew when I was young that I was different from other boys. Throughout my early school years, I think many people knew that I was gay. Did I know? Yes and no. I knew I was attracted to men; however, it wasn't until the end of medical school that I came out, initially to my family, who were supportive. My parents and sisters pretty much knew already but we never spoke about it, until I addressed it with them. If I was ever to write an autobiography, it would be called *Hidden in Plain Sight* because that has been me all along, out, but spending the majority of my working life in the straight medical and business world.

Growing up as a gay and Jewish man in South Africa during apartheid, I personally witnessed the Black–White issue as the main focus of overt oppression, however homosexuality was also outlawed, and it was an anti-Semitic country. The majority of the Afrikaans were members of the very conservative Dutch Reform Church, and their hatred was targeted first and foremost at the Blacks, then at the Jews, and then homosexuals. The police often raided the gay bars, something I personally witnessed, very similar to what was happening in the United States in the 1970s which prompted the Stonewall movement. I left the country soon after finishing my medical training as I did not want to serve in the apartheid government military.

I: One of the major things in hiding in plain sight is that people see what they choose to see or what they want to see rather than what's in front of them. Did you go to medical school in Johannesburg?

SL: Yes, University of Witwatersrand, Medical School.

I: What attracted you to medicine?

SL: I was an enquiring and empathetic kid. My mother wanted her only son to become a doctor and pushed for me to go to medical school. I always wanted to take care of people, especially those who were most vulnerable: the sick, the downtrodden, and the disadvantaged. So to me, it was natural that I would pursue medicine. However, I had a deep love for building design and architecture at an early age and I still love amazing architectural buildings. While architecture was in my blood, it was my second choice. That love was in the family as my baby sister did go into architecture. Rounding out my siblings, my older sister also went into medicine and then law, and my second sister went into the counselling field.

I: Why did you choose psychiatry and when?

SL: Actually, I was first attracted to psychiatry as a medical student. In the first year, as part of a sociology course project, I read a book by Elizabeth Kubler-Ross, a pioneer in near-death studies. At the time, 'hospice' was not even a word used in South Africa. I read the book and persuaded my medical school colleagues to pursue this as a group project, in what was then called thanatology. We produced a video focusing on a person's final resting place, what a dying person thinks about their demise, and what comes after death. It was after that project that I felt a calling to care for terminally ill patients. Working with a pharmacist and with some oncology nurses, we started the first hospice in South Africa. Professor Selma Brody was the sociology professor and guiding faculty member who helped us with our project, and as I proceeded through medical school, I became one of the primary hospice experts in South Africa.

During my training, I worked with some of my medical school team to both conduct a study and write an article on hospice care which was then published in the peer-reviewed *South African Medical Journal.* The article was read right round the world. When I was planning to come to the United States I went to see Professor Edwin Schneidman at UCLA, a Holocaust survivor and world-renowned expert in suicide and leader in the field of thanatology, and he became my mentor. When I was trying to decide whether to go to UCLA or Sacramento where my sister lived, he said: 'Saul, I learned from the concentration camp that (in order) to survive you come to crossroads every minute of your life and you have to choose a path, and no matter which path you choose, there will always be another crossroad leading to another path, and then another crossroad.' I think that has been my whole philosophy in life (in good times and bad times). As I became more involved in thanatology, there were no thanatology or hospice residency positions because the field had yet to be developed. So, psychiatry seemed like the ideal specialty for me to pursue.

What drew me to psychiatry was personal in that I always wanted to know why people behaved and responded in different ways to both the good and bad in their lives. I was also curious as to what causes mental illness and how we can effectively treat it. I wanted to know more about what causes the differences within some families where one child can socially adapt and academically flourish while the other siblings end up getting into trouble or going down a path where mental illness and substance use become part of their lives.

I: Do you have any regrets about going into psychiatry or choosing psychiatry?

SL: Oh no, no! No!! I have loved psychiatry. It is a professional decision I have never regretted. My colleagues are my heroes. I believe that caring for those with mental health or substance use problems, where the brain and mind are so complex, it is the 'last frontier' of medicine. And today, we are just in our early adulthood in solving the workings of the brain and mind. I envy the young psychiatry residents (registrars) for the future they will have because we are just beginning to imagine the treatments and cures that they will have at their fingertips for illnesses that we now grapple with in psychiatry.

I became politically active because of my family background. I saw that medical and professional organizations can bring about sustained and greater change, be it medical, social, or scientific. So, I chose to become a part of that. In my residency, I was the President of the California Association of Interns and Residents (CAIRS) which at that time was the Residents and Fellows Union.

On the clinical side, I was also doing a lot with borderline personality disorder and narcissistic disorder groups. Dr Otto Kernberg was my hero, along with Dr Gunderson, both experts in the field of personality disorders in the United States. I loved the work and loved caring for my patients, but in the end, it was not my career pathway destiny. I have always thought about change and how and who can affect change. I believe that it is in systems that effective change occurs. Systems are able to help people who need care and systems effect lasting changes. Hence, my career moved from the clinical and research side into policy, political, and organizational positions that allowed me to help psychiatrists and all medical professionals have the opportunity to access equal resources and education, and the ability to care for all patients.

I: Over the years as you moved into administration and leadership roles, do you miss seeing patients?

SL: For a while, I did not. But interestingly, in the last few years I have begun to miss seeing patients. After earning my master's degree in public administration from Harvard, I opened my own health consulting company, which I ran for 10 years, and then, when given the opportunity to head up the MESAB and the anti-apartheid educational trust that gave scholarships to Black South African students, I had no choice but to say yes. I am proud to say that the MESAB helped more than 20,000 students through scholarships to enter the medical, dental, nursing, and many other disciplines in the healthcare system. So, as you can see, I gradually moved further and further away from clinical care as I led these organizations. I do sometimes think that I'd love to go back to clinical care, but it is just a dream. As the APA's CEO and Medical Director, I continue to read the journals and keep up to date, but hands-on clinical work is different. So, my longing will just have to remain a longing at this moment. My deep experience and knowledge are now in the administrative, policy, political, organizational, and academic arenas.

I: You talked about Dr Schniedman and Otto Kernberg. Are there any other heroes or people you feel are role models for you?

SL: The first one is Professor Phillip Tobias who became the Dean of the Medical School I went to. He was world-renowned in palaeontology (study of ancient life from algae to the biggest dinosaurs and our first human ancestors through study of fossils) and his mentor, Professor Raymond Dart, found the skull of the Taung Child. Professor Tobias was an exciting lecturer, a brilliant clinician and teacher, and we bonded over palaeontology and hospice care. There was one point when I wanted to drop out of medical school, and he was the person who stopped me from doing so. He helped me, deeply and profoundly, in times of doubt and stood silently smiling in the wings in times of success. He was like you, and you like him, Dinesh—a man of honour, a great mentor, a friend, and above all a leader, who has profoundly impacted my life in many ways.

I: There have been generations of clinicians who were probably gay. For whatever reason, they sublimated their energy into the profession rather than relationships. Is this what it was like for you at medical school?

SL: Correct, and rather than focusing on work-life balance I chose work.

I: And was there anyone else after these two men?

SL: The other major hero of mine was Nelson Mandela. By his own and others' accounts, his vision, fortitude, and resilience helped him in his darkest hours to retain his vision of a society free of racism, where equality for all was the end goal. I have read a lot about him and I met him twice. He made the judgement that it is better to bring people together. He was the one who taught me that even if you disagree with someone, it is important to sit at a table together and work through the problem or issue for the betterment of all, rather than stand on the sidelines causing dissension.

It is important that APA as an organization, and other psychiatric associations world-wide, and all of us as individuals struggle and learn to become anti-racist. Mandela believed that while the struggle to bring people together may have been hard, even violent at times, we need to work towards that goal.

I think Philip Tobias believed that, as well. He always said, 'You have to bring people together and sit and talk about things. Demonizing one group to another is never good and only prolongs the pain and the journey to finally getting to peace and equality.'

I: I am interested in the people who have influenced you. It is the story that you were describing earlier about Schniedman and how at every step, we make a decision regarding which direction we are going to take, and then you have to make another decision, and so on. In a way that is a very philosophical yet quite pragmatic response. Were there other people that you can think of that you feel indebted to? That you wouldn't have achieved what you have done were it not for them?

SL: Oh yes. One never walks alone. Just as I joined the department of psychiatry as a resident in the University of California, Davis, Professor Joseph Tupin was the Chair. He went on to become the Dean and the Medical Director of the whole hospital system of Sacramento UCD Medical Centre. We were at times at odds with one another over residents' work conditions as I became more and more involved with medical politics. But he understood that while I was good at clinical care, I excelled at the political—administration—policy side of medicine and psychiatry. I was on the Council of the California Medical Association representing all the residents in California. At the AMA, I became a delegate for California and later for APA to the House of Delegates (the AMA's deliberative body creating policy), and at APA, where I sat on numerous Councils and Committees over the years. Joseph Tupin realized that psychiatry would help me to understand people's natures and learn from them, but my ultimate calling was in organized medicine. He was a great Chair who understood his residents and faculty strengths. There were times when some of my colleagues in the department would get little irritated about how many meetings I was going to, but he would always intervene and support me. He was a terrific mentor. Even now when I see him at APA Annual Meetings, he will always come and tell me that he knew I would excel and thank me for the work I have done for psychiatry, APA members, and patients as the CEO and Medical Director. I would also thank Fredrick (Fred) Goodwin who was then the Administrator of the Alcohol, Drug Abuse and Mental Health Administration at HHS (US Department of Health and Human Services) which is the equivalent now of SAMHSA (the Substance Abuse and Mental Health Services Administration) and the associated institutes which included NIMH (National Institute of Mental Health) and National Institute on Drug Abuse (NIDA). He offered me a job when my career was still in its early years as his special assistant for Medical Professional Affairs because he wanted to get the government more involved in the professional associations. He mentored me in my administrative and organizational career. Dr Benny Primm was another mentor as head of the Office for Treatment Improvement (later called the SAMHSA Center for Substance abuse Treatment (CSAT). They both knew I was into collaboration between primary care and mental health and substance use care, and between him and Fred Goodwin, they gave me the opportunity to create a huge US national initiative of linking and integrating the health systems. Today many of the collaborative clinics came out of the seed money from my Linkage office as demonstration grants.

Mentors come in and out of one's life, usually at the perfect time. So, as I moved through my career another gentleman who has been a great mentor to me appeared. He was the President of Royal College of Psychiatrists (RCP), then the President of the World Psychiatric Association (WPA), then became the President of British Medical Association (BMA). He has been an exceptional mentor to me. He showed me that in spite of adversity, one needs to keep the vision front and centre, and continue to keep online with the message you're giving do the best you can, and that friendship above all else is to be cherished. He is Professor Dinesh Bhugra, a man from India who rose in the psychiatric profession against incredible odds and showed me the vision of always doing your best and remaining true to who you are.

I: Over the years, that you have been involved in psychiatry, how has it changed?

SL: When I came into psychiatry, I preferred community psychiatry. I missed the era of the psychoanalytic movement. I would postulate that biological psychiatry is the future and is the unknown territory soon to be explored that will help us leap forward in the science of psychiatry, however the art of psychiatry still continues in the psychotherapy arm of psychiatry which it has to. Each of these excites and interests me. We now see the sequelae of COVID-19 in terms of brain and neurocognitive issues that we are only just beginning to recognize. This is why at APA, we started a registry to collect anonymized large data series where we have the opportunity to learn more about mental illness and substance use disorders. I have always been keen to adapt to new technologies. I think that's what my father taught me. One should move with the times. What is past is gone—it was good for the time, but science and knowledge move forward every day. What we now have is the new brain frontier that is biological, but it will always have a psychological dimension.

I always say to the medical students who are thinking of going into psychiatry that I envy them because when they look back 20 years from now at what they see today, it will seem like the Middle Ages of psychiatry. That is exactly what happened to me when I started my training. In the late 1980s there were the tricyclic and monoamine oxidase inhibitor types of antidepressants and then the first SSRIs (selective serotonin reuptake inhibitors) came out and these revolutionized treatments in psychiatry. This made me think about the changes that were still to come as technology and knowledge began to expand, using new diagnostics and the science of the brain and mind.

I: I know, I agree, and I think that's exactly how I feel. I tell my students the same thing: I feel quite envious but it's not because they are young. I think psychiatry is at that stage where medicine was about 150 years ago. You had tuberculosis but nobody knew what caused it; you were sent off into sanitorium and given good diet and hopefully you recovered, or you didn't. Then BCG was discovered. Then antitubercular treatment came along, and tuberculosis became a relatively but eminently treatable disease. The same thing is happening with bipolar disorder and gut bacteria. Who knows what lies ahead? Are you optimistic about changes in psychiatry? What do you think about the current state of psychiatry?

SL: I think that here, in the United States, we are unfortunate because for the past two decades and longer, the government has not provided the same funding for mental health and substance use research funding as it has for other illnesses, cancer for example. Yes, some may say that federal funding for NIMH, NIDA, and NIAAA (the National Alcoholism Institute) has increased, but it is a drop in the ocean compared to the other National Institutes of Health (NIH). We are constantly lobbying for more money for health and mental health research. In some ways, there still is a stigma surrounding mental health and substance use illnesses. We need a moonshot mental health and substance use initiative. We have never been given a dedicated budget like cancer or diabetes or some of the other institutes. This has now changed but the research budget is still below where we should be comparable to the other institutes. COVID-19 has shown the after-effect of us not having the resources or the advanced knowledge that has been developed for other medical diseases and conditions.

I have always said that this has placed psychiatry at least 10 to 15 years behind while we could have been in research. Because of COVID-19, things are changing, and with people in quarantine or working from home, people are beginning to realize that anyone or everyone can become depressed or anxious. I am hoping that this groundswell of opinion will begin to really resonate not only with the politicians who appropriate the funding allocations but also with the Biden Administration and government departments, as well as with the public, so that we will view these illnesses like all other illnesses. Some of the illnesses we will be able to cure and others will just become a chronic illness, but the person will have a life just like others with any chronic illness. I am hopeful, but I think we all are in a hiatus right now, regarding how we get the needed resources. President Biden has spoken about 'moonshot' initiative' in cancer; I think we need a moonshot in mental illness and substance use disorders. We need the money and investment both within the government and in the private sectors to truly get us to where mental illnesses (including substance use disorders) are just like any other diseases be they acute, chronic, or curable.

I: Apart from funding, what else do you see as a problem in psychiatry?

SL: If I could phrase the question differently, 'What has been a problem in psychiatry and how to correct it?' Psychiatry has been represented by a vast majority of White persons (disproportionality men) since its inception as a profession, both here in the United States as well as around the world. The Black Lives Matter campaign that followed the death of George Floyd has placed a spotlight onto the problem nationally but also on our profession. That horrendous murder that we all witnessed sparked a worldwide movement. We must repair what was done to the Black and minority populations and communities around the world, wherever they are, and create an equitable and non-discriminatory system.

I think what's going to happen is a change which we are seeing in psychiatry today. More women are joining medicine and psychiatry. We are seeing women, and particularly more Asian women, going into psychiatry. We clearly need to increase representation of all the minority groups in psychiatry. We also need to look at other under-represented groups, International Medical Graduates (IMGs) that travel to and work in all the nations of the world as education becomes more standardized regarding how to create a system of care of prevention, early intervention, treatment, and recovery services. LGBTQI (Lesbian, Gay, Bisexual, Transsexual, Queer, and Intersex) is clearly still a minority group that remains highly stigmatized even today (some equity advances have occurred, but an underlying homophobia remains). The United States saw our past-President, at the stroke of a pen, say that all transgender people must leave the military even though many were interpreters in the war that has been going on in the Middle East. While President Biden has rescinded those executive orders, the people forced out have since moved on, leaving a vacuum of good people who shouldn't have been discriminated against to start. We have not quite won the battle for equal rights, even though people may think so.

I am an IMG. In this country, and around the world, there is still a stigma regarding foreigners as people often view people with accents very differently. We are a global world now, through both the Internet and airplanes. COVID has clearly shown us that. Isn't it time for us to realize that we are all one species no matter what our colour or what our religion or sexual orientation, or what accents we have? Knowledge is becoming available to all, including medical knowledge and training of physicians and other health professionals. I am certainly hopeful for the future. I hope that by the end of my life, I will see a lot more equity, inclusion, diversity for all regardless of their race, ethnicity, sexual orientation, accent, etc.

I: How would you improve recruitment in psychiatry? Is that an issue in the United States?

SL: Yes, although we have been doing really well recently in filling our slots of residency training programmes. I have to thank the residency training directors and the chairs of departments of psychiatry but also the mental health consumer organizations who have really helped us. One of the most amazing advertisements I have ever seen and will always remember was the Royal College media ad to recruit medical students with their wonderful video of 'Choose Psychiatry' through the eyes of the general public and those who have a mental health or substance use addictions, and the psychiatrists, from trainees, practitioners, and professors.

I looked at that and I said, 'Wow!' Even though I had gone into psychiatry, seeing that video would have really made me understand the potential of psychiatry and what a psychiatrist can do to help their patients and the larger community. I think that's what we are beginning to show in the United States. We have gone into middle and high schools encouraging and supporting students who have a vision of wanting to go to medical school. Unfortunately, young African-American men are not going into medical school or pursuing psychiatry. To address this, we established a stream in our programme for them at APA through our Foundation and we have extended this programme to include Hispanic/Latinos, and Indigenous people. We find that today's younger generation is a lot more open to psychiatry and show a desire to help those with mental health and substance use disorders. We say to them, 'think of medicine and psychiatry as a life-long profession of helping and healing both the body and the mind'.

I: What do you see as characteristic of a good psychiatrist?

SL: I'd say first, good training, and second, understanding both the mind and the brain in mental health and substance use illnesses. Understanding that mental health/ substance use illnesses are both influenced by biological and psychological factors is necessary. Being aware of research and the potential research to unlock the workings of the brain and mind is important. Psychiatric research is reaching its young adulthood and it will progress exponentially into the future. Young medical students and residents can see that. Technology will change things. With our smartphones and our PDAs (personal digital assistants) giving us additional resources, a good psychiatrist will also be open to and embrace change. The future, which we have only begun to understand, will be a three-way relationship between patients, psychiatrists, and new technologies. If we expect our patients to change then it is important that all psychiatrists are open to change as well. I believe they will embrace the new treatments and technologies of the future.

I: Earlier you alluded to gaps in the practice of psychiatry and the shift from psychoanalysis, and within that I think you talked about biological and psychological factors but not social ones.

SL: Obviously, socio-political, economic, and environmental factors are a major issue. I was also drawn to psychiatry because the social, economic, and environmental issues of apartheid in South Africa were acute, and you saw the big differences between Blacks and Whites. Many of the Black South African medical students who studied with me and were my friends are now in the new South Africa in leadership positions. There were not that many people of colour in my class because the government would not pay for them to go to medical school, so they needed to get bursaries or scholarships. Those who got into medical school clearly were the most determined, and they would go home to study in candlelight because they did not have electricity. They would have to walk home or catch a bus; the roads in their areas were not paved and the food available to them was not abundant. I think more attention is being paid to social determinants of health and mental health in particular. I have always believed in the model of psychiatry that looks at biological, psychological, social, and environmental factors. You must look at all of those to understand where the patient who walks through your doors is coming from, and what their life experiences are, and the disadvantages the system has set up over generations upon generations. Another broader level is climate change and our environment. There could be a lot of hardship for humanity if we don't address this quickly. If we take the wrong route, it will hurt the poor, vulnerable, and the disadvantaged and desperate even more than it hurts others. For example, South Africa has large populations who lack access to housing, food, and healthcare, and they are facing disasters such as flooding or droughts. Similar conditions exist for many patients with mental illness in the United States. We must begin to look at that broader picture to see what role we as individuals and psychiatry as a profession must play in correcting these inequities.

I: What do you see as the gaps in training in psychiatry?

SL: I think the big gap is that in the United States, we do not have diverse representation in the medical schools and residency programmes. We need to make psychiatry enticing to people from all underrepresented groups, including Black, Hispanic, Asians, Indigenous peoples, Women, and the LGBTQI medical students. They need to see psychiatry as one of medicine's last frontiers—the brain and mind, where science and new technologies are showing us different things every day. The diversity gap is one we all need to actively close by recruiting, mentoring, sponsoring, and helping different groups of people.

How do we change a nation to start thinking differently about psychiatry? As the population continues to grow, we must ensure that more psychiatrists are trained which takes more than seven years in the United Kingdom, with additional time for additional specialization. Here in the United States, we have four years of undergraduate learning, four years of medical school, and then three to four years of specialty training. So how do we train more people? I believe more people would come into psychiatry if we had the training slots available. We also need to ensure that the different specialties and subspecialties within psychiatry continue to grow. I believe that in the end, science will show us some of the solutions. There will always be a need for talking therapies because people want to talk to someone who can help them. But I think those are the gaps.

I: What's your view about psychiatry's social contract and how we can achieve that? I don't know what it's like in America but in this country, the rates of compulsory treatment and detention among African Caribbean, African, and Asian groups are much higher than in the White British population. That raises the question of another part of the social contract.

SL: In the United State we too have disproportionate numbers of Black and Hispanic men in our jails and prisons. As a society, we need to look inward to explain this disproportionate incarceration and seek to ensure that judicial, societal, and health equity is afforded to everyone. Everyone should be able to receive culturally competent and sensitive healthcare. The cultural formulation that we have with the DSM (*Diagnostic and Statistical Manual*) is a way to help the majority psychiatrists to understand the impact of culture on mental health and illnesses. In other cultures, races, and ethnicities. But the question remains: how do we really make it 'a prime directive'—if I can use a term from Star Trek. Americans speak very differently from the British and South Africans and from the many other nations of the world. Even now when I say something, sometimes people still look at me in a strange way and comment on my accent, even though I have been in the USA for more than 30 years. Everyone has a different accent depending on where one grew up regionally. How do we begin to help individuals from other cultures, and countries? Maybe the way to do it is getting role models to normalize, accept, and respect our differences, to understand how the social context is important in understanding different racial and ethnic groups.

I: Looking back, what would you tell your younger self?

SL: Exercise more and do not be as work driven (laughs).

I: Great. Just that?

SL: What would I tell my younger self? You are who you are, embrace being gay, embrace being an International Medical Graduate; be true to your faith and the Hippocratic Oath; and always strive to do what's best for your profession, your co-workers, and the people you represent and above all your patients and their families. Last, but by no means least, fully embrace your mentors, teachers, and the leaders whom you will be guided and taught by.

I: So again, it goes back to having role models.

SL: It was my role models who stepped up and helped me embrace who I am, even to this day. A part of helping people is also having people around you to help you. You need to 'pay it forward' by offering the same help to others later on in your life. This job, as CEO and Medical Director, has given me the opportunity to help medical students, residents, early career psychiatrists, general members, and those that have retired show the worth and light that I see in them, in their helping patients and their colleagues. Isn't that what we all should be doing every day?

I: And what would your advice be to the trainees of today, to the residents?

SL: Stick with it!! Talk to your mentors when times are tough, and also when times are good, and play it forward. As I said a little earlier, the future of psychiatry is so bright that you will be the leaders of tomorrow because of the changes in treatment and recovery for our patients. Also, choose wisely in the profession (of psychiatry) that you are in or are thinking of going into. Remember that there are plenty of different disciplines within psychiatry and that you *will* find the thing you love the most and spend want your career in. This may be cellular biology or population-based research or different subspecialties of psychiatry, or in my case the administrative side and a leadership career. There will always be an avenue for you to find that will keep that flame alive inside you. Get involved and never say 'oh, someone else will do that'. Most importantly, remember that everyone's opinion matters and needs to be heard.

I: What would you like to be remembered for?

SL: I think those who really know me would say I am kind, loyal, have overcome adversity, and tried to do good, that I was as hard on myself as on others, and in the end, I left the world a little bit improved.

I: Which you have and in lots of ways. I'm not just flattering you as I think in terms of your achievements, and not only within APA, the AMA, the DC Department of Health, and MESAB but also the people who have seen you in action speak very fondly of you. So yes, your kindness and loyalty speak for themselves. Which of your achievements are you most proud?

SL: I think starting the formation of the first hospice in South Africa, with a pharmacist and a sociologist, and all the oncology nurses who showed me gentleness, kindness, courage in the face of obstacles, discrimination, and dying. MESAB, and APA and with the support of the Boards of Trustees, and the Assembly (our Parliament/Congress), and all the members, we are all helping to move an organization into the twenty-first century.

I: One of the most impressive and stunning things that you did as a medical student was that sociology project, taking it forward into a much more practical and pragmatic way. Because policies are one thing but actually doing something makes it much more important.

SL: I can give you a quick anecdote of how the threads of life, education, and a profession tie things together. When I was doing the initial sociology project in that first year in medical school, I went into the cancer centres to interview those getting chemotherapy. There was an elderly British woman who was dying. She knew she was dying; the chemotherapy wasn't working, and I had the opportunity to record a video interview with her. We talked about circles of life. We were talking about it because in hospice you never know how a patient is going to react when you finally get the diagnosis of a terminal disease. Some people say 'I will fight it till the end', and others say 'I'm not fighting it anymore'. Some say, 'I never want treatment', and others will say 'I want all the treatment I can get'. She finally said to me, 'I've had enough, Saul. I have tried, it's over for me now, it's time for me to go. I have had a charmed life even when I was a baby."

Her language intrigued me. Why did she say 'even as a baby'? So I asked her to tell me a bit about her life? She replied, 'You know I nearly died as a young kid.' 'Oh,' I said, 'from what?' She replied, 'I got a terrible infection, and was dying but my father was the dentist to the King of England. One day the King asked my father about the family and how were they doing because my father was looking out of sorts. My father explained that it was really tough for him at that time as his little daughter was dying because of a blood infection and no treatments were working. The King said, 'Hold on, I just heard about a new possible medication that they've just discovered that apparently kills blood infections. Let me talk to the person who knows about this.' And the next thing she told me was that her father got a call and the person said, 'Listen, we are doing this trial on a drug called penicillin. We don't know if it works or not. We have no clue about the dosage. We have never done it on a child but we are happy to give it to your daughter.' They gave it to her and obviously gave her enough that she survived.

I always remember that story. She said, 'You know you have to be lucky in life.'

When we were doing the filming of the movie CURED at the Smithsonian in 2020, (a film about being a gay psychiatrist in America, the pathologizing of gays and lesbians as mentally ill by the APA in the DSM, and APA's removal of homosexuality from the DSM in 1973), the archivist showed me some of the artifacts the Smithsonian had collected.

After the filming ended, she said, 'I have something here that I bet you would be really interested in.' She ushered me into a side room and went to the closet in a separately air-conditioned room and pulled out a petri dish. She said, 'This is part of the original Fleming penicillin petri-dish samples that we have in storage.' All I could think of was that wonderful lady, my patient, and I was taken back to the reason I went into medicine and psychiatry. It was because of the care of patients and listening to them and seeking advances in medicine. What makes me excited about the future for psychiatry, the APA, and medicine is all the advances that are still to come.

I: Thanks very much Saul. That is really moving and wonderful. Is there anything else you wish to add?

SL: No, thanks.

I: Thank you for sharing your fascinating experiences and your story.

10
Mario Maj

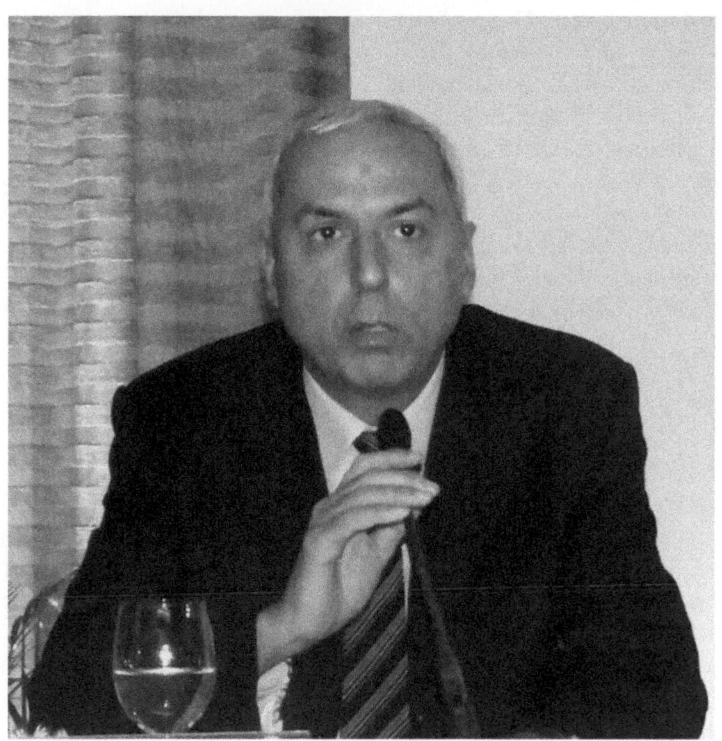

Biography

Professor Mario Maj was born in Naples in Italy, trained in medicine and psychiatry, was awarded qualifications at the University of Naples, and subsequently obtained his PhD from the University of Umeå, Sweden in 1986. He is currently Professor of Psychiatry and Chairman, Department of Psychiatry, University of Naples (1992–present) having previously been Professor of Mental Hygiene, University of Naples (1985–1992). He was President of the World Psychiatric Association (WPA) (2008–2011), prior to which he was WPA Secretary for Publications (1999-2005). He has also been President of the European Psychiatric Association (2003–2004). He chaired the Section on Neuropsychiatry of the Global Programme on AIDS of the World Health Organization in Geneva (1989–1991). He chaired a joint task force between Association of European Psychiatrists (now known as European Psychiatry

Association), European Union of Medical Specialists (UEMS), World Health Organization (WHO), and WPA. He coordinated a European Community Project on Burden on the Families of Patients with Schizophrenia (1994–1997) and a European Community Project on the Implementation of Psychoeducational Interventions for Families of Patients with Schizophrenia (2000–2004). He is the founder and the editor of *World Psychiatry*, the official journal of the WPA (impact factor 49.548, ranking number 1 among psychiatric journals and among all journals included in the Social Sciences Citation Index). He has been awarded several honorary fellowships from organizations around the world. He has been President of the Italian Psychiatric Association (2000–2002), the Council of Italian Professors of Psychiatry (1997–2000), the Italian Society of Biological Psychiatry (1991–present), and the Italian Society of Psychopathology (2007–2013). He is currently the Director of WHO Collaborating Center for Research and Training in Mental Health, Naples, Italy (1992–present). He has been a member of the Workgroup on Mood Disorders for the DSM-5 (the *Diagnostic and Statistical Manual* 5th edition), and a member of the International Advisory Group and Chairperson of the Workgroup on Mood and Anxiety Disorders for the Chapter on Mental Disorders of the ICD-11 (International Classification of Diseases).

Interview

I: Why did you choose psychiatry?

MM: Like many colleagues of my generation, at least in my country, the main factors that led me to choose psychiatry were my interest in psychoanalysis (I was greedily reading Freud's and Jung's books from when I was 14 years old), and the perception that community mental healthcare could become a crucial element of social progress (the years of my medical training coincided with the peak of the movement that generated the Italian mental health reform of the year 1978) (Basaglia reforms which led to closure of psychiatric institutions). Notably, the relationship between psychiatry and neurosciences was much less clear for young people like me at that time, at least in Italy.

I: Who were your role models?

MM: I was very lucky to have begun my work at the international level when I was in my early 30s. I was working with Carlo Perris in Sweden in the early 1980s, and I had the opportunity to meet eminent leaders such as Karl Leonhard and George Winokur. At the same time, I started my collaboration with the World Health Organization (WHO) which brought me into contact with Norman Sartorius, Paul Kielholz, and John Wing. Slightly later on, my interest and clinical experience in the use of lithium in the prophylaxis of bipolar disorder led me to form a very close relationship with Jules Angst and Mogens Schou. These prominent psychiatrists became my main role models.

I: What are the memorable occasions in your practice or research in psychiatry?

MM: In the early 1980s, a network of WHO Collaborating Centres in Mental Health was established which became very active in organizing exchanges of visits and multicentre studies. I remember my involvement in that network, in representation of the Naples Collaborating Center, as a very stimulating opportunity for learning, interacting with many colleagues, and getting a global view of the development of our discipline. My experience in establishing and leading one of the first centres for the long-term management of bipolar disorder in my country was also extremely useful to me especially in conducting some long-term follow-up studies in large samples of patients. In the late 1980s, my appointment as the person responsible for the Neuropsychiatric Branch of the Global Programme on AIDS of the WHO in Geneva gave me the opportunity to contribute to the characterization of HIV-associated dementia, which was a memorable experience. Subsequently, my long-term involvement in the activities of the European Psychiatric Association and the World Psychiatric Association, where I had the honour to serve as President, led me to become familiar with the situation of psychiatry and mental healthcare in a number of different regions, including Eastern Europe, Central Asia, and Sub-Saharan Africa, and to establish contacts with hundreds of clinicians and researchers in many countries. I would also like to mention my participation in the development of the ICD-10 and ICD-11 (in the latter case as the Chairperson of the Workgroup on Mood and Anxiety Disorders and as a member of the International Advisory Board) as well as of the DSM-5 (as a member of the Work Group on Mood Disorders), which offered me an important opportunity to interact with many prominent colleagues.

I: How has psychiatry changed in your time?

MM: When I started my research and practice in psychiatry, in the late 1970s, there was a widespread expectation that mental disorders would turn out to be disease entities exactly as conditions studied by the other branches of medicine, and that a precise and reliable diagnosis of those disorders would automatically lead to the identification of a specific aetiology and pathogenesis for each of them, and that this would spearhead the development and implementation of effective treatments. Throughout the decades of my experience within the discipline, that optimistic view has gradually vanished. We know today that the vast majority of patterns of mental disorder are unlikely to represent natural kinds (unlikely to be exclusively biological causation) and that diagnosis in itself is insufficient to guide the formulation of the management plan and the prognosis. We know that a variety of factors influence the outcome of all psychiatric treatments. These include response to pharmacotherapies. A multitude of vulnerability and protective factors are involved in the aetiology of all patterns of mental disorder, the majority of which are non-specific. The perception of this complexity can easily generate a sense of defeatism, and this is something that we have to fight against actively.

I: What are your views on the current state of psychiatry?

MM: The above evolution is currently reinforcing some sceptical or even hostile attitudes towards our discipline that have been always present along the decades. The future of our profession will depend upon our ability to convince the general public that the complexity of mental disorders requires an equally complex biopsychosocial approach that only our discipline is able to provide. The existence of a biological, a psychological, and a social component in our discipline is not a weakness but evidence of its peculiar integrative nature, and it should be perceived, presented, and promoted as such. Rather than denigrating each other, the proponents of the different approaches should look for synergies and cross-fertilization. We also have to refine our public image and promote it. In addition to treating competently a broad range of mental disorders that are very common in the population, today we provide counselling in schools, in the workplace, in prisons. We are asked by colleagues from other medical disciplines to provide advice for the emotional problems of their patients. We interact on a continuing basis with user and carer organizations. This new reality of our profession is not well known but is also probably not sufficiently developed in several regions of the world. We have to build up this new image and make it public. At the same time, we have to ensure that psychiatric practice worldwide are equal to this new image.

I: Which of your achievements are you most proud of?

MM: I am proud to have founded and to be the editor of a scientific journal, *World Psychiatry*, which has become the world's number one journal in terms of impact factor not only of all psychiatric journals but also of all journals included in the Social Science Citation Index. *World Psychiatry* is the first psychiatric journal to reach an impact factor of 20, 30, and then 40. At the same time, it is the most widespread psychiatric journal, it is available free of charge, it is published in several languages, and it is widely perceived by psychiatrists as a tool that is relevant to their everyday clinical practice and useful to foster their professional growth.

I am proud of having relaunched the European Psychiatric Association. It was about to go bankrupt just before my presidency, during which time we started to have an annual congress and itinerant educational courses and activities for young psychiatrists. I am proud to have contributed to make the World Psychiatric Association an active, respected, and truly international organization.

I am proud never in my career to have succumbed to fads in the field, never to have brought political or ideological interests into my professional activity, and never to have received money from pharmaceutical companies for myself or my family.

11
Felice Lieh Mak

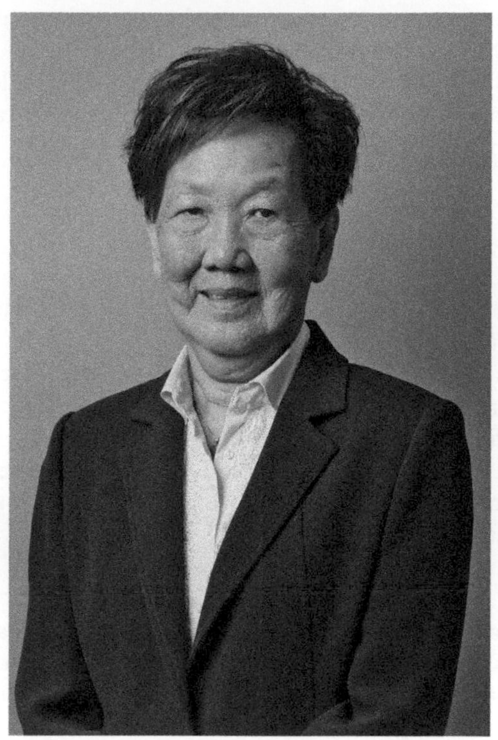

Biography

Felice Lieh Mak comes from a diverse cultural background. She was born of Chinese parents in the Philippines, where she completed medical school. She was trained in psychiatry in the United Kingdom and became a medical academic in Hong Kong.

She was appointed chair professor in psychiatry at the University of Hong Kong. During her tenure she nurtured the development of psychiatry which was in its infancy in Hong Kong at that time. While serving as dean of the medical school, she initiated the reform in the medical curriculum and broadened the teaching and learning of psychiatry.

In 1993 she was elected as the first woman President of the World Psychiatric Association. During her term she organized the visit to the then USSR to investigate the abuse of psychiatry for political purposes, reformed the governance of the

Association to ensure that it is fit for purpose as an international organization, and formulated the template for the teaching and learning of psychiatry in undergraduate medical education.

During the four years leading up to the handover of Hong Kong to the People's Republic of China, she was a member of the Executive Counsel of Lord Patten, the last Governor of Hong Kong.

From 1997 to 2012, she served as Chairman of the Medical Council of Hong Kong. In the course of her chairmanship she reformed its procedures and composition to guarantee that its primary role is to protect the public.

She was awarded Commander of the British Empire (CBE) for her services to psychiatry. After the handover she was awarded the Gold Bauhinia Star in 2012 for services to psychiatry and education.

Interview

I: Thanks very much Felice, for making the time. Can we start with your early life and your childhood? What was it like?

FLM: (laughs) Totally different from what it is now. I was born during the war (World War II) so my parents and some friends were living in the deep, I wouldn't call it a jungle but it's a forest in the south of the Philippines.

Some of my earliest memories of my childhood are running through the cornfields, chasing monkeys, planting trees, swimming in the stream, digging up sweet potatoes. So that's my childhood.

I: When did your schooling start? How did you find your way into medicine and psychiatry?

FLM: When the war ended I came back to the city with my parents in the Philippines.

My father started to work as a principal in a Chinese school. It was a primary and secondary school, my mum was teaching at the primary school, and we lived on the campus of the school. So my dad was a dreamy sort of a person. He liked poetry, he liked to read, and in fact his English teacher in Nanking, where he did his university degree, was Pearl Buck. The first book I was introduced to was hers. That was my Dad's influence, the literature, the books, the poetry in Chinese and English. He emphasized that I should not only learn English but also Chinese, which to my regret now I didn't take seriously. So my Chinese is really poor. I am barely articulate in Chinese, especially in writing. My first desire was to be a writer, my father encouraged that. My mother was a different kind of person. She came from a quite well-off family, her father had three wives and, very cleverly, he sent one wife to Canton to look after business, another wife to Hong Kong to look after the business, and one to the Philippines. And so my mother spent a lot of her time in the Philippines because she was the daughter of the third wife. Coming from a business background, she was a very good businesswoman. She thought it was a very bad idea to be a writer. She told me that I could never make a living and I had to stop wanting to become one. It was not a good thing.

I: Unless you are Agatha Christie.

FLM: Or Pearl Buck (laughs). My mother said this very subtly. She had always wanted to be a doctor. Unfortunately, coming from a big family and being a woman, she never got into medical school. She was sent to study home economics at the university. It's a good thing that she was sent to university even if only to study home economics. She took me along with her whenever she went to the doctor for follow-ups and chats with her GP and she kept saying, 'Oh what a great man he is, helping people'. Lo and behold, her cousin was married to an ENT surgeon and they came to set up a practice very near where we lived. In summer I was asked to go to his clinic to help him. I must have been 12. I watched him do adenoids and tonsillectomy and helped fetching instruments. So, I said one day, 'That's interesting. Medicine is interesting.' My mother was happy, she encouraged me, and in secondary school I loved biology. I loved chemistry but I still liked history and literature. I nurtured both at high school. I also liked sports. I was a bit of a rebel, organizing insurrections against the nuns for being very unfair and showing favouritism to some students and as a result, I was kicked out of the convent school. By that time my parents were already in business, they had a business of their own. They sent me to the school where my father was the principal, so I ended up with two years of Chinese which was good, and Chinese and English literature. I brushed up on my Chinese language, so that was good. I wrote plays and directed my classmates in those plays. I liked being on stage and liked public speaking, so this was early exposure to that skill. Because my mother was a bit shy, whenever there were any speeches that she needed to make to the primary school parents she would send me to do it for her. My father was very influential in helping me shape my presentations. He got me to focus on one topic and not make any more than three or four points, which I then developed. He was pretty good at teaching me logical thinking and logical presentation and I enjoyed that. I loved biology. When I was in senior high school, there was a very strange disease affecting Filipino men. They were dying in their sleep and no-one could find any cause, but it appeared that they were having nightmares, and then they would die. This was called Bangungot by the Filipinos. I found it really interesting. I did some research when I was in third year of high school and came up with a theory that that the disease was caused by a stress problem that led to an overwhelming secretion of gastric juice causing death. I went on to explore how stress affected the body and caused death. I sent the report to the Chief Medical Examiner in Manila, asking him to look into it. He thanked me for my ideas, and that was all I heard. I started reading, I think, by the age of six or seven. I spent a lot of time reading, especially in the summer during which I would read through the entire public library. But you know, I still had time to go out with friends and do things like swimming, catching fish and all that. Then I was sent away to the university. Since there was no medical school where I lived, I had to go to Manila. When I was in pre-med, my favourite subject was logic. We had a wonderful logic teacher. He was very unusual for a Filipino because he was brought up in a public school in the United Kingdom as well as at Cambridge University. He spoke with a plummy accent and introduced us to logic. He kept us inspired. There were my other teachers. I found chemistry boring but the teacher was really good. She was German, and even inspired some of us to learn the German language. I had another influential teacher who was superb. He taught an optional course on rational psychology, which included religious aspects of psychology. He had a great sense of humour.

I: Rational or relational?

FLM: Rational. It's rational psychology. He taught us about contributions of Thomas Aquinas and theology. It was the intellectual stimulation that I was interested in. In the second year of my pre-med, the Chief Medical Examiner came to where I was staying and he said, 'Oh, I read your article. I would like you to come and spend some time in my lab.' He was not only a medical examiner but also a great medical historian, and we would sit down and he would introduce me to Montessini and Parto. I would go with the ambulances collecting dead bodies, watch pathologists do autopsies. It is terrible when someone dies via medical malpractice, For example, doctors tore someone's uterus and she died of exsanguination. Drownings are pretty awful as well; the stench. I saw a lot of them in the first year. In med school, anatomy was easier for me because of this exposure to autopsies. Medical school was fun! It was challenging, it was interesting. The professor asked me to do research projects for her, so that helped me a lot. I liked the clinical years. They were fun because we had great teachers. One of our teachers taught us internal medicine. She introduced us to medical semiology. In those days that was impressive, it was just clinical science and symptoms, she called it semiology. It was amazing.

I: Were there many female students? What was it like at that time?

FLM: There were. It was a Dominican medical university, so was dominated by Spanish, that was why we were required to learn Spanish. I also picked up Filipino, and other languages from friends and domestic helpers, nannies, etc. Most of us grew up in that kind of environment with English and Chinese as a base and then other languages like German, Spanish. It was a big school, 500 students I think, separated into different classes.

I: Five hundred in total or in each year?

FLM: In total. It was a big school. We were forty in a class. Because it was run by Dominicans, males and females were separated.

I: You were in separate classes?

FLM: Yes, and we were not even allowed to use the same stairs. There was an elite class for the males and elite class for the females. I was in one of those elite classes in the upper bracket. Again, it was great fun. We had friends who loved music, whose parents loved music. My friend's parents were musical and sent her to learn classical music and we would go there and listen to Mahler. There was a lot of naughtiness, of course, like not going to lectures, hiding in the female toilets so that the male teachers could not find us, and all those things. We met up with a group of students from another university, the University of Philippines who were writers. There was also a Jesuit priest there who encouraged intellectual discussions and was an amazing psychologist. We became a loose group of people who became his disciples. He was very articulate and wrote very well. I got on well with him and on campus, he became known as Jean-Paul Sartre and I was known as Simone de Beauvoir (laughs). And we used to spend our days talking about existentialism and Albert Camus. We thought we were very brave because we read *The Naked Lunch* by William Burroughs, pretty radical because the book was so highly sexualized. 'I had a pretty standard student life, going to parties, meeting up with different groups of people, playing sports.'

I: How much psychiatry were you exposed to and how did you end up choosing psychiatry?

FLM: My introduction to psychiatry was very early in my studies. When my family came back from the forest to the city there was a hospital close by. The head of the public hospital became very good friends with my parents so we were able to go to the hospital and visit him. Later, when I was in med school, in the summer I would do some work there. From my childhood I remember a story about a woman who was described as crazy. She was probably psychotic. She was naked and chained by her neck to a post. Some of my friends threw stones at her. I was horrified. I said, 'That is a human being. What's wrong with her? She might have been terribly traumatized by something.' That woman stayed in my mind. Why was she like that? Why do people become like that? So that's where my interest started. Of course, philosophy and psychology played a role too. I went through the medical school, I liked different subjects, and I thought I would be a pathologist because of my experience working with Medical Examiner, doing slides for him. But I realized I wanted involvement with people so when the internal medicine specialist taught us semiology, I began to think that internal medicine couldn't be all that bad. Perhaps I would end up being a gastrointestinal specialist. Then I came across a great teacher in Neurology who made neurology simple and showed me how fascinating the brain is. He really inspired me. We had a psychiatry teacher who was a good teacher but he was a bit strange. He would come in to lectures wearing a Panama hat, take it off and put it on a chair, and in the middle of the lecture he would forget that the hat was there and would sit on it. At that time t as here was quite a lot of interest in psychoanalysis as therapeutic intervention, I wasn't really attracted to it as a field of study because I thought it was unrealistic but I thought it was really great for films; we were into art-house films—Ingmar Bergman and others. We had a one-week placement in a huge mental hospital. I didn't pay too much attention to the placement; I was just doing rounds, seeing patients, not taking it very seriously. So when it came to choosing a specialty, I thought Neurology would be fine but after a while when I was in Queen Square as a paying student, I discovered people like Russell Brain, who was absolutely brilliant. When patients walked in, experts like him could reach a diagnosis quickly, telling them they had ataxia, etc. I started thinking that this was great as an intellectual exercise but may not work in management partly as very few drugs were available. The question was what could be done. I liked the intellectual exercise but not the lack of treatment and so I turned my sights on psychiatry. The reason was that it included a lot of aspects of study that I really liked: philosophy, sociology, history, patient contact; far better than gastroenterology, for example. Why did I go to the United Kingdom? Most of my classmates from the Philippines went to the United States. A few would go to Denmark and a few would go to England, but only a very few. The two reasons I went to the United Kingdom were that my father was an Anglophile and I didn't want to be doing just psychoanalysis and the UK brand of psychiatry was more eclectic—it was social, biological. So I opted for that. After doing my internship in assorted places I ended up in the Littlemore Hospital in Oxford. My first placement was in a therapeutic community and that was fun although it was chaotic and I like things to be more ordered. So, after this I went to join a more traditional team looking after patients where I did most of my psychiatry training.

I: Right. Did you do your Diploma in Psychological Medicine (DPM) and returned to Philippines? How did you end up in Hong Kong?

FLM: I failed my DPM. I thought that while I was waiting, to retake the exams I would go to the United States and take up Neurology again. I applied to a number of places. Yale accepted me but I needed a Green Card for the fellowship residency post, so I had to wait for a year before that came through. I did not know what to do while waiting, then my father very cleverly suggested that I go to Hong Kong. Back when I was at Oxford, I met my future husband's sister and her husband. It is a small Chinese community there so we used to cook and have dinners together. We used to gather at the home of a particular family on weekends, and the wife's brother was living in Hong Kong where I met him eventually, and married him.

I: When did you get your specialty qualification?

FLM: After I got married. I went back to the United Kingdom and did my attachment at the Warneford Hospital with Michael Gelder who was Professor of Psychiatry at Oxford. I did my clinical attachments learning about EEGs as well as adult and child psychiatry. Then I sat my exams. A consultant I had worked with at the Littlemore Hospital was my examiner, a great coincidence, and I got through my membership.

I: How did you get your professorship at Hong Kong University? How difficult was it for a woman at that particular time to get to that level?

FLM: It wasn't difficult at all. They were short of psychiatrists. There was no department of psychiatry, no Chinese University of Hong Kong at that stage. I worked at the Castle Peak Hospital. After a month I couldn't take it; it was really chaotic and it was an asylum. It was very different from the experience in Littlemore Hospital (in Oxford) and that really put me off. I resigned and then, luckily, PM Yap, first professor at Hong Kong University, recruited me.

I: Was he the person who wrote about Culture Bound Syndromes?

FLM: Yes, that's right. He heard about me and asked me to join him. I had always thought I might like being an academic because my father was academically inclined. So I joined the department which consisted of three people, two lecturers and one professor. That's how my academic career started.

I: Over the years, in your view how has psychiatry changed? Has it changed for the better or has it declined?

FLM: It has changed a lot. In Hong Kong I think we set up the first general hospital psychiatric unit and also the first one to have a child psychiatric unit. It was tough, I think it was tougher for PM Yap than for me. It was tougher for him as he was such a scholar and a gentleman, up against the big professors in the big clinical departments in the University who thought psychiatry was useless. They gave him a hard time. He wanted more time to teach and to practise; at that time psychiatry was only given ten lectures and a one-week placement. PM (Yap) was fighting against this and the attitude that if you treat crazy people, they must be crazy, and because you treat them, you must be crazy too. This was the attitude he was up against and he found it really difficult because he was not aggressive not assertive at all. He was a great scholar and couldn't cope with these people. They were really rough on him. He hated faculty meetings. Colleagues would ignore what he said and they would say, 'You know, we don't want our students to be doing something which is not very useful.' Basically, they were selfish. Nobody wanted to give us curriculum time. So poor PM (Yap) got very stressed out. He was very sad. He tried to hide all this from us and thought that we did not know about it. He went to Mexico City for a World Psychiatry Association (WPA) meeting and he died there.

I: From what?

FLM: A couple of days before he left, there was a very acrimonious heads of department meeting where he was belittled. We think that he died from the stress. Anyway, after he passed away there was somebody more senior than me who became a sort of acting head of the department. So I stayed. Then we got lucky. We were allocated a number of beds for patients who now descended on the wards. The hospital was up in arms. It did not know why all the mad people were coming into our wards. Staff worried about whether these mad people would pull drips out of other patients. Anyway, there we were, three of us looking after fifteen beds. Then one night there was an urgent call. A very senior academic administrative staff member wanted a psychiatrist because his daughter was behaving hysterically and was probably on drugs. I had to go to their home and I sorted everything out. I managed to persuade the daughter to take some medication and gave her an injection. In this way I got this very senior academic administrative staff member on our side. Then a few weeks later, maybe a few months but within that year, a very senior academic developed delirium tremens (DTs). An urgent call came in to let me know a patient was climbing out of his bed and was trying to strangle a nurse. I was asked to come and assess and advise. I had seen such cases as Littlemore so I treated him and he calmed down. I explained the situation to him and all that was done to him. This patient didn't like being followed up; he loved his whisky! So what could we do but treat him when he presented? After this, we got more respect, we started getting more referrals, took people into our wards, and people would walk up and say, 'Hey, being a psychiatrist, having a psychiatric service, is not such a bad idea.' We had another senior academic whose mother became depressed, so we were also treating bread-and-butter depression. Another case comes to mind who was the son of a senior academic developed a transient psychotic episode while he was on a flight. He tried to rush into the cockpit and was arrested. Of course, the academic and his son came to Hong Kong and saw me. I treated the boy and he got better and went back to school. Last time I heard, he was happily married and living in London. All this made our colleagues and the hospital value psychiatry and psychiatrists. So when the professor retired, I planned and built up the unit and took charge. In the meantime, the medical curriculum underwent reforms. So, we got ten weeks where we could train students full-time.

I: Our training in India was only two weeks in the fourth year and virtually everybody went on holidays then. Do you have any regrets in choosing psychiatry?

FLM: No, it was fun. No regrets.

I: What are your views on the current state of psychiatry?

FLM: I'm an optimist. I think psychiatry is improving. To say that psychiatry will disappear is silly; it won't because there are loads of patients that need psychiatric care and nobody will look after them apart from a psychiatrist. The demand is there.

I: And demand is increasing

FLM: Yes. That is because people are becoming aware of what psychiatry can do now. Stigma appears to be going down as well.

I: Do you have any thoughts about what makes a good psychiatrist?

FLM: Basically, it's the love of the job that determines everything. If you love your job, you are interested and fascinated by it. And that's the general approach to things, enjoy and do well.

I: Switching tracks slightly, you were the first woman to head the department, then become President of the Hong Kong College of Psychiatrists and then of the World Psychiatric Association. What was that like?

FLM: Maybe I'm in denial (laughs). I'm not sure, but really it is nothing more than you need to be a good clinician, you have to prove yourself. If you're a good clinician then you treat VIPs and that helps your profile, but you have to be good to start with. I attracted a lot of interest because I was the first person to publish a paper on autism in the Chinese population in Hong Kong when people said there was no such problem. I was also the first person to publish a study on child abuse among the Chinese people in Hong Kong. That led to my getting some government recognition and becoming interested in families of children with autism and running clinics for them. I had a mentor at the university who was the professor of Obstetrics and Gynecology. She was very friendly with the (Hong Kong) Governor's wife because of her work in family planning. The Governor's wife was also very interested in services for the mentally challenged. My mentor introduced us. We managed to work together in a number of fields related to children, families and mental health. She really had a good heart and intentions and we worked very well. I took over as the Chair of a voluntary agency and the Governor got to know about it and I was given an Honour. The voluntary organization helped conduct workshops set up half way homes etc thus influencing policy in a number of ways. The next governor of Hong Kong thought that I was always criticizing the government. I was interviewed on the radio saying that the government was not caring for the mentally ill, that mental hospitals were in a bad state, that the government was not looking after or planning for the elderly at a time when the percentage of the population that is ageing is increasing dramatically. I got into trouble with several policy-makers. Very cleverly, being the colonial government, they appointed me to the Social Welfare Advisory Group. So now I was in the tent, not shouting from the outside (laughs). You know by accepting it, I ended up troubleshooting for the government whether it was dealing with non-governmental or governmental organisations, welfare services or children's services. A close colleague who was very astute official helped very effectively behind the scenes. The Governor, the Chief Secretary and the Financial Secretary were in the Central Policy Unit to which I was co-opted. It also had two outstanding barristers one was also a great theologian, a very interesting guy, a and the other barrister who eventually became our first Chief Justice. Another member was the CEO of Hang Seng Bank, which is the subsidiary of Hong Kong Shanghai Bank (HSBC) and also CEOs of, at that time it was called, Hong Kong Electric and that of HSBC. So it was a collection of academic people, business people, professionals. We produced reports on specific topics requested by the Governor and the financial secretary. It was great fun because from the beginning it was a very interesting time. The Joint Declaration for the return of Hong Kong to China was already signed with Beijing and we were sold down the river. And before that happened, Governor Wilson said I have done enough for welfare and appointed me to the Legislative Council. But that was all a waste of time. There was a lot of political posturing by many members. However, the most interesting time was when Tiananmen happened. I was very friendly with the democrats you know partly; all my values are democratic apart from financial aspects on which I am a conservative. I did not think that communism worked. I am like my mother very pragmatic about money, so that's when we see eye to eye. But anyway, the leader who was a very articulate barrister, Martin Lee, could not make it, so they asked me because my English is better than most of the others. I had to go with them to Westminster to lobby for passports. That was how I ended up in London meeting Paddy Ashdown and others and being interviewed on the BBC. So those were my political activities.

I: So how did you get interested in WPA and what was that like? You don't need to give any secrets over here.

FLM: No, no secrets at all. WPA was another phase in my life. I'll tell you all the time I've been very lucky. There were all those people who helped me. So at that time there was some meeting in Bangkok, and I was giving a presentation. But anyway Alfred Freedman came and he wanted me to join the Section on Education in WPA. I knew about the WPA because one of our consultants was the Secretary General of the WPA, in the old old days. So I know the WPA. And Alfred s invited me to join and I did saying why not. So that's it. So then of course becoming the President was the neutral choice because there was this great battle between the Russians and the Americans, about abuse of psychiatry. So the Russians had their candidate and the Americans wanted to present somebody but not American, so I was their choice. I was a woman, I was Asian, I was pretty good in English, and I knew the WPA. And I was neutral, I didn't really care for the politics. So I was elected and the Americans backed me.

I: Looking back at your career now are there things that you think, you could've, should've done differently?

FLM: Thinking back, nothing of significance. Because it seems so, maybe again I'm in denial, because everything seemed to just flow so naturally and I think that worked. I had a broad knowledge base and I was articulate, I was aware of social issues about medicine, about good governance. In fact, I wrote the ordinance for the organization of the mentally challenged individuals. I was really very keen on good governance.

I: And if you were writing to your younger self, what would you say?

FLM: Enjoy what you're doing, just have fun.

I: Do you think that we are getting the right kind of people coming into psychiatry, how do we improve recruitment?

FLM: Recruiting is a mixture, there's some weird people, then there are weirder people, I think other specialties also have some weird people, so we can't say that. I think we are getting good people, specially few years ago when Linda (Lam) (Chapter 8) was instrumental and encouraging to lot of good people, but I think it's the training that is far too short, the training is not good enough.

I: And you were saying earlier that being a good clinician is important to achieve all other things and therefore it links quite nicely with good training as it is all about clinical skills.

FLM: Yes.

I: And as a leader what kind of skills you think are necessary with your own experience. You have really been an exceptional leader in lots of ways and lots of levels, you've achieved a lot, so what skills would you say are essential for that?

FLM: Well, first is people skills, you have to like people, you know you've to like them. And I guess empathy because we all say right, especially when I give expert advice, I would like to know what judges are like, so it's always good to see what that person is like. Some of the politicians I would like to know what's behind them.

What their agenda is? So, understanding people not only empathy but understanding. What makes them tick? Third is having integrity, I'm not being idealistic or anything or purposely trying for integrity, because I'm lazy.

I: Because you're lazy? I don't believe that!

FLM: Yes, because it's too much trouble to be lying, it's too much trouble hiding things. So why not just be honest, be open, you don't have the burden, you don't have to look over your shoulders.

I: In your career, what are the achievements you're most proud of?

FLM: Okay, I think I'm most proud of having treated patients. Of course, there are sad things like patients committing suicide.

I: Okay, obviously you have had major impact on policy particularly in Hong Kong and on ethics globally. What would you like to be most remembered for?

FLM: I think mostly about Hong Kong, when my name is mentioned it's on personal integrity.

I: Okay, Thank you very much for your time. It has been great hearing your story.

FLM: Thank you.

12
M. Sarada Menon

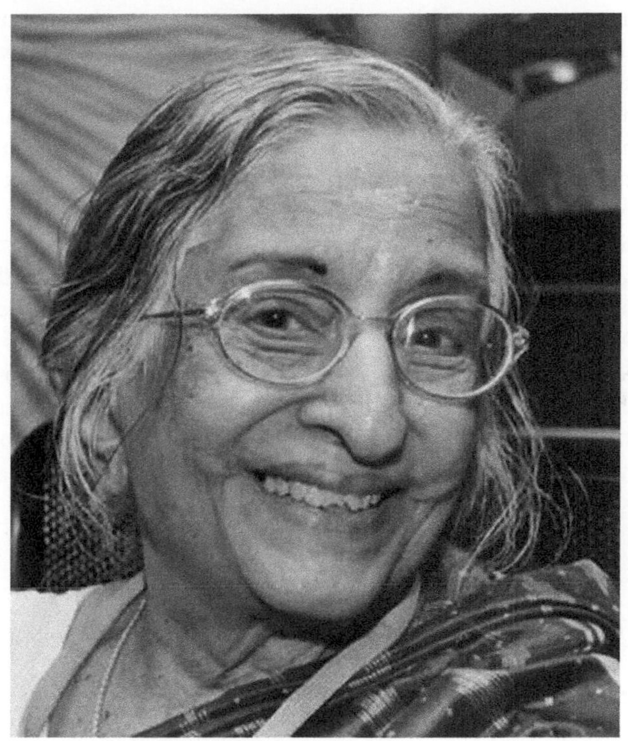

Biography

Dr Sarada Menon, graduating in 1947 with a postgraduate degree in Medicine, displayed her willingness to walk the untrodden path by choosing a career in psychiatry when prevailing social attitudes were notoriously negative not only towards the mentally ill but also towards mental health professionals. Joining the state government services in Madras (now Tamil Nadu, India) as a junior doctor, Dr Menon witnessed the evolution of modern psychiatry, from non—neuroleptic custodial era to the present age of brain and recovery. Dr Menon was promoted as the Superintendent of the state-run Madras Mental Hospital (now known as the Institute of Mental Health) in 1961 and to say that the era of psychosocial rehabilitation was born with this is no exaggeration. She saw with great foresight, that interactions among social workers, the patient's family, and the patient were the key to the patient's recovery, educating them about illness and treatments. She introduced outpatients' services and occupational therapy after the acute phase of the illness, Dr Menon started the Industrial Therapy Centre which, at the time of its inception, was the first of its kind in the entire country. She was also responsible for starting postgraduate courses in psychological medicine to train medical personnel and other mental health professionals including nurses and social workers. She helped establish psychiatric clinics in all the district general hospitals in Tamil Nadu.

Dr Menon was instrumental in establishing the premier voluntary non-profit organization, the Schizophrenia Research Foundation (SCARF), in Tamil Nadu for working towards a better future for the mentally ill and led it for 23 years. It continues to offer vocational training, social skills training, family consultation services, sheltered workshops, and job placement. Financial support is given for children of patients with schizophrenia to enable them to continue their school education, family education classes to remove the stigma attached to mental illness, and community-based rehabilitation. She also set up a halfway home (residential centre for limited period accommodation) and a home for those with intellectual disability. She held key positions in the Red Cross and was responsible for the work on cyclone shelters during the 1970s. Mobile dispensaries to rural areas were started and programs in disaster preparedness were conducted under her supervision. She was honoured with the Padma Bhushan (third highest civilian award) by the Government of India in 1992. Till her death at the age of 98, she continued to see patients, attend conferences and mentored young psychiatrists. She passed away on 5th December, 2021.

Interview

I: Thanks very much for your time. You came from a very large family. What was that like growing up?

SM: I am the eighth of the family of 11, six sisters and one brother older than me, and two sisters and one brother younger. I was born in Mangalore, Madras Presidency in that period, called Karnataka state now. My father was in the judiciary and liable for frequent transfers. In those days, daughters were not too welcome, sons were preferred (now it's different). When my sisters, who had come home from the school in the afternoon and were told there was a new baby in the house, they asked: 'boy or girl?' My grandmother, with a grunt, said 'girl'. Boys were welcome and were the light of my mother's life. However, I was my father's pet. I was a happy-go-lucky person. I never liked to go to the school. When my sisters were leaving for school, I would pretend to be sick and escape with my father's permission. In the afternoon, I would be hale and hearty again (laughs). When I was about 6 years old my father was transferred to Chinglepet (now called Chengelpattu) about 35 miles from Madras. I had the pleasure of participating in the wedding of two of my sisters, great fun and each a real gala event. Then my father had to arrange all the education of the junior members of the family. My elder brother had to go to a school run by priests in Yercaud. I had to join a convent school in Madras (now Chennai). I stayed with one of my sisters in Madras, and attended the Presentation Convent for five years.

When I was admitted to this school, I had to be tested to ascertain which class I could join. I was deemed fit for the second standard and was immediately sent to the class. After welcoming me, the class continued. Just before the lunch break, the nun in charge said, 'Come on dearie, you must sing a song or recite a poem for us'. I was struck speechless and scared. All the others in the class were much older and more confident than me. I was unable to do anything. After a while the nun said, 'All right. We will give you time. Tomorrow you will sing for us or else I will kill you.'

I went home, did not tell anyone, but decided to solve the problem myself. The next day, I went to the school and settled down in the first standard. When the nun in charge came to me and asked why I was there in that class and not second standard, I replied, 'I can't go into that class because the nun there said she would kill me'. She let me continue in the first standard, having understood the situation. I completed five years at that convent. Since my father had transfers to other places for brief spells, I also studied in other schools for short periods.

I joined the Good Shepherd Convent and was admitted into the fifth standard. There were only five or six students with me. When I passed that I reached the sixth standard, and so it went until we reached the Junior Cambridge class (Eighth Standard equivalent). After clearing the exam, all the other students left because they had finished their education and were supposed to 'settle down' but I wanted to continue. The Convent could not hold a class for one student alone so I had to seek admission elsewhere. Therefore, I went to the Church Park Convent, and requested admission into the Senior Cambridge classes. I completed the course and passed the examinations and as soon as the results were out, I immediately applied for my college studies to the Women's Christian college, selecting physics, chemistry, and natural science as my subjects, which would qualify me for admission for medicine.

I: So you were a true pioneer at that time.

SM: While I was at the Good Shepherd Convent, two lady doctors came to stay with us at home with my parents. They were my mother's friends. They took me to the Maternity Hospital in Chennai where they were working. I started feeling very unhappy seeing the suffering of the women at that hospital. This exposure stayed with me and started the desire to become a doctor. After Senior Cambridge, I spent my days in Jodhpur where my father was working as Minister for Justice to the Maharaja of Jodhpur. I had five or six months before joining college. My father was insistent that I should engage with something useful during this period while waiting. He appointed a mathematics professor to teach me mathematics and an office secretary to teach me typing. I was busy studying but also found time to watch polo. There were two polo grounds near our house where the Maharaja used to play twice a week. My sisters and brothers were with me during that time.

I set out for Madras when it was time for me to join the college. Father and I reported to the college, but unfortunately they had admitted me into the wrong group of studies and nothing I could do helped me to change to the selection I wanted. I therefore decided to join in the group available (chemistry, natural sciences, logic). With the subjects that I had taken for the Intermediate course, I could not enter the medical college. My father, who was not keen on my studying medicine, was happy about this and he secured a place for me doing zoology honours at another college. But I had my mind set on studying medicine. I requested permission to study physics alone, completing a two-year course in one year. She granted me permission to do this. After I passed my physics examination, I was fully qualified to join the medical college. Securing admission into the medical college was not a problem in those days. At that time, women students were given stipends and scholarships so by the time I was admitted it was free. After five-and-a-half years, I qualified for the MBBS.

During the last year of MBBS we visited the mental hospital. In a class taken by the professor of mental diseases, we gathered in a hall, and on the stage saw a number of persons, ill clad, gesturing, posturing, laughing, and totally unaware of themselves and surroundings. No-one could explain the cause of or treatment for the problems these people were clearly encountering. They were locked up, chained sometimes, sedated with painful injections, and given food which they might or might not eat as no-one was checking. I found the scene to be very traumatic. These people needed help. I was moved and motivated to do something, but how?

I had to complete my course and undertake some training before I could do something to help. After my MBBS, my father suggested that I go to Delhi (where he was working) to do my house surgeon job (equivalent to first year training) for one-and-a-half years at Irwin Hospital, now known as Maulana Azad Medical College. After another one-and-a-half years of work in a mission hospital in Andhra Pradesh, I joined the Madras Medical Service and applied for my post-graduate specialisation (MD) in internal medicine. My brother who was in England then, had tried to secure a place for me for training in psychiatry in the United Kingdom but the Dean of Studies in Madras Medical College advised me to do my general medicine postgraduate training first before starting psychiatry training.

I joined the medical service, for the degree of MD in General Medicine, completed my training and received my postgraduate qualification in 1953. I spent a couple of years looking for a training centre in psychiatry. During this time I chanced upon seeing a young girl in a special ward, in a bed with railings. She was very violent, could not be controlled and had to be sedated with a painful injection. She was sent home because we could not help her any further. This incident turned out to be another motivation for me to pursue psychiatry.

I went to London in 1955 and stayed with my brother who was working with Professor Cecil Powell in Bristol. I tried to get a job in Addenbrookes in Cambridge, but settled down at the Maudsley in London. The clinics were held at Cane Hill Hospital which was on the outskirts of London and the teaching at the Maudsley in south London. I liked being at Cane Hill Hospital even though the distance and the uphill climb to it was very tiresome after the long bus ride from central London. Unfortunately my father had a stroke in India and I had to return. I cancelled my leave from the medical service in Madras (now Chennai), and was posted to the Stanley Medical College as an assistant physician in the Department of Medicine. After a year, the government was deputing candidates to the All-India Institute of Mental Health, now known as NIMHANS, in Bangalore (now Bengaluru) for two years, for training in psychiatry. I joined and completed my two years training and returned to Madras (now Chennai) and was posted to the Government Mental Hospital where I worked from 1959 to 1978.

I was appointed as superintendent at that hospital in 1961. Patients outnumbered staff in significant numbers: 2,800 patients, only one or two qualified staff, no qualified nurses—that was the situation in the hospital then. There was no outpatient service. The patients were seen in a small room. When they were brought in, staff would take down their name and address and the patient would be admitted without further questions.

I was first put in charge of the female section. I thought the first thing to do was to start the outpatients services. I vacated a ward and converted it into an outpatients department. Subsequently, I got permission from the government to build an outpatients centre on hospital grounds on the other side of the road from the main building with all the necessary facilities. It is still there and still functioning. Then I had to plan what to do for the patients. I had no experience in administration, I only knew clinical work. Anyway, for me, the first priority was patient comfort, ensuring that they had proper accommodation, food, clothing, care, and medications. So I increased the accommodation provision and improved the staff/patient ratio. I set up a Day Hospital too and because the outpatients and day hospital were functioning well, the pressure on inpatient beds was reduced. The purpose was to treat as many patients as possible as outpatients. There were criteria for admission: nobody was to be admitted who lived within a five-mile radius unless they could not be managed at home because of violent behaviour or suicide attempt occurred. In that way I managed to bring down the inpatient numbers.

There were no social workers and there were no schools of social work then. The Red Cross trained people for nine months in general social work. They were all only educated to the tenth class standard. They received training for six months and given some basic knowledge in social work. I took them and I employed them and I trained them further. I found them very good as they had the mental make-up for this sort of work. In those days the training in English was very good and my trainees' command of the language was good. They took very good patient histories. I found that very useful. Then the Madras School for Social Work started up and I was able to appoint more social workers. Apart from taking a patient's history the social workers were also responsible for keeping in touch with the patient's family. By keeping in touch with the families and supporting them, it was easier to discharge patients from the wards so I could again bring down the number of inpatients.

I had to improve training programmes for medical officers, paramedics, etc. I started the Diploma in Psychological Medicine (DPM) course. All the other staff, like auxiliary nurses and midwives, needed training. I used to teach nurses in particular, running classes for them, and all other categories of employees. From improving the staff numbers and qualifications starting the DPM and training, it was a Herculean effort to get things going.

I: At that time did you have to fight a lot for resources?

SM: No, I don't think so. I used to send proposals to the government for any improvements in the hospital and then follow this up by personally going to the government officer concerned, explaining the need, using the required influence, and securing what I wanted. In this way I was able to hold on to a large piece of land for the hospital which would otherwise be handed over to other organisations. I had to assert myself, and all my requests were met. I used to trudge up and down the government Secretariat, seeing the Ministers and the secretaries of health and that's how I got what I wanted.

I: In those times, did it matter that you were a woman?

SM: No, I never had any problems.

I: Looking back, you had a magnificent career and you have done wonderful pioneering things. What prompted you to set up SCARF?

SM: The government mental hospital had an excellent occupational therapy section with all essential types of work being encouraged. The results were very helpful for the hospital. Spinning, weaving, tailoring, mattress making, mat making, book binding, carpentry, gardening—the patients were regular in their attendance and they worked very well too. However, there was hardly any communication or incentives for the patients and community. I took the best of the patients into a separate unit, which I called the Industrial Therapy Unit. There I arranged a different environment, with a focus on punctuality, self-identification, socialization, training, the offer of incentives, etc. We started manufacturing many marketable goods, and the money thus made was invested in the unit itself to improve services further. The most recent addition was the bakery. We supplied fresh bread to two government hospitals and to achieve this, I had to go to the relevant person in the government department and ask him to accept my tender though a little more expensive than other tenders, because the bread was being made by the disabled mentally ill.

Throughout all this time, I watched improvements being made in patients' symptoms, communication, socialization, interest in recreational activities, participating in games and indoor/outdoor activities, playing and listening to music, watching movies, and remunerative work. I took the bold step of finding out whether patients were capable of living independently. To facilitate this, I refurbished a small building, which was earlier used by a staff member, and housed four patients, giving them instructions on how to manage their lives. They would stay there and maintain the building and premises, food would be supplied, and they would go to work in the Industrial Therapy Centre daily. After a week, we found all four of them back in the ward! That was my Waterloo moment. By that time, I knew what needed to be done for the patients to help them stay independent, but I was to retire from the service soon.

After retirement, I was asked to serve in the Red Cross and I did so for five years. At the same time, I worked under the university teacher's retirement scheme, where I taught postgraduate students of psychiatry and started a new psychiatric OPD in the Port Trust. At the same time I carried out a small research project looking at personality profile of parents of schizophrenia patients using the Cattell's 16 Personality Factors Questionnaire.

At the time, I used to visit the psychiatric department in the General Hospital regularly. With the experience gained from the Government Mental Hospital (subsequently Institute for Mental Health IMH), and constant pleadings from parents and guardians of people with schizophrenia whose health had improved and who had become manageable but totally inactive at their young age, I thought we should give some thought and effort to the last leg of treatment. The psychiatric

OPD in General Hospital at that time, was run by Dr Rajkumar, a young, dynamic, and well-qualified psychiatrist, and Dr Thara, a promising young research assistant, engaged in a study in schizophrenia by the Indian Council for Medical Research (ICMR). We combined forces to try to do something in the OPD itself, but later decided to form an organization to achieve our goals. The preliminaries of forming an organization were completed and we had to choose a name. Since my interest was care and rehabilitation, I suggested the 'Schizophrenia Care and Rehabilitation Foundation'. The name had to incorporate research as well, so we decided on the Schizophrenia Care and Research Foundation. Over the years, the word 'Care' was dropped and it became the 'Schizophrenia Research Foundation'. Subsequently, there were several suggestions that the foundation should be named the Mental Health Foundation. But I was keen that the term 'Schizophrenia' was retained in the title, and so it has survived until today! The objectives were and are care and rehabilitation, public education, and research.

We faced initial obstacles of working in a small single-room office and then a two bedroom apartment. We are now in the present building, which is our own, thanks to the foresight and benevolence of the government of Tamil Nadu. Dr Rajkumar left for Australia, I left owing to health reasons but remain connected closely with the work. Dr Thara was an excellent fundraiser and researcher and really built up the foundation. I feel the rehabilitation component of the foundation needs to be further strengthened, studied, and expanded.

Psychiatrists and allied professionals in India at least are often not very interested in or aware of the concepts of rehabilitation and recovery models in psychiatry. After the long struggle with the treatment of a patient and achieving manageability, staff get tired and feel that their work is done. Caregivers also become quickly worn out with the thankless job they perform. Social workers and other para-professionals become dissatisfied with lack of patient improvement and wonder when the end of their involvement will come. The treatment, commitment, and interest in the patient often stop too early. The object of treatment is to remove symptoms, restore patient to his or her original state of functioning, and accepting what the patient sees as their role in life. Disability that continues after mental illness and the secondary symptoms of schizophrenia have not received much attention over the years. I was thinking of this when I started SCARF. Rehabilitation is not an easy task. It requires the support and help of the family, other non-governmental organizations (NGOs) involved in similar work, people to liaise with government and society. This means a lot of integrated interdisciplinary coordination and work. I am looking forward to a time when SCARF will be known for its excellence in research into biopsychosocial causes of this disability and planning effective interventions to correct them, and restoring the patient to his original state of functioning and role in society.

I: Looking back, 70+ years of your life have been committed to psychiatry. What do you think of the state of psychiatry now? What are the positives and negatives about it today? What have we done right, what have we done wrong?

SM: Psychiatrists are working well, but after postgraduate training, many of them settle down to 'business as usual'. They lose interest in the quality of their service and have little desire to extend their services and keep up-to-date with the growing demands of the field. They do not try to improve their knowledge and they stop working on innovative ideas. There are so many areas within the field, like women's mental health, addiction, liaison psychiatry, forensic psychiatry, disability, and many others which need more input. But the more we learn and the greater the advances in treatment find us losing sight of the most important aspect of care, namely personalized care for the patient.

I would not say psychiatry has gone wrong but it has changed; society has changed, lifestyles have changed, environmental demands need adjustment, technological advancements require internalizing, and with all this comes changes. The understanding of mental illness is changing. Treatment and management have to follow this understanding. Thus, in order to provide focused and targeted care, then the psychiatrist has to alter her approaches to look at things in a different way. They will have to change attitudes, methods of assessments and approaches, which will make a psychiatrist a different person. Today's psychiatrist considers their practice a business rather than a service. With their expertise in touchscreen gadgets, which they feel will advance their career, present-day psychiatrists have become more and more dependent on them.

Today's psychiatrists seem to be losing their original skills, personal characteristics of compassion, empathy, sympathy, consideration, and kindness. They do not consider physical health and its innumerable requisites and that is very often overlooked. Psychiatrists do not mingle with other medical professionals and do not sell psychiatry to them. They stigmatize themselves. I would like to see the day when the Professor of Psychiatry joins ward rounds with the Professor of Medicine and offers input as relevant. They need to join the hospital case discussion groups, present cases or papers and improve the consultation liaison psychiatry concept and practice.

Another lacuna, as I have mentioned before, is the lack of awareness of and less inclination to provide the critical inputs in rehabilitation and recovery for patients with schizophrenia who may or may not have achieved some symptom control.

I: What was your two months at the Maudsley like?

SM: Cane Hill Hospital was so far away. I was just breathless climbing up that hill to the hospital daily! The classes were held in the afternoon in the Maudsley, the teaching was good, and the clinics were at Cane Hill Hospital. It was nice but I hardly had the time to appreciate, work on it and enjoy the whole thing because I had to return to India owing to my father's ill health.

I: I feel that we have stopped holding on to the patient's hope and we don't contain their or the team's anxiety either. We tend to get even more anxious rather than saying things will be fine. How do we train the next generation of psychiatrists?

SM: First of all, undergraduate education requires a total overhaul. I think I have written in detail about that.

I: I agree with you. I think we have to start with undergraduate education and if I had the power to change the curriculum, I would start by teaching psychiatry from day 1 in an integrated way rather than just offering two weeks in the fourth year. I mean all you see as an undergraduate is chronic patients.

SM: I am reminded of my discussion with the late Professor JS Neki, in Chandigarh Post-graduate Institute of Medical Education and Research (PGI). We thought that the student ought to be exposed to some subject or aspect that relates to psychiatry during every year of medical school so that it should not feel totally unconnected to their regular studies. For example, studying the limbic system and autonomic nervous system could be linked to mood disorders and anxiety disorders, the psychopathology and psychopharmacology of these being discussed at the earliest opportunity. Clinical psychiatry should start in the third year with a short outpatients posting, a longer clinical posting in the fourth year, and at least one full month of internship in psychiatry. Psychiatry should be included in the final clinical exam, to be assessed by a professor of psychiatry. Every student who qualifies for the MBBS must be able to treat simple cases in psychiatry. Instead, what we have is psychiatry being introduced as a new thing, like an alien coming into the student's life somewhere in their medical training.

I: Once upon a time, patients were called aliens and we were called alienists.

SM: Yes, it looked like that. Even when I was working with the outpatients, I was in charge of the outpatients in the general hospital when I joined. I worked for two hours, 10 a.m. to noon three days a week. I couldn't even see one patient properly in that time. So I changed to work 9 a.m. to 5 p.m. for six days a week. In those days, inpatient beds were scattered in the general wards of medicine, so they would have three beds here, three beds there. I would admit a patient there, and one day he gives some trouble, and the physician in-charge asks the nurse to inform me and to transfer the patient to the mental hospital. I couldn't quarrel with him so I suggested that they are brought to my outpatients clinic at 9 a.m. They will be in my OP while I'm seeing other patients. Once the physicians leave after their rounds, the patients can be sent back so it won't disturb the physicians!' So I continued like that.

I: So that must have meant you had to work incredibly hard.

SM: Yes, we had to work hard, overcome these barriers, find a way.

I: What drives you? Why did you work so incredibly hard? You worked on research and policy proposals and getting accommodation sorted and outpatients. What was the motivation?

SM: I really don't know. When I was interested in something and I wanted to do it, I would go all out to do it. I always thought it was no use blaming the other person if something didn't work. I have always had to take the initiative to get things done. The effort was to get these mentally ill people back to a functional status. So every opportunity I got, I used, and I used all my efforts to get to that goal without hurting anybody. That is very important. I'm not a leader, I'm a worker.

I: I think you are a leader in the sense that you have the passion and the courage and the vision to deliver. That's what good leaders do. As a worker you can see the other side and that makes it easier to incorporate that into your vision. You studied for your MD in general medicine. How do you think it helped you? Should we be encouraging young psychiatrists to do medicine before they come into psychiatry?

SM: I feel that exposure to general medicine before attempting psychiatry is very helpful. It helps in the overall approach to a psychiatric case if you have a background in medicine to support your understanding of the case. This is also why, while drawing up the training programme for DPM in the Institute of Mental Health, I included three months' rotation in internal medicine and neurology in two years. The same thinking made me designate one of the psychiatric consultants in our staff as the physician, but this was objected to by others in the hospital who stated that every doctor in the hospital was a physician.

I: There was a time when you couldn't get into the Maudsley training programme unless you had your MRCP and somewhere along the line, early to mid-1980s they stopped that. I think this has created a problem because partly because if you have that background, you are much more confident as a psychiatrist.

SM: Yes, correct.

I: You know that asking the right questions but also linking physical and mental health in a much better and cohesive way works.

SM: Yes, I feel that way. The suggestion is good, it would help very much if you had some training in internal medicine and neurology.

I: Looking back, what are you most proud of?

SM: (laughs) I had a goal of working towards improving the status of the mentally ill and I didn't change that goal, I kept working towards it. During these years of work, I did not focus on any other objectives or posts. I didn't want to be the head of an organization. At some stage I got a telegram saying that my name had been put forward for the presidency of the Indian Psychiatric Society. I turned it down.

I'm very happy because rehabilitation is now recognized as possible. If psychiatry is the Cinderella of medicine then rehabilitation is the Cinderella of psychiatry. I got the Rehabilitation Section recognized under the Indian Psychiatric Society. The other satisfying work that I can recall has been the recognition of the importance of women's mental health. The third relates to the opportunity to discharge and reintegrate inter-state patients who have recovered and returned to their homes or domicile states with effective networking with NGOs across India—through the pioneering work of Mr Mohammed Rafi, with his NGO ANBAGAM in Chennai, and Shraddha in Pune being notable examples.

I: Over the years, do you think stigma against psychiatry, psychiatrists, and psychiatry patients, has changed?

SM: Rather than stigma, the word 'discrimination', as suggested by you, I think, is more appropriate to describe the attitudes and behaviour towards the mentally ill. Stigma is much less now than when I entered the profession in 1959. A greater number of patients are willing to be seen by psychiatrists. More families are accepting treatment by the psychiatrist and patients are being taken to shops and restaurants, so there is more acceptance. People with disabilities are recognised and accepted in schools, offices, and by the general public, and I am sure this will improve further. The stigma against mental illnesses will be eradicated in the future. But irrespective of caste, creed, or socio-economic status, there are still some people who are reluctant to visit a psychiatrist. They won't acknowledge or accept the mentally ill or mental illness, and are not keen on marrying into a family with a history of a relative with mental illness. It is difficult to remove or correct these attitudes.

When I first started, after I treated a patient and they were getting married, his or her father would come to me and say gently, 'I'm giving you the invitation to this wedding but please don't come.' If I went to any meeting or any conference or a party or something, I will hear somebody asking, 'How do you know her?' Those days I was ignored if this happened, knowing me must have meant that the connection was someone with a mental illness. It is not like that now. I will be acknowledged as someone's doctor. But still, and sometimes in the higher echelons of society, mental illness still carries a stigma.

I: If you were starting again what would you change? For example, before I went into psychiatry I was advised to do medicine and emergency medicine, not psychiatry. In hindsight I wasted two or three years doing this whereas I should have just done what I wanted and gone straight into psychiatry.

SM: That was what happened to me as well. My parents never wanted me to become a doctor and my professors didn't want me to go to psychiatry. Against all that advice, I went to the Maudsley because this was in my mind: medicine first, then psychiatry. I wouldn't tell my younger self to do things differently!

I: What would you like to be remembered for?

SM: (laughs). That I can quote Robert Frost.

I: SCARF is your legacy and through SCARF, making rehabilitation important and recognizable, but now rehabilitation has been transformed into recovery which is inevitable because these things change and evolve and fashions come and fashions go. So in 100 years' time, if somebody looked you up in Wikipedia, what would you like them to find?.

SM: The principles of rehabilitation and the individual's journey in their recovery process from the clutches of mental illness, I think, will remain, irrespective of whatever advances may come in neuroscience and therapeutics. The efforts that we all had put in at this time could be considered as the foundation on which much needs to be built and will be built for years to come. I can't hope for everyone to recover, everyone to be 100% normal but the acceptance of disability by society, I hope, will be universal. It will be so nice to see that.

I: Thank you so much for sharing your life story. It is truly inspirational.

13
Driss Moussaoui

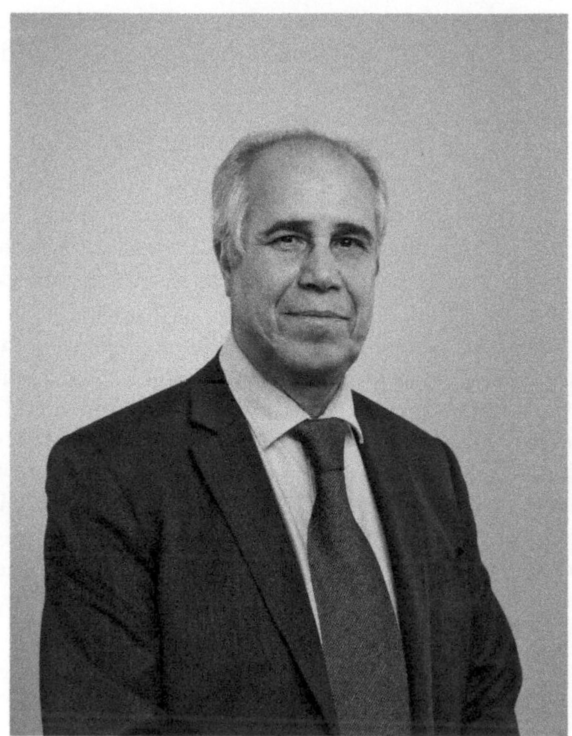

Biography

Driss Moussaoui is Professor Emeritus, Faculty of Medicine, Casablanca, Morocco. He was the founder and chairman of the Ibn Rushd University Psychiatric Centre in Casablanca from 1979 to 2013. He was also director of the Casablanca World Health Organization (WHO) Collaborating Centre in Mental Health from 1992 to 2013.

He was President of the Moroccan Society of Psychiatry and of the Arab Federation of Psychiatrists. He has edited or co-edited 10 books and published more than 150 papers in international journals.

With the World Psychiatric Association (WPA) Executive Committee he helped establish the Jean Delay Prize (1999) and is the scientific director of the WPA series

'International Anthologies of Classic Psychiatric Texts' (French, German, Spanish, Italian, Greek, and Russian, in preparation).

Driss Moussaoui is past-President of the World Association of Social Psychiatry (WASP, 2010–2013) and member of the French Academy of Medicine. He is WPA and WASP Honorary Member, and currently President of the International Federation for Psychotherapy (2018–2022).

Interview

I: Could you tell us about your childhood and growing up?

DM: I was born in 1949 in Marrakesh. At that time, it was a small town of about 100,000 people. I spent my first 17 years there until I joined the Faculty of Medicine of Rabat, which was the only one in Morocco in the capital of the country. I spent seven years there in my undergraduate studies and became resident (first grade) before going to Paris for my postgraduate training in Psychiatry at Sainte Anne Hospital. I lost my father when I was four years old; my mother and her four children had very little money to live on. Despite this, she was one of life's battlers and managed to have two children who became professors of medicine and two who became ambassadors in the diplomatic corps. So one of the sources of energy and knowledge of life came from the teachings of my mother.

I: What attracted you to medicine?

DM: It was by chance, as I had a '*baccalaureate*' in literature and not in science. When my brother asked me what kind of studies I would like to pursue, I told him it was economics. He said, 'Why don't you go for longer studies, such as medicine?' And I said that I wouldn't be accepted because of the kind of '*baccalaureate*' I had achieved. He said he would take care of that because he knew somebody who allowed me to enter the Faculty of Medicine of Rabat. This Faculty opened in 1962 and I became a student there at the age of 17 in 1966. I was one of the first medical students in Morocco trained in the country, not abroad.

I: Why did you choose psychiatry?

DM: I thought it was a rational choice, because entering a medical specialty where no other Moroccan was trained (the head of department was a neurologist and assistant professor) meant that I could thrive. But a cousin of mine came to see me when I returned to Casablanca in 1979 and said, 'Do you remember when we were children, we used to play, and one day you said, "Let's play psychology; I will try to guess your thoughts"?' I was 11 at that time, so that desire to think about other people remained in me and influenced my decision to go into psychiatry. Now, if I had to choose again, I would make exactly the same choice and cherish the same profession. I think it is the most extraordinary profession one can have in a lifetime.

I: No you have any regrets? In choosing psychiatry

DM: Not at all. I have loved what I do, I still love it, and if I had to marry a profession, it would be this one.

I: Who were your role models, heroes, or heroines?

DM: I was very lucky to be accepted in Sainte-Anne Hospital, which was the Mecca of psychiatry in France and one of the main centres in Europe. In 1973, I got accepted by the Department of Psychiatry of Professor Pierre Pichot, who was one of the students of Jean Delay, the Founder of the World Psychiatric Association. Pierre Pichot was the secretary of the First World Congress of Psychiatry in 1950 and he was a remarkable man, very cultivated. He was also a psychologist, and he introduced quantitative psychopathology into France. He was also the very first to introduce behavioural therapy in France. I had a great relationship with him. He was a really hospitable man; he helped me a lot throughout my career and I owe a lot to him.

The second man who made a difference in my professional life is Norman Sartorius (see Chapter 19). I met him for the first time in 1982 and I learnt classic psychiatry with Professor Pichot and mental health in the context of society with Norman Sartorius which was also very important. However, my medical thesis in 1973 in the Faculty of Medicine of Rabat was on the relationship between psychiatry and the cultural way of raising children in Moroccan families. We already had social psychiatry before we knew anything about social psychiatry.

I: Do you have any particular impressions about any patients that you have seen?

DM: I could write books on my relationships with patients. They were true teachers to me. I learned so much from them and I continue to do so today. When you learn something from a patient, make sure you thank them. I treated or contributed to the treatment of about 20,000 patients and they all taught me a lot. The same goes for students. I taught about 12,000 students in Morocco, both undergraduates and postgraduates, and I learned a lot from their questions.

I: What do you think psychiatry needs today?

DM: It is very clear that research needs money, but all those who say that you cannot do research because of a lack of money are wrong. You can do great research with paper and pens or pencils. The most important thing is to have a good idea. The most important thing is to motivate people around you, to make them join your research study. And if you have a great idea, you will find money for that. We worked, for example, on abnormal involuntary movements in people with schizophrenia, in people with schizophrenia who had never been medicated, and with people we knew in Portland, Oregon. The National Institute of Mental Health (Bethesda, MD) gave us a grant of almost half a million US dollars. In 1979, when I created the Department of Psychiatry in Casablanca, I was the only psychiatrist in the public and academic sectors catering to four cities and 5 million inhabitants and I had only one resident with me. When I told my team members that we needed to undertake research because research is very important, they looked at me as if I was crazy. They thought: 'How come you can say this when you don't even have chlorpromazine for your patients. How dare you say that you're going to do research?' But we did. Among the very first research studies conducted in the Casablanca Department of Psychiatry we did WHO collaborative studies on biological psychiatry and psychopharmacology (the dexamethasone suppression test in depression, haloperidol doses in schizophrenia, eye movements in people with schizophrenia). The first contact with WHO was made through Pierre Pichot in 1980, and the head of the Division of Mental Health at that time was Norman Sartorius. Even though for years it had been very hard from the institutional point of view to carry out research but we did so. We presented research studies in international congresses and published in journals. Each of these international interactions was like oxygen for us when we felt we were suffocating under mountains of all kinds of difficulties. Relationship with the outside world, and I'm saying this to mental health workers from low- and middle-income countries, is essential and the network we build outside our own country is as important as the one we build inside the country. It was indeed oxygen for me to go to WHO meetings, to WPA meetings, to go to congresses, to meet people, to tell them what we were doing, and to listen to what they were doing. Don't sit and weep in misery over your lack of funding and human resources; find a way to open your work to society and the outside world. It is also extremely important to open up to civil society, to non-governmental organizations (NGOs), to the media, and to talk about difficulties and problems that you are encountering. Of course, the Minister of Health in your country will not be happy, the administration will not be happy, but it doesn't matter, just do it.

I: Through your fruitful years of experience, how has psychiatry changed in your time?

DM: At the end of 1970 and the beginning of 1971 I was the resident who had the best grade in the exam and when I chose psychiatry, people said I was crazy. They said, 'You could choose cardiology, you could choose surgery', but my choice was psychiatry. At that time, treatment with insulin coma was widely used in Rabat. We had 10 to 15 patients in one room, injected with insulin. Next room, we had 15 to 20 patients every day receiving electroshock without anaesthesia, one near the other and watching what happened to the neighbouring patients. The situation was really very, very, very, bad. In 1979, there were 18 million Moroccans and we had fewer than 10 psychiatrists for the whole country. The situation was really disastrous. In Casablanca, I had 50 beds and I received least 50 patients in acute psychotic state needing hospitalization every day. When medical students (some were older than me; I was 29 in 1979) saw such a violent environment with aggressive patients and degrading treatment, it is no wonder they didn't want to join psychiatry. It took me years to improve the environment in order to make the students feel safe enough to choose psychiatry.

I'll give you two examples; the first one was in 1979 when I arrived, we didn't have a single window with glass. During winter time, people entered with acute psychotic episodes and died because of pneumonia. So I asked the administration to put in glass in the windows, but they said no, 'because they might be broken by your patients. We are going to put just wooden frames.' I refused the offer because we needed light in the corridors otherwise the place would seem worse than a prison. They ended up putting in window glass, 22 glass windows on the first day. The following day at 8 a.m., all the administration staff were waiting at the entrance of the ward because during the night, one patient broke 13 windows. They said, 'You see, this is terrible. We're going to put in wood and we told you we would.' I replied, 'Before 12 noon today all the glass will be replaced. Please continue your work.' I didn't know how to do it but I managed to find a parent of one of the patients who was less poor than the others and who accepted to buy the glass. And the work was all done before 12 noon. This is how we continued to improve the department.

ANOTHER STORY: we had very young secretary in 1979. She was 18 years old and not very tall, and we had patients who were often physically dominant, sometimes very violent. She managed to calm down frightened patients who were on the ward after having taken street drugs and being under the influence. The fact that she could calm them was an important lesson. This example was helpful to all of us. But still, I had to persuade every single person to stay on, despite this very difficult atmosphere. It was a day-to-day work in order to improve. Once when I entered the locked ward for males at 2 a.m. and I heard silence with everybody sleeping, I realised that it had taken two years to start to win the battle and maybe the war. This took a permanent effort. At the beginning of this adventure, I could only go to the National Pharmacy every second week to obtain one or two boxes of chlorpromazine or some needles to inject levomepromazine to patients, not to speak about all out-of-stock other medications, especially long acting neuroleptics. Stock of medicines was perpetually low.

Keeping things running was a daily battle, and I could have easily left, saying that doing so was completely impossible. Somebody said: 'We didn't know it was impossible to do, so we did it.' That rings true for me. I started as the chairman of that department at the age of 29 and I was probably foolish enough not to consider that running things smoothly was almost impossible to do. But fortunately, with the team, we made it. In 1979, 1980, and 1981, I saw up to 73 patients in one afternoon's consultation session. And if I didn't see them (most of them were either bipolar or people with schizophrenia), if they stopped medications, you could expect to see them agitated, violent, with a relapse two or three weeks later and coming back with families seeking rehospitalization. After these sessions I would return home and not have the strength to eat. I slept like a stone until early morning the following day, rising to start the battle again. You were asking about evolution of psychiatry in Casablanca and Morocco; when I retired in 2013, we had eight professors of psychiatry and 51 residents and 104 beds, of which 100 beds were built from scratch, funded by donors and benefactors of the association I created in 1979. In 1992, we obtained the title of WHO Collaborating Centre in Mental Health and Neurosciences. This was an enormous achievement, made possible by dealing with problems in a smart way and by collaborating with good people, inside as well as outside the institution.

I: What are your views on the current state of psychiatry?

DM: In Morocco, we have done 5% of what we should do. I spent 35 years fighting for psychiatry and mental health. When you see that the treatment gap for people with schizophrenia in the United States, the most powerful country in the world, is 50%; when you see that the largest psychiatric hospital in the United States is the County Jail of Los Angeles (4,000 people); when you see that about only 1% of the budget of WHO is given to its mental health division; you know that psychiatry is not doing terribly well throughout the world. There is civil war between various trends in psychiatry and mental health; you have biological psychiatrists, social psychiatrists, psychotherapists, and clinical psychiatrists, each using a different language and attacking those in other camps, for ideology and resources not to mention the tensions with other mental health professionals. This is very destructive. We need to build bridges between various components of mental health work. I am fighting for this all the way; this is one of my fights on the international scene.

What I see is that we do not involve enough patients and families. We do not do enough epidemiological studies in prisons and jails. We do not work enough in transgenerational psychiatry; when there is one mentally ill person it acts negatively on the health of all family members, and sometimes the whole neighbourhood is affected. When you have a person with paranoid schizophrenia spending all day walking the streets armed with a knife, everybody feels unsafe and nervous. When this person shouts throughout the night, nobody can sleep. When the house is destroyed by violence because of substance abuse or delusions, the distress of the family is immense. This is to say that when we think we treat a patient but we do not address the suffering of those around the patient, the children, the family, and the neighbourhood. We need to work hand-in-hand with social workers. We need to have a psychotherapist for children, seeing those who are in difficult situations. We need to have more mental healthcare in schools. There are taboos and stigma yet to be overcome. What do we do with that? How can we prevent it?

What is called burnout, probably a mix of depression and anxiety, among doctors, among residents, even in psychiatry, is a huge problem. Do we help the people who are supposed to help the patients? No. Do we deal enough with mental illnesses in India, China, Indonesia? No. You have, for example, one of the most beautiful spots in the world, Bali. It's heaven on earth. There, hundreds of patients in villages with psychosis are chained up with no treatment. It's full of tourists, it's full of money, and yet these problems remain. So there is a plan to improve psychiatry and mental health but it remains on paper, not fully implemented. The WHO is very good at planning.

I: From your point of view, is psychiatry brainless or mindless?

DM: Unfortunately, it's both. And we do need to put brain in mind and mind in brain. I have seen this civil war going on and on for decades between people working in biological aspects of mental ill health with others working on psychosocial aspects. But even in psychotherapy you have a kind of intolerance towards different techniques and theories, and people often use one tool rather than from a number of options available to help people in need of mental health support. Human beings are complex creatures; mentally ill patients are even more complex and it would be stupid to think that only one therapeutic approach fits all patients. According to the biopsychosocial model, the more integrated the therapeutic approach, the better. Also, this means that psychiatrists have to be as modest as possible. Psychiatry is probably the most complex profession and we deal with complex problems everyday.

You had earlier asked me who are the people who influenced me in my professional life. I mentioned Professor Pichot, who was my teacher. I mentioned Norman Sartorius. I need to mention two other people. One is Professor Alfred Freedman, who was the founder of the *Comprehensive Textbook of Psychiatry*. He was the President of the American Psychiatric Association and in 1973 he was the one who ousted homosexuality from DSM II. A few months before his death, the *New York Times* wrote an article about him, saying that this decision to remove the category of homosexuality from the list of mental disorders was one of the ten most important decisions taken in the twentieth century. He was a very dear friend, a real humanist, and a role model for me.

The other person I would like to mention is Professor Leon Eisenberg from Harvard. He was an extraordinary man who did many important things in his life. He was one of the strongest advocates for the biopsychosocial model. He also created an association called Physicians for Human Rights, and this association received the Nobel Peace Prize in 1997. His wife, Carola Eisenberg, who was also a psychiatrist, delivered the speech in Oslo before receiving this prize. Leon Eisenberg held a Chair of social medicine at Harvard because he thought that social components and the social aspects of psychiatry were important for medicine as a whole. He also trained in Child Psychiatry and child development (also see Chapter 14, interview with Carol Nadelson) and was one of the founders of social psychiatry in the world. He was very involved in the discussion about mindless and brainless psychiatry. He published on the topic in various journals.

I: What do you see as problems with psychiatry?

DM: Autism. Psychiatry is autistic. Psychiatrists believe in their techniques, in their theories, and have difficulty looking outside their own specialist area. The world is bigger than just psychiatry. What happened in 1952 with the discovery of chlorpromazine by Delay and (Pierre) Deniker led to the destruction of the walls of the asylums and to the reintegration of patients into the community. But on the contrary, at the present time psychiatrists are imprisoning themselves in psychiatry and not looking at the society. This is one of the reasons why there is stigma and discrimination against patients, against psychiatric medications, psychiatric institutions, against families and patients, and against psychiatrists themselves. Psychiatrists do not talk up enough about their specialty, they do not explain enough about what they do. They are not positive enough about the subject and the profession. They consider that they work in a complex field and that they cannot share it, which is wrong, because even the most complex fields can be simplified and explained. And once public understand, they are less frightened. The walls of asylums may have been destroyed but there is today a kind of psychological wall around psychiatry and psychiatrists, separating them from the rest of the community. It is the responsibility of psychiatrists to break down those walls.

I: How would you improve recruitment in psychiatry?

DM: There is only one solution: to take care in the best possible way of undergraduates. When I was Chair of the Department in Casablanca I told my collaborators that there is nothing more important than a medical student who is with us for two months. They should be taken care of. And they should be helped to overcome the fear many people have of mentally ill patients. They should also understand that studying psychiatry is important for their own personal development. If they understand that, then there will be plenty of students who will become postgraduates in psychiatry. These two months of rotation are crucial for the future of psychiatry worldwide. If we don't bother to take care of our students and treat them with respect, forget about it, nothing will happen.

I: What do you see as characteristics of a good psychiatrist?

DM: A good psychiatrist must be happy, first. You cannot help others if you in trouble, in difficulty yourself. We all have difficult moments that we need to overcome in order to be able to help others overcome their difficulties. The second thing is to ask oneself if you really care about your patients. If you don't like them, please leave, you can't help them. It's a matter of love and your patients feel it; if you like them, if you are really fighting in the best possible way to help them out of the dark place they find themselves in, they will know it. There is knowledge of the subject and there is a moral obligation and authority as a psychiatrist. Knowledge can be acquired through a number of sources including the internet but gaining experience by looking after patients is crucial. A good psychiatrist is one who always learns from others; from colleagues, from congresses, from patients, from families, and from people who work in the wards. You know how I diagnosed my first case of rabies? It was from a man who cleaned the floor who told me: that the patient had been bitten by a dog. I asked for a glass of water and started to drink and the patient became very agitated because of hydrophobia.

It was the uneducated man who cleaned the floors who taught me to spot rabies. It is very important to retain one's humility, and to know that we must keep learning all our lives, from all kinds of people and situations. Our certainties are false until otherwise demonstrated. We need to be aware that what we think is the truth might be proved wrong weeks or months later, as happens in all medical fields and in life as well.

I: What do you see as gaps in psychiatric practices or in the practice of psychiatry?

DM: What do we need to improve? Education, If I remember well, Nietzsche said: When we solve all problems, there will remain one unsolved problem: education. We can always improve on the education we receive. I used to say that mental health is too important to leave it in the hands of mental health professionals. It belongs to everybody; everybody should be involved.

I: Mentioning education, what do you see as gaps in training in psychiatry?

DM: Seeing patients in prisons, working with non-governmental organizations (NGOs), taking care of street children, taking care of women abandoned and abused physically, and so on; working with civil society is very important. Learning about what happens in the private sector is also important and learning how to convey what it is that you are doing. You can have very smart ideas but if you do not express yourself in a clear and understandable way, it is pointless. It is important to be a good communicator with the patients, with the families, with poor people, with illiterate people, with politicians, and with colleagues in other specialties. Of course, there are some people who are talented at communication by nature, but there are communications techniques that can be taught and learnt. Because we work in an intimidating field, we need more than any other specialty to convey the right messages in the right way.

I: How to do you think the social contract psychiatry has with society can be delivered?

DM: This is an important question. The social contract must be written and agreed upon locally. We see large differences from one country to another, from one region to another. I saw a policeman in uniform inside the department of psychiatry, in a rich Western country. I would never have accepted the presence of a policeman outside my department in Casablanca. In other cities in Morocco, police can sometimes be found inside the departments, but not mine. It is important to be a good lobbyist for the psychiatric cause. When people say wrong or stupid things about psychiatry or psychotropic medications, we should not accept it. When people say seclusion, even for a few hours, is unethical, this is not right. Laing you may have heard of was seen as an anti-psychiatry psychiatrist in the UK had said," If I throw my family's money out of the window, lock me up". Psychiatrists are often put on the defensive. Some people say that psychiatrists are bad, almost criminals, when they use psychotropic medications or force towards patients. If a patient with religious delusions believes that he is a prophet and asserts that whether you believe him or he will start killing people, how are you going to convince him that he is wrong other than treating him with antipsychotic medications against his will? If we do not do act in this way, the people who will pay a very high price are first the patient and then their families and carers. The same people who attack psychiatry and psychiatrists claiming they are not humane will sue us if there is a homicide or a suicide. There is huge ambivalence in this social contract that is highly harmful to psychiatrists, psychiatry, patients, families, and society at large.

I: What would you tell your younger self?

DM: Be happy, you will make it.

I: And what is your advice to trainees of today?

DM: To take care of your family, very important. To be happy. To enjoy working, and never stop working. When you stop working, you die.

I: What would you like to be remembered for?

DM: For helping a few patients.

I: Finally, which of your achievements are the ones you are the proudest?

DM: I have received three medals in my life of which I am very proud. One is the gold medal of blood donor. I have given my blood for about 35 years. I am O negative group. I was very happy to receive that medal. The second 'medal' is a pen given to me by the Moroccan Association of Users in Psychiatry when I left in 2013 and I am very proud of it. The third one is a watch that was given to me by the staff of my department when I left in 2013. So, when your staff say, we love you and when your patients say we love you and I have helped save a few people with my blood, then what else. I won't speak about my family; this is another story.

I: Thank you so much for your time and sharing your life story and experiences.

14
Carol C. Nadelson

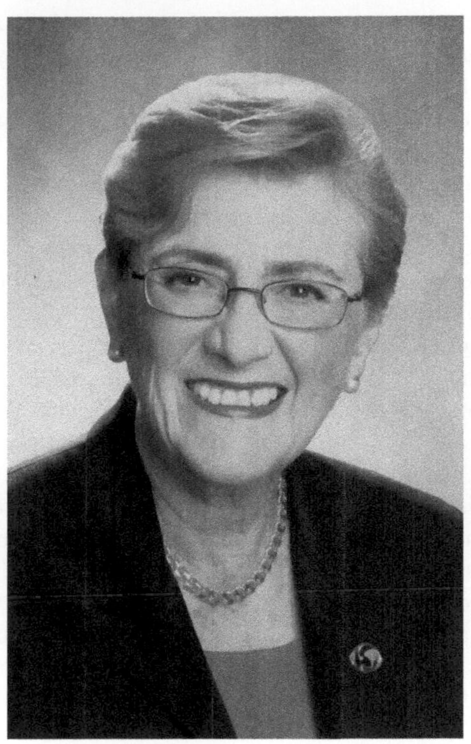

Biography

Professor Carol C. Nadelson is a national and international leader in psychiatry. She is the Founding Director of the Partners and Brigham/Women's Hospital Office for Women's Careers (OWC) and Professor of Psychiatry at Harvard Medical School. She has also been Professor of Psychiatry and Vice Chair of the Psychiatry Department at Tufts University School of Medicine. She has been a powerful influence on policy related to women in medicine since her academic career began at the Massachusetts Mental Health Center and Boston's Beth Israel Hospital. She is a Phi Beta Kappa graduate of Brooklyn College and in 1961 earned her MD from the University of Rochester School of Medicine, where she was elected to Alpha Omega Alpha, the national medical honorary society.

Dr Nadelson was the first woman President of the Massachusetts Psychiatric Society and the American Psychiatric Association. She has been President of the Association for Academic Psychiatry, the Group for the Advancement of Psychiatry, the American College of Psychoanalysts, and she was as Editor-in-Chief and CEO of American Psychiatric Press, Inc. She has served on several boards, including the Menninger Foundation, the Society for Women's Health Research, and the American College of Psychiatrists. She currently serves on the Boards of American Psychiatric Association and the Foundation for the History of Women in Medicine.

Dr Nadelson pioneered the development of programs to advance women's careers, working to facilitate leadership development and mentoring to advance the promotions of women faculty and to ensure benefits for women MDs and PhDs, making OWC a national and international leader in medical education. She is recognized widely as an authority on women's mental health and she was a founder of the first day care centre for women professionals in Brookline, MA, and a rape crisis centre at Beth Israel Hospital in Boston, MA.

As a leader in many medical and scientific organizations, Dr Nadelson has been honoured with numerous awards, including the Alma Dea Morani Renaissance Woman Award from the Foundation for the History of Women in Medicine; Changing the Face of Medicine from the National Institutes of Health; and the Elizabeth Blackwell Award for leadership in the advancement of women in medicine. She was awarded a Macy Fellowship at the Radcliffe Institute and a Fellowship at the Center Advanced Study in the Behavioral Sciences at Stanford University. She received an honorary DSc from Brooklyn College and is a Fellow of the American Academy of Arts and Sciences.

Dr Nadelson has published more than 300 scientific articles, books and developed non-print materials and delivered over 1,000 lectures on medical and psychiatric topics nationally and internationally.

Interview

I: May I begin by asking what your childhood was like?

CN: I grew up in Brooklyn, New York, when it was a middle-class suburb of New York City. My family, including my younger sister, lived in a small house. I did all my schooling nearby until I went to college, which was located in a different part of Brooklyn. I don't remember that the word psychiatry was ever mentioned in my home when I was a child because my parents thought it meant the patients in the state mental hospital about three or four streets away. We were not supposed to go near that area because the people in the mental state hospital might hurt us.

My parents' main concern was that I get a good education and find a worthwhile career. At that time and place, girls had very little choice. If you were middle class, as I was, the options were to become a teacher, a nurse, or a secretary. That was not what I wanted. I was nine or ten years old when I began thinking about becoming a doctor. My parents thought that was not a reasonable goal and were not supportive of my going in this direction.

At that time I was very close to my grandfather who was suffering with lung cancer. I often visited him in the afternoons after school, talking and reading to him. I began to think that maybe I could become a doctor and cure cancer. My fifth grade teacher and my uncle were very supportive. I thought more seriously about it and shared the idea with my friends and they announced in the ninth grade yearbook. So, I went to high school and took many science classes and started a research project with my biology teacher, who thought my doing medicine was a good idea. At the end of high school I began studying at Brooklyn College because it was free if you lived in New York City and my parents could not afford to send me elsewhere. It was then that I began to talk about going to medical school very seriously and to take pre-med courses. My parents continued to object, but my uncle, my mother's brother who was a lawyer, and his wife, with whom I was very close, defended my position. My parents agreed and I spent my college years as the only woman pre-med. In my class it was one woman out of 200 men.

I: Wow!

CN: I was a somewhat shy student but I ran and was elected President of the Biomedical Society. I was surprised at how comfortable I felt in that role and my academic performance continued to make me eligible to be elected to Phi Beta Kappa (Honour Society). There was less questioning of my goal by that stage and I graduated top of the class. I was very encouraged by my teachers and my premedical advisor. I applied to a great many schools, about 24 in all. My advisor thought it would be difficult to get in and the men in my class usually applied to half that number. I did get accepted and was overjoyed.

The finances were difficult but I was able to find a Foundation that was supportive of women's careers. As a result of their support I did not have to pay any tuition fees. I had a terrible time with interviews because people were often rude and demeaning but I was eventually accepted.

I was in the second year doing very well, but in the middle of the year I became engaged to marry one of my college classmates. Being young to get married was not unusual at that time and we thought that one of the schools would admit one of us. The University of Rochester accepted me as a transfer student and I spent the rest of medical school there. Medical school in Rochester spent four years apologizing to me for not having accepted me in the first instance. Being at the university was a rewarding experience and I loved it. It was a great place to be and the course orientation was towards psychiatry. Although I had not thought of psychiatry for my career I had the good fortune that two of the leaders of US psychiatry, John Romano and George Engel were teaching. Engel was instrumental in developing the biopsychosocial model. We had a very good and close relationship. We were able to disagree and argue with each other and come out as friends. They supported and encouraged me. As I rotated through many medical specialties, I became increasingly more interested in George Engels' emphasis on medical psychiatry. He was an internist and a psychiatrist and he was the vice-chairman of the department, a notable figure in psychiatry. The culmination of this was that I decided to become an endocrinologist, but I won the prize in psychiatry. I thought this might be telling me something. I had interviewed at all the most sought-after programmes, as my advisors had encouraged me. This was the beginning of the couples matching programmes where married couple could be matched to rotation schemes together and as both my husband and I were matched together.

At the end of my interviews around the country, I came back feeling demoralized partly because questions that I was asked in interviews were inappropriate and rude. I explained this to my advisor who was shocked at this. I felt helpless to do anything because my interviewers were professors and I was a student applying for a position that women did not generally apply for. When I finished crying, my advisor said, 'Why don't we work out something? Why don't the two of you stay here and be interns? We will put you first on a match for placement for training and you put us first and we are done. So let's do it that way because we would love to have you stay.' So my husband and I did just that. We were both interns in medicine but I was still thinking about psychiatry, and during that year I decided to go into that field.

My husband and I decided we would move to Boston. He was accepted into a programme in medicine followed by a fellowship in cardiology. I was accepted for a residency at Massachusetts Mental Health Center. I didn't know much about it or its history but it was seen as the very best place to go. I had never lived in Boston but I liked the city so we moved there. I was at Mass Mental Health Center and my husband was at Beth Israel Hospital.

At this time, our marriage broke up and we continued on our own. For me, Mass Mental was a wonderful experience, although as usual women were very much in the minority. There were only four women out of 24 positions, but the atmosphere was welcoming and it was a great place to be. At the end my time at Mass Mental, I still wanted to do more in medical psychiatry. Mass Mental didn't have a medical unit and it also had a limited patient population. I wanted to learn more about psychotherapy. I thought that Beth Israel Hospital was the ideal place to be, which it probably was, and the chair of the department was a woman, the first female professor and chair at Harvard. So, I went to Beth Israel hospital and the atmosphere was very different from Mass Mental. We saw a lot of cases of medical psychiatry and undertook a lot of consultation psychiatry. We also did a lot of psychotherapy because by this time the Boston Psychoanalytic Institute was established in town and many of the people working there were supervisors in psychotherapy. When I left Mass Mental, Jack Ewalt, the chief of the hospital, said to me that he was really sorry that I had chosen to leave because he wanted me to stay on, become the Chief Resident, because they never had a female Chief Resident. He thought I was the right person for the role but understood and said that if I wanted to leave he would support me. He promised to stand behind me, whatever direction I chose. The fact that he was willing to support me was a remarkable experience. It allowed me to get to know how psychiatry worked, what the organizations were, and what the politics were. I knew that Jack was Professor of Psychiatry at Harvard Medical School and had been a President of the American Psychiatric Association. The issue of the place of women in medicine and psychiatry was important to him, and he always encouraged me to keep going.

At Beth Israel, having a role model like Grete Bibring was amazing to me. She was an Austrian emigrée to the United States, at the forefront of psychoanalysis and very involved in psychiatry, including in its role as a medical specialty. She had built a very good relationship with the chair of medicine at the hospital and we had a strong interaction with the department of medicine. Beth Israel Hospital was friendly to women. I became the consultation person for the obstetrics and gynaecology department and the head of the medical student education programme. I developed my major interests in medical student education and consultation/liaison psychiatry. I met Leon Eisenberg who had been recruited to be the chair of psychiatry at the Children's Hospital in Boston and got to know him. I began to develop courses in teaching psychotherapy, human sexuality, and many aspects of medical student education. At that time I also met Malkah Notman who became my co-author and friend for life. I became more involved in Harvard Medical School activities. Leon Eisenberg became the chair of the admissions committee and he was dedicated to including more women and underserved minority students. So he asked me to chair a sub-committee that would challenge the existing model and patterns of recruitment and improve our record on recruitment of women and underserved populations. This was a very exciting experience for me. I was taken aback to be asked to take this appointment up, me being a very lowly assistant professor. I sought advice from people from different fields of medicine who were also committed to the goal of improving the diversity of the student body. We developed guidelines including how to conduct unbiased interviews, eliminating asking personal questions or commenting on dress, and what to include in reports. The Committee submitted evaluations of applicants without mentioning their gender, race or identity. When the data was unveiled it became clear that ha lf of our group were women. The committee noted and acknowledged a significant improvement. This was a very exciting time. At the present time most medical schools in the United States have more women than men applicants and acceptances and the recruitment of underserved minority students has improved substantially. In addition to my work within the psychiatry department at Beth Israel hospital, I often did work in the Emergency Room and was often called for two problems.

In the emergency room, we began to see many young women, often college students, who had been raped, and we had no resources to help them and no person with expertise. Malkah Notman developed a rape crisis centre which enabled schools to obtain a consultation from us. They could send people to the emergency room so that we could take care of them. This was the first real hospital-organized programme in the city. The other area we began to consult about was reproductive psychiatry. We came across secret abortions. We saw women in the emergency room and elsewhere having undergone illegal and unsterile procedures because abortion, unless it was considered therapeutic, was illegal in our state (Massachusetts). This was a medical problem that we had to solve, so psychiatry got involved and consulted with the obstetrics and gynaecology department. We developed a rape crisis centre that included abortion counselling with the obstetrics and gynaecology department which was very grateful to have our input. We developed a programme for psychiatrists to evaluate women who applied for abortions and to consider their mental state. We developed criteria for therapeutic abortion at the hospital that could be used as guidelines for other hospitals and clinics too. But why was all this happening? What was the outcome? We formed a working group with obstetrics and gynaecology, the clergy, and psychiatrists to study what was going on and to make recommendations for improvement.

That was my early career. By this time it was the late 1970s and I was recruited to become the vice-chair of psychiatry at Tufts Medical School. At approximately the same time, one of my supervisors, Leston Havens from Mass Mental Health Center, encouraged me to run for office in the Massachusetts Psychiatric Society. It was a long-standing society which had never had women on the executive committee and very few women members. He thought I was competent and would do a good job so they invited me to consider running for secretary and so I did. I was elected and began my political career in psychiatry. I went to Tufts as a vice-chair of psychiatry and the Director of Education, two quasi-political positions. In the Massachusetts Psychiatric Society, I rose to become the vice-chair of the society and then I was encouraged to run for President. It was the past-Presidents who really pushed me to seriously think about it. I became the first woman President of the Massachusetts Psychiatric Association. At Tufts, I was the first woman training director and vice-chair and I became Professor of Psychiatry there. That's the earlier part of my history. Do you want me to go on?

I: Yes please. Then you moved nationally, didn't you?

CN: Yes. As a district branch President I got to sit in on many APA meetings so I got to know active members and became one of them.

I: What was that like?

CN: I was appointed to many committees and task forces of the APA. At that time in the APA's history there had never been a woman President, it was 143 years old before I was elected President. First, I ran for Vice-President. I was encouraged to run for the post which have led to President position. I didn't win that election but I learned how one runs for that office. By the next time I ran, won with the help of a huge number of the women psychiatrists as well as men who wanted to expand membership and have women officers. Everybody was very supportive. I was on the Board of Trustees when the question of running for APA President came up. It was early in the 1980s. I remember very vividly sitting in a room with two of my close friends who were also involved at the senior level in psychiatry and they also subsequently became APA Presidents. We talked for a whole evening and they encouraged and supported me. Men who had been my supervisors and even more casual acquaintances were enthusiastic as well. We decided that I should run a campaign against a very popular and competent person who had been Vice-President earlier and was well known and a friend of mine. He and I spent a lot of time talking about it. Bob Pasnau made an agreement about how we would run the campaign. It was a wonderful experience. We each went to different areas and we called all district branches. Because the United States is so large, some states have more than one district branch so there is a large land mass and population of psychiatrists to reach. We agreed that would not speak badly about our opponent but instead focus on what we thought we could bring to the APA. So I travelled around the country and tried not to be discouraged since many people I met thought that my opponent would win easily and my run was seen as a 'practice run'.

I conquered my fear of speaking in public, I learned how to handle questions. I had a group of friends who couldn't have been kinder and more helpful. I decided to ask one senior woman in each district branch to help. This gave me a national team representing different states and different areas. I received a lot of positive feedback. Colleagues were warm and welcoming. They set up meetings for me so I could present a talk to them. Since I was on academic lists, some activities in areas that were of interest to psychiatrists, I often conducted grand rounds, or a university presentation.

I: What was it like breaking that glass ceiling?

CN: Well, it was both frightening and exhilarating. I had remarried. My husband was a psychiatrist who was in my department at Beth Israel Hospital and I had two children. My husband couldn't have been more supportive. He was always supportive and enormously helpful. He was not challenged by rigid sex roles. He was the chief of consultation liaison psychiatry at Beth Israel and along the way he was recruited to become the chief of psychiatry at the Boston Veteran's hospital.

Let me give you a few examples of what became routine during my Presidential year. I travelled widely that year throughout the country and internationally. We were at a WPA (World Psychiatric Association) meeting in Mexico City and all the Presidents of the psychiatric societies around the world were introducing themselves. I was at the end of the line (I was used to being there) and when they got to me the lights went out in the auditorium. I was on stage, the message was clear, I wasn't considered one of them by whomever put the lights out. I didn't look like a president. Another event was related to sex role stereotypes. We were at a meeting in Germany with the German Psychiatric Society. We had a big dinner and the German Society gave gifts to each of the representatives of the APA. At that time I was the President Elect of the APA, and I was a woman. They gave books of Freud's writings and other major works in psychiatry to all of the men in the room and all of the women received dishes. One could take it as a joke, but it wasn't. They knew I was soon to be the President of the APA, another person had been President of the Royal Australian New Zealand College of Medicine, Judy Gold was the President of the Canadian Psychiatric Association, and Astrid Heiberg in Norway was a major figure in the hierarchy of the Norwegian Psychiatric Association. The World Psychiatric Association had elected its first woman President, Felice Lieh-Mak (See Chapter 11). The APA has had 12 women Presidents since then. I feel pleased about that.

I: You opened the doors for a lot of women to rise and get elected but there is still an element of misogyny around. How do you think psychiatry has changed over the course of your career?

CN: The field has opened up. When I was beginning, there was a very strong view that intensive psychotherapy was the best overall treatment. Biological psychiatry, neuropsychiatry, and psychopharmacology were in their infancies.

Respect for psychiatry was spotty. Biological psychiatry was considered second class. I love teaching residents now. I supervise psychotherapy at Brigham and Women's Hospital. I became the editor and chief of the American Psychiatric Publishing Inc (APPI) when it was very young. Initially I had to convince Mel Sabshin and others on the committee that I had the qualifications to be the Editor-in-Chief of the Press (APPI), a newly formed publishing enterprise of the APA.

Initially he was surprised. He told me that he hadn't thought of me for the role, that he had another APA member in his mind, but to his credit, he gave me the job. I grew the American Psychiatric Press from four books in its beginning to well over 1,000 and it was a thriving enterprise by the time I stopped being the Editor-in-Chief. I felt we had much to offer the field.

I: What do you think of the current state of psychiatry?

CN: I think that the field is in reasonably good shape. I think people respect psychiatry. One doesn't hear people question their judgement when they choose psychiatry as their specialty. I think the problem is more the way our community and our society do not know of our problems with funding and resources. What is available is insufficient.

I: What do you see as the characteristics of a good psychiatrist?

CN: The pandemic has revealed new issues to consider. Being aware of biological, psychological, social and environmental factors. The integration of psychotherapy with psychopharmacology has improved. Other improvements include the robustness of our research and integration with other fields and the needs of patients and families, as well as innovation in techniques and new types of therapeutic approaches as well as the roles of various mental health experts with different areas of expertise as funding, site, organizational structure, environment, and resources.

I: And what do you see as gaps in training?

CN: Currently there has been some change because of the pandemic. The roles and responsibilities of residents will need to be assessed in the light of their experiences.

I: Moving on to psychiatry's contract with society, is it possible to deliver on that, do you think?

CN: The US healthcare system differs from healthcare systems in most other high-income countries. It is not primarily a government system as it is not uniform and it does have a private profit motive as well as public non-profit components. Psychiatry is underserved and under resourced. So the social contract is also different.

I: What would your advice be to trainees/residents when you teach them?

CN: Residents need to learn about the field, research, clinical work, and emerging areas in order to make decisions. They need to know where their heart is. We should be able to help them do this. They should have the opportunity to explore through fellowships, electives, and supervision.

I: And what would you tell your younger self?

CN: I think I would have done what I did (laughs). I have never been sorry that I took up psychiatry. I did have a period of questioning whether I should have gone into other fields but I learned enough about psychiatry in my early training to believe that I made the right choice. I think we need to be more active in medical psychiatry and work with medical people at all levels. There's so much to be done there and the COVID pandemic has made it clear that the need for psychiatric input is enormous.

I: You have achieved a tremendous amount and I think psychiatry's gain has been endocrinology's loss. Which of your achievements are you most proud of?

CN: That's a very difficult question. What stands out is entering my career with a glass ceiling challenging me. It has been an honour to meet the challenges in the field. Psychiatry has expanded and been increasingly productive by including the talents of women who have assumed leadership roles and have contributed so much to research, education, and clinical work. It is fulfilling and exciting to have been part of this revolution.

I: Thanks very much for your time and sharing your life-story. Really appreciate it.

15
Ahmed Okasha

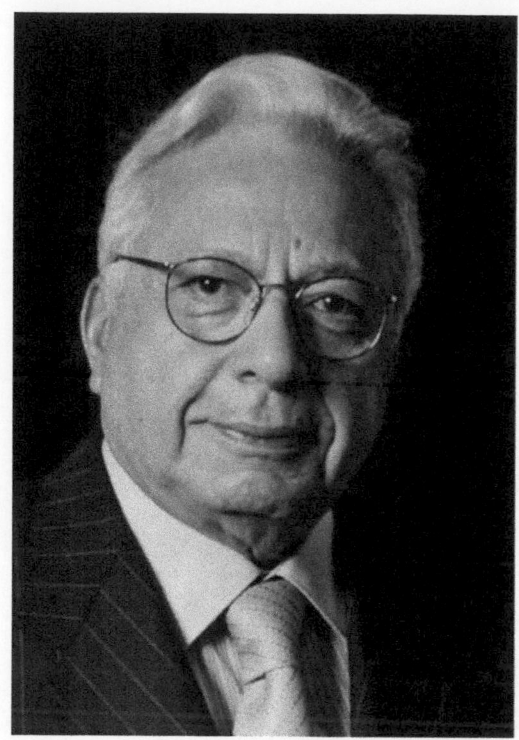

Biography

Professor Ahmed Okasha trained in the United Kingdom and on his return to Cairo established the psychiatry unit at the Faculty of Medicine Ain Shams University in 1964, then founded the Okasha Institute of Psychiatry in 1990. He is also Director of the World Health Organization (WHO) Collaborating Center for Training and Research in Mental Health, Institute of Psychiatry–Ain Shams University, Cairo, Egypt. He was President of the World Psychiatric Association (2002–2005). He has been President of the Egyptian Society of Biological Psychiatry and of World Federation of Societies of Biological Psychiatry. Currently he is Honorary President of the Arab Federation of Psychiatrists and Egyptian Psychiatric Association. He is also a member of the Executive Committees of the Academy of Science and Technology, Committee of the Science and Technology Development Fund, National

Investment Charity Education Fund, and the Egyptian Presidential Council of Distinguished Scientists. He is adviser to the Egyptian President of Mental Health and Community Integration. He has published widely both in national and international journals and is on the Editorial Advisory Boards of 23 international scientific journals. He is a Member of National Mental Health Council, the Supreme Council of Culture, the Supreme Council of Health, and the National Council Addressing Fundamentalism and Terrorism in Egypt. He chairs the scientific committees of fellowship of the Egyptian Board of Psychiatry, fellowship of Child and Adolescent Psychiatry, and fellowship of Egyptian Board of Addiction Psychiatry. He has received honorary degrees from the International School of Postgraduate Medical Education (ISPME) in Lausanne, Munich and national awards from the Government of Egypt.

Interview

I: Could you tell us about your childhood and growing up?

AO: I think I was lucky; I had a happy childhood. My childhood was enriched both environmentally and genetically. My father was a senior general in the army, so I learnt discipline, perfectionism, feeling responsible, and respecting the elderly from my childhood. From my mother's side, I was exposed to many cultural, artistic, and social aspects of life. My uncles, her brothers, were very important people in Egyptian politics. During my childhood there was no television, no computers; we only had the radio and sitting in the social set-up of the family for entertainment. I was exposed to family gatherings from the age of two or three, with prime ministers and ministers and heads of political parties from my mother's side. Thirdly, I was very lucky to have as my elder brother Dr Tharwat Okasha, who was the vice premier in Egypt during Nasser's time. He was also the Minister of Culture and he taught me as if he was my private tutor, taught me about music, about literature, about art, about museums. When I was growing up, he was studying for his doctorate in Paris where he used to take me to the Louvre every day on his way to his office. He used to tell me that you have to study in this hall in the Louvre, the Pharaonic Hall, the Greek Hall, the Roman Hall, and so on. When he was an ambassador in Italy, he sent me to the museums there with his secretaries. When I was about seven or eight years old, a symphonic recording consisted of about 10 vinyl discs, not like the single CD of today. My brother used to read and he would ask me to change the disc every three minutes or so. He was very generous and was always explaining that Rimsky-Korsakov's music means this, Tchaikovsky's means that, Beethoven said so and so. When he started to write his encyclopaedia on art in Arabic, we used to have discussions three or four times a week. I lost him four years ago; he was my best friend. You can see inscribed on his photo what he wrote to me in Arabic; I'll try and translate it. 'To my dear brother, Ahmed Okasha, I hope God will give you more health to be the best brother I had in my life. A renowned scientist, whose advice I'm very happy to have who is a dear friend, and I am always enlightened by his experience. To you, with love, appreciation, and great admiration,

Tharwat Okasha.' There were 16 years between us but he always treated me as a mature adult, never as a child.

I: What attracted you to medicine?

AO: My grandfather was a mayor of one of the cities of Egypt. My paternal grandfather was very angry that I didn't want to be like the other members of my family and join the army or the police, or be part of anything in which I didn't have to take money from people. He was very angry that I would be charging fees after I examined a patient. He thought that this was a disgrace to our family. He did not consider that to be honourable. But my maternal uncle was Professor Mohammed Talaat, the head and father of physiology in Egypt and across the Arab world. He worked as a dean in the Medical School of Alexandria, in Cairo, and also in Baghdad. He had written books on physiology. He would come to visit his elderly sister, my mother, and I was very attracted to his wisdom, his sincerity and dedication, and his speaking about patients as if they were real members of his family. I found it very humane. I think one of his first books was a translation of a book by Dr Henry Link called *Return to Faith* in which a psychiatrist lost his faith and gradually realized that faith plays a very crucial role in the psyche of an individual. I read it when I was 13 or 14 years old. This probably embedded something inside me which affected my future. The second thing is that I was always interested in mankind, in humans. I was very interested to see this creation of God, a human being, and I wanted to take care of them, wherever they came from, anywhere in the world, from any religion or any race. This gave me satisfaction more than anything else.

I: Why did you choose psychiatry?

AO: Psychiatry is the most humanistic branch in medicine and is the most scientific branch in human sciences. This attracted me tremendously. It is the only medical specialty that can let you see the person as a whole. Now, 50 to 60 years later, there is psychiatry for the patient, not just medicine to treat the patient. Psychiatry was the only subject that was for the person, not for the organs. When I was a physician and the surgeon used to tell us that he would like to do thyroidectomy, appendectomy, or treatment for hernia or piles, I used to ask him the name of the patient. He used to smile and ask me, 'What do you mean, by name? The registrar would start and have the case ready and even open the wound or incision. I don't have to see the patient's face or know his name to treat him.' I went to work in ophthalmology and the same thing happened. We would prepare a patient for glaucoma or cataract surgery, and again, no-one mentioned the name of the patient. I found that the doctors were extrapolating the person to an organ, to an appendix, to an eye, to piles, to an extent that I used to laugh with my professor and say so this patient is called 'Ali Hernia' and the other is called 'Mohammed Appendix, because he has no name. From the surgeon's point of view, he's just an organ. And I was very afraid, trying to choose a speciality for my residency because I was one of the only five people who graduated with highest honour in medical school. At that time all psychiatrists graduating from Egypt did not have very high grades in their final years of school. Actually, it was those with the lowest grades who specialized in psychiatry.

So, when I went home the dean had told my mother, being her relative, that despite the fact that I was one of the top five graduates, I wanted to work in something related to madness. My parents asked me if I was serious and why, and I replied with what I have just told you. They accepted me wanting to start something new, especially at that university where there was nothing except a neurology department; there was no psychiatric department. And so I was the first one in my speciality to ask for a scientific scholarship to go on a government scholarship to Britain, where I stayed from 1959 to 1964, and where I took my membership in medicine. At that time, the Royal College of Psychiatrists did not exist so I had to go to Edinburgh, where I had to study half medicine and half psychiatry because all specialties existed in Edinburgh, such as cardiology, neurology, etc. So actually this is why I chose psychiatry because it sees a person as an individual.

I: Do you have any regrets?

AO: Well, as I told you earlier, during my childhood, I was very lucky. My father never told me that I had to study; I took that responsibility myself since childhood. I'm a planner; I never do anything without planning. I planned studying psychiatry; I planned how to take scholarship from the government during Nasser's time as it was very difficult as governmental financial educational grants were limited. I went there and I planned to be a good psychiatrist. I obtained all my degrees at my first attempt; all memberships, all fellowships, and all diplomas. I had a plan that I would earn these degrees and go back to Egypt. I was offered a place in Britain, Australia, in New Zealand, in America, and in Canada, very high-ranking posts. I was very young then. I finished my education at the age of 27, I had all these degrees, diplomas, and memberships. I preferred to finish my timetable of my studies than have any leisure time, studying was my priority. So even back then I was planning on how I could succeed, because I felt I had to succeed every day. That's what I always tell young people: 'Don't wait to study a month before the exams. Fill your timetable every day and know that you have finished, so that you succeed every day. So you have all the joy, the pleasure, the endorphins, the encephalins, the benzodiazepines, and the GABA, all of them are working so you can succeed and then you will be happy every night before you sleep.'

I: Who were your role models, heroes, or heroines?

AO: Well, my elder brother, Dr Tharwat Okasha, was a real model for culture, art, appreciation of beauty, tasting beauty in all respects, and this affected me tremendously. From the scientific point of view, a role model I remember was Professor Paul Galiongy who was the head of the medical department and a professor of medicine and endocrinology. He was very interested in medicine in ancient Egypt and wrote a book in English after he studied many papyri. He was elected to the Royal Society of Great Britain because of this book. One day, when I was a youngster just returning from my scholarship, I was still a lecturer, I found him calling me over the telephone and asking me to visit him at his home. I was surprised because this was not the custom in Egypt. So I went there and he told me that he was reading the Ebers Papyrus. This papyrus was about the heart. He would ask me: 'What's this, Ahmed?' and I would say, 'This is schizophrenia' and 'This is depression' and 'This is dementia'. And he told me that it was obvious that I now had a goal in life. I asked him what that was and he said, 'To study mental disorders in ancient Egypt'. Ancient Egyptians believed that all psychiatric disorders originated from the heart, so there was no stigma from mental illness and it was viewed as a physical disorder. The stigma only appeared when the psyche was differentiated from the soma, but when ancient Egyptians treated psychiatric disorders they were treated in the same place, with the same respect as patients with physical disorders, using interpretation of dreams, herbal treatment and essence. He gave me his book 'Medicine in Ancient Egypt' to read. I was the first person to study mental disorders in ancient Egypt. I remember I was once invited by Professor Sabshin, in the United States, who was the Secretary General of the American Psychiatric Association, to give the plenary lecture about mental disorders in Pharaonic Egypt. I pointed out that the Egyptians used to diagnose personality according to the size and colour of the heart; for example a black-hearted person or white-hearted person, someone with a large heart, or a restricted heart. One's personality depended upon the nature of his heart. There was also in the Kahun Papyrus which included a citation about the uterus, about hysteria. It was not the Greeks who described hysteria but it was in ancient Egypt where Hippocrates read about how they used to treat hysterical symptoms with vapours that can expel or repel the uterus, because ancient Egyptians believed that all these symptoms; conversion symptoms or dissociative symptoms, are secondary to the churning movements of the uterus which was searching for humidity. When I went to Britain to the Institute of Psychiatry I met Sir Aubrey Lewis, who was the head of the department at the time. And, as you know, we usually ask our professors which textbooks they prefer. He referred me to two small books before we started discussing psychiatric disorders; he told me to read *The Castle* and *The Trial* by Kafka. I went back to him, a bit angry and told him that I didn't want to stay in England, I wanted to go back to my country as soon as possible, finish my training and my degrees because I was not in England to read stories. He smiled at me patiently and told me to read the novels and get back to him. The language was very difficult, it was disconnected and abstract, as if the writer had something wrong with him. I went back and told him that I read them. He asked me what I thought of them. I told him that the writing was disconnected and Kafka went from one topic to another without finishing the first, so the association is loose. He burst out laughing and said, 'You'll be a very good physician; this is a schizophrenic thought disorder.' From that time, he drew me to everything related to culture and art. For instance, he was the person who told me that if one reads Shakespeare, you will see that he had known all mental disorders, before psychiatry was born. Aubrey Lewis told me that psychiatry was 150 years old when we were in the 1960s because before this all mental disorders were treated by philosophers and religious healers.

I: Do you have any lasting impression about patients?

AO: My experience, which extends well over 55 years now in psychiatry, has taught me that psychiatric patients are completely different from what others think about them. Don't believe that they are violent, or they cannot work, or cannot marry, don't believe that it is lack of faith or magic, or it is because of the evil eye. Psychiatric patients in my opinion are the most humane and sensitive creatures of God because they feel emotions and motivations, thoughts, in a superior way that makes them suffer. The mental suffering especially involving thought disorder is unique for humans it's very rare to find animals with mental sufferings. Animals are very faithful but that is because we, human beings, take care of them, feed them, shelter them, and the like. They don't have genuine affection for us. The loyalty of patients is great and the most loyal patients are psychiatric patients. The impression they left on me was that they taught me modesty, empathy, reality, and understanding of their pain.

I: Any memorable occasions in the practice or the research in psychiatry?

AO: My practice and research in psychiatry taught me something that was not understood. We used to say here in Egypt that living in rural areas gives you freedom, purity, cleanliness, and a more peaceful life. But I was astonished during my epidemiological work that depression in rural areas is more widespread and deeper than in urban areas. It is more prevalent in overpopulated areas where unemployment and poverty are predominant. So it's not true that living in the countryside will make you happier than living in urban areas. The second thing which is very interesting is that Post-Traumatic Stress Disorder (PTSD) is sometimes used for political gain. When the tsunami in Phuket, Thailand occurred in 2004, I was at that time President of the World Psychiatric Association and got in touch with the World Health Organization (WHO) because there were 400 children who had lost their parents on an island which was severely damaged during the tsunami. We had agreed to send some psychiatrists to help these children with PTSD. By the time we found the personnel and finances and sent them, I was shocked when they called me and said there were no PTSD (symptoms) in these children; the majority of the families who had survived the tsunami had adopted the parentless children. We found them playing football, happy and laughing. This is a very religious area, an island in Indonesia, predominantly Muslim, not fundamentalist, but very conservative. They believe in God and they believed the tsunami was the wrath of God because they were not virtuous. I was shocked and told our colleagues in Europe that it was ridiculous to claim that PTSD doesn't exist there, as I'd been told. The other item is the medicalization of normality. Until 1980 we had something that we cherished in our culture which is shyness. Now we call it avoidant personality disorder or social anxiety and there are drugs to treat it. People lived with this honourable shyness, and they were very happy and virtuous, but now it is called a mental illness. It is just like we described gender identity disorder as a part of psychiatric classification, but classificatory systems are now trying to remove it. Now the DSM and ICD systems are classifying so many transitionary symptoms as mental disorders, calling them specific and nonspecific disorders, which means any symptom can be treated medically for the sake of the pharma industry. This has made me aware after so many years that we are the victim and subject of the influence of the industry, creating psychiatric disorders to serve the pharmaceutical industry. Today, so many psychiatric disorders have the same aetiology, the same outcome, the same pathology, the same physiology, and the same neuroimaging, treatable with the same medicine. We will discover not drugs but a sort of modulation of the neural circuits that are disrupted, downgraded, dysregulated, or desynchronized in different illnesses.

I: How has psychiatry changed in your time?

AO: I think I have mentioned before, as I suspected this will be a question that medicalization of normality is a real factor and we're going to see more people in urban communities, more elderly people living longer, all having more psychiatric disorders. According to what can be observed now, there is an increase in depression in the global population. By 2030, depression will be ranked number one in DALYs (disability adjusted for life years) according to the WHO, before heart disease, accidents, respiratory diseases, and so on. I expect there to be a complete change because of the use of information technology, telepsychiatry, digital psychiatry, the use of nanotechnology in psychiatry, treating people in remote locations without the presence of psychiatrists by the Internet or telephone; this will be the future of psychiatry. In the future, there will be primary care psychiatrists who practise in primary healthcare centres; you won't need to go to a psychiatric clinic or hospital but can simply visit the primary care psychiatrist or physician, something that should be welcomes particularly if we realize that 40% of somatic symptoms are secondary to psychiatric disorders. Primary care psychiatrist will change how hospitals and clinics are run.

I: What are your views on the current state of psychiatry?

AO: It is going in the right direction after the study of different connections in the brain called the 'connectome project'. I think that all drug companies have stopped developing new medications because it seems that targeting neurotransmitters is not the only way to treat psychiatric disorders. Now we are beginning to look at the connectivity between the grey and white matter or brain circuits. This will completely change the management, treatment, and even the stigma behind mental illnesses.

I: Is psychiatry brainless or mindless?

AO: No, neither anymore. This completely stopped after we discovered so many disconnectivities that are present in all our psychiatric disorders and that they are very similar, so diagnosis itself will now be different. It is no longer dependent on the symptoms but will depend upon a real pathology of the brain itself, the neural circuits. I'm expecting quite a change in this discussion of brainless and mindless soon.

I: What do you see as problems with psychiatry?

AO: The problem is that some people are reductionistic; they think the mind is different from the brain. Some people think there is nothing called mind, it's only a brain, although the mind is the highest function of the brain. That is why some people like to say that psychiatry is behavioural neurology and neurology is organic neurology, and it's better to call psychiatry clinical neuroscience. I believe that we must place more emphasis on basic sciences, neurosciences, neurophysiology, and the like, and this will help us discover a lot of things about psychiatric disorders.

I: How can you improve recruitment in psychiatry now?

AO: I think in order to recruit young psychiatrists to psychiatry that undergraduate teaching for medical students should be done by charismatic psychiatric professors to act as role models for these students. This, I believe will increase interest and recruitment to psychiatry as a speciality. However, as long as psychiatry is seen as a secondary or non-important branch and professors and teachers of psychiatry try and make students laugh and be sarcastic about psychiatric patient, I don't think you can ever recruit them. I think by studying the connectome and pharmacogenomics and gaining better outcomes for our patients than all other medical illnesses, then we will recruit better psychiatrists. It is simply untrue that psychiatric patients can never recover. Diabetic patients don't recover, coronary heart patients don't recover, cancer patients don't recover, and liver cirrhosis doesn't recover, but in psychiatry we have 30–40% of people who can stop their medication and recover completely. Why are we getting gloomy? We have to give be optimistic about the future.

I: What do you see as the characteristics of a good psychiatrist?

AO: He should love psychiatry and his patients. He should be charismatic and emphatic and should be communicative. You can gain knowledge from computers but to having communication with patients and their families is the only thing that will enhance the psychiatrist's reputation.

I: What do you see as gaps in the practice of psychiatry?

AO: The gap I see is that psychiatry is being practised mostly by psychologists; not that they don't have an important role, but psychiatrists also have an important role. Psychiatrists now are working as social workers and psychologists should respect other specialties and should keep their behavioural neurology in perspective. This is the only way psychiatry will get a chance to develop further.

I: What do you see as gaps in training in psychiatry?

AO: I strongly believe that you teach psychiatry as a module in the first year, which is now present in so many medical schools. You see a patient who has cancer and teach the related topics in pathology, physiology, surgery, and oncology. We need to realize that 30–40% cancer patients have depression so psychiatry should be included in training too. The same thing should happen with Parkinson's, with myocardial infarction, etc. If you teach psychiatry in a modular way, that is to say showing its relation to other disorders as well as looking at the aetiology in a psycho-socio-biological approach, this will help to keep psychiatry continually progressing and in touch with other branches of medicine.

I: How do you think psychiatry's social contract can be delivered?

AO: Psychiatrists should believe that they are part of the society and part of the social network. Until they have better communication with policy-makers and with people in administrative jobs, and unless we give them a model to study and practise, we will never build the social contract that is required. This is because the people who make decisions about the economy and budgets for psychiatry and mental health are politicians, not psychiatrists. We should always communicate with them as they don't understand the extent of mental health problems in the community; they need to be told again and again that one in every four people suffers from mental illness; they need to be shown the research from the London School of Economics that has shown that if you treat depression, the years lost in employment without treatment could increase the country's economy by 2–3% at least.

I: What would you tell your younger self?

AO: I would tell him that I'm not getting older, I'm just growing. So when you ask me how old I am, I will not say I'm 80 years old. I will say that I'm 80 years young, not old.

I: What is your advice to trainees of today?

AO: Humility is more important than knowledge, and communication is more important than knowledge, and most importantly, sincerity and dedication is more important than knowledge. I can have a basic knowledge, but that I can attain even by sitting with my computer, from which I can get any information about the world. I used to get references by going to libraries, to find books for reference, and now you can find the same in five minutes with a computer.

I: A doctor and a psychiatrist usually keep on studying for a life time? Is that tue?

AO: Even at my age I read psychiatric journals, books about culture, newspapers, and I enjoy watching football matches and listening to music. Don't focus on running your life solely in one direction; you may end up being more successful, but you won't be happy unless you have a multitude of interests in your life.

I: What would you like to be remembered for?

AO: I have tried all my life to fight against the stigma of mental illness and I have already managed to be a continuous member of this project along with the World Psychiatric Association. From the first moment I came back in Egypt from the UK after my scholarship the image of psychiatry and psychiatrists was very bad. I was the first psychiatrist to appear in the media and on television in the Arab world. TV was black and white at that time and I appeared on the most important programme called 'A Star is Born' or something like that. And I told them that I was not a star, that I was just a lecturer at a university. But they told me that I was the only Psychiatrist) that was educated abroad and who returned. I think fighting the stigma of mental illness is important. When I came back, people did not know the difference between the words psychiatrist and psychologist because in Arabic it is the same thing, 'Nafsia', so I changed the term to psychological medicine 'Alteb Al Nafsy'; this was in 1964 and now in all departments across the Arab world it is called psychological medicine and not psychiatry. I'm now preparing a campaign to fight stigma in Egypt with several partners: firstly, Misr-Al-khair, which is the biggest charity organization in Egypt, secondly, of the Egyptian Psychiatric Association and thirdly, the Arab Federation of Psychiatrists. I managed to secure finances to raise awareness, reduce stigma, and flawed beliefs about psychiatry among the population and patients.

I: Which of your achievements are you most proud of?

AO: My life, thanks to God, is full of achievements, but if I had to pick one it would be my work with the World Psychiatric Association, which lasted for 16 years and ended by my becoming the first President not from Europe or the United States but from an Arab nation, a Middle-Eastern country, and also a Muslim. I was elected unopposed first time in the history of WPA, against all the odds. I'm so proud of this, of having the appreciation of so many psychiatric associations across the world, of having honorary fellowships in many countries, and more or less achieving the highest merit prizes in Egypt; the most prestigious one is called the Nile Merit Prize. Apart from this, I also won the highest medal in art and science in in Egypt. I'm also proud of my publications. But I am also proud of something which means much more: almost all our professors in Egypt are those whom I have trained and examined or I promoted them. They are all my sons and students. This is my greatest achievement; my continuity lies in them.

16
Tarek Okasha

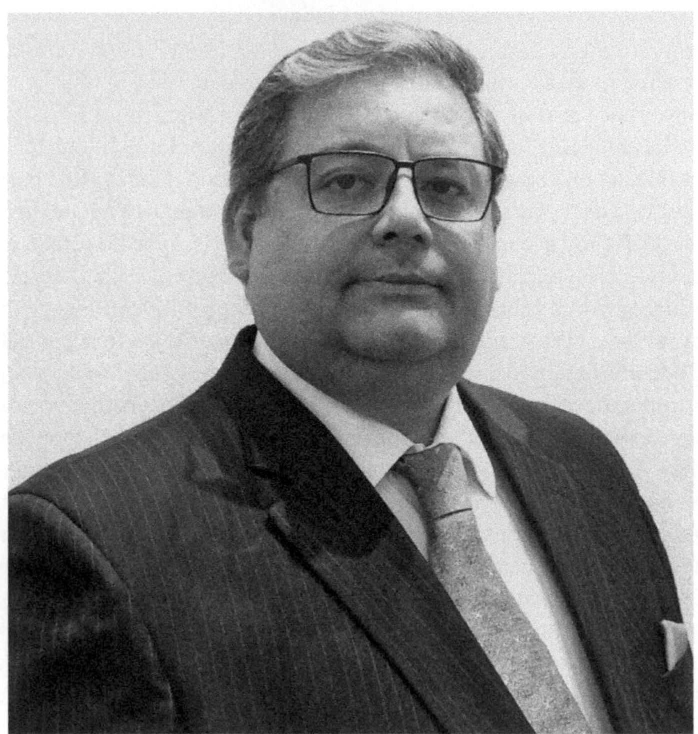

Biography

Professor Tarek Okasha is Professor of Psychiatry, Okasha Institute of Psychiatry, Faculty of Medicine Ain Shams University in Cairo, Egypt. He is also Director of the World Psychiatric Association (WPA) Collaborating Centre in Research and Training in Psychiatry. At present he is President of the Egyptian Alzheimer Society and past-President of the Arab Board of Psychiatry. He trained in psychiatry in the United States and in Egypt. He was an Executive Committee member World Psychiatric Association (WPA) and Secretary for Scientific Meetings World Psychiatric Association and in this role chaired the WPA Operational Committee on Scientific Meetings (2008–2014). He is also chair of the Higher Council of Universities Committee in Egypt. He has published widely and is Editor-in-Chief of the *Middle East Current Psychiatry Journal*. He established the psychiatry unit, Faculty of Medicine, Misr University for Science and Technology, 6th of October City. He is visiting Professor of Psychiatry to the Psychology Department Faculty of Arts, Cairo University, and Executive Committee member of several organizations such as the Egyptian Psychiatric Association and the Egyptian Society of Biological Psychiatry. He is on the Editorial Board of many international and national journals and has published widely.

Interview

I: Could you tell us about your childhood and growing up?

TO: I believe that I had a very balanced childhood. I went to an English-speaking school where I learnt English, Arabic, and a little bit of French. During my childhood, aside from going to school and getting good grades, my parents were insistent that I also play sports and they wanted me to play two types of sports; individual sports and group sports. For individual sports, I played squash and for the team sport, I took part in swimming and, later, water polo. I believe that playing sports during my childhood and adolescence had a positive influence on my personality; to have persistence, to complete something, to want to achieve, to want to win, to become better, to try and improve oneself, to be comfortable being a part of a team, and to have peers that you wanted to be like and peers that you didn't want to be like, sports taught me all this. I grew up in an ordinary household comprising my father, who is also a psychiatrist, my mother, my younger brother, and me. We enjoyed family time and travelling together. My father, being a psychiatrist, used his knowledge to create a safe, healthy, and enriching environment for my brother and me. My mother, being British, gave me the opportunity to experience both Egyptian and British culture and traditions. My parents were very keen on me getting a good education and on increasing and widening my horizon of knowledge. We used to travel every year in the summer to different countries to visit relatives and friends. I believe this had an influence on my development since I was exposed to different cultures, apart from my Egyptian heritage and background.

I: What attracted you to medicine?

TO: I was very good in biology in school and I enjoyed all the sciences, whether biology, chemistry, or physics, more than history and geography. I was also better in biology than in physics or chemistry and was lucky that three or four years during my schooling, I had teachers who encouraged me to take this interest forward. Since biology was my favourite subject, the logical choice to pursue my interest was to go into medicine. There were no other options and when I reached high school, my aim and target was to go to medical school. I don't think I ever thought of going into any other college or university other than medical school. I had no interest in engineering or any of the other social sciences.

I: Why did you choose psychiatry?

TO: When I finished medical school, I found that I enjoyed medicine more than surgery. I did not want to specialize in anything related to surgery. The two sub-branches of medicine that I liked very much were cardiology and neuro-psychiatry. Until I finished my house officer year, I was trying to choose between them both; cardiology was very intriguing to me. When I was house officer, cardiac catheterization had just been introduced and that was a revolution and everyone was talking about how cardiologists would now become the new scientific gods, if you'd like to use the term. Cardiology seemed to be the branch of medicine to be in. At the same time, I was very interested in psychiatry, maybe subconsciously because my father had talked about psychiatry so much and I had seen him working, studying, writing, seeing patients, and heard his stories about them. So maybe this also helped. Finally I decided to take psychiatry and I think I made the right choice.

I: Do you have any regrets?

TO: Actually I don't have any regrets. If I went back again, I would choose neuropsychiatry or psychiatry as a speciality. I wouldn't choose any other branch, definitely not surgery.

I: Who were your role models, heroes, or heroines?

TO: My key role model while growing up was my father, as a physician, as a professor, as a psychiatrist, and as a teacher. Another role model was my uncle; he was completely the opposite. He was a person who worked with art; he wrote 42 different books related to different cultures; for example Japanese art, Chinese art, Pharaonic art, Islamic art, and he also undertook an extensive study on various Italian periods and styles such as the Renaissance and the rococo. He was an artist, a historian, and a researcher. He was also a very patriotic person and was extremely passionate about everything he did. I learnt a lot from him, what it means to be a patriot, and how important it is to be passionate about what you do. I also learnt that I have to love and enjoy whatever it is that I am doing, and that success and money have to be accompanied by self-satisfaction and a feeling of purpose. Another person who influenced me is my mother because she is very caring and very giving. She will always go out of her way to do things to make other people happy without expecting anything in return. She taught me empathy and compassion.

I: Do you have any lasting impression about patients?

TO: There are two patients that left a lasting impression on me; the first patient was very well-educated and had achieved a high status in his work. He was the director of one of the most important sporting clubs in Egypt. He came to see me when I was a junior doctor, working as an assistant to a professor. This patient was severely depressed. It was very strange for me then, to see a person who had so much power, money, and influence and had so much control over the entire sporting club, with so many people working under him, suffering from depression. As a result of the depression all his achievements lost their meaning and his lack of motivation and lack of energy were the only things apparent; it was as if his soul had been taken away from him. Seeing this was an eye-opener for me and helped me reach a deeper understand of the suffering of a patient with depression. After his improvement he was discharged from the hospital and he came back to follow-up three or four times. Unfortunately, he stopped following up and stopped taking his medications. Six months later I learnt that he committed suicide by burning himself. This was a personal shift in my understanding of depression and how a person can be so demoralized that he reaches such a state. As a young doctor this experience motivated me to focus and specialize in mood disorders.

The second patient was suffering from schizophrenia; he was delusional and had the belief that aliens were withdrawing his blood. I watched the patient in the ward, saw how scared he was, always making sure that he was standing next to a wall not next to a window so that he was safe, and how his behaviour was altered. We would call it bizarre behaviour but for this patient it was not bizarre, he was genuinely afraid that aliens would take his blood. So when he went to the bathroom he would stand away from the windows, shower away from the windows, walking in corridors he used to crawl to avoid windows. All his behaviour reflected the fact that he was living in his own reality. The concept of psychosis changing someone character so much was for me, in my early years, shocking and it showed me the extent of the deep suffering of mental patients. Although in schizophrenia the rapport with the patient is weak, these patients are suffering just as much as patients with other disorders.

I: Are there any memorable occasions in the practice or the research of psychiatry apart from these patients?

TO: I have a lot of nice and memorable occasions. The most important of all was in 1997 when I had the chance to travel to the University of California in San Diego and I worked in the international mood centre whose director then was Professor Hagop Akiskal who was the one leading researchers in mood disorders, more specifically in bipolar disorders. I had the opportunity to go and work with him and learn from him. At that time he was constructing the temperament scale and I helped him translate the scale from English into Arabic. It was a memorable experience for me. I got to experience the process of research hands-on, how it starts with an idea, and how different people connect with each other like cogs in a machine in order to produce research. In Egypt, we don't have this system, so the researcher himself has to be the writer, the translator, the person who collects samples. I learnt the entire process of how to set up a research unit. I'm very lucky that I went there when I was very young, just after I had finished my doctorate, and it made me realize that I must implement this process if I ever wanted to work in research and get published.

I: How has psychiatry changed in your time?

TO: I'm not very old so it hasn't changed that much, but at least when I started working, I witnessed moving from the old method of delivering ECT to the new method of monitored ECT via machines that monitor EEG, ECG, and EMG. The concept of giving adequate or inadequate seizure to all parameters related to it was also taken into consideration. The introduction of other physical therapies such as rapid transcranial magnetic stimulation was also being introduced at the time. I also think one of the most important things was the decrease of stigma. I heard about the stigma about psychiatry that was present in the 1950s, 1960s, and the 1970s and then I watched its gradual decrease in the 1980s, 1990s, and the new Millennium, and how people's acceptance of the terms 'mental illness' and 'psychological problems' has changed for the better, but still needs improvement. I believe change is taking place currently at a fast pace, whether it is related to pharmacogenomics or the connectome; psychiatry will change and will improve, and I hope that I will at least be able to witness the early parts of this change.

I: What are your views on the current state of psychiatry?

TO: I think currently psychiatry has a problem. Other specialities are becoming involved in treatment methodologies of psychiatry. The pharmacologists are interested in psychopharmacology. Some psychologists are interested in prescribing medication, while others are working with different forms of psychotherapy. Life coaches are now saying that they can do things better than psychiatrists. So psychiatrists have to find their identity, they have to find something that others cannot do for themselves. If you talk about psychotherapy, psychologists will say they can take this on; if you talk about ECT then an anaesthetist might say that they can take this on. We have to find or redefine ourselves. I think one of the biggest mistakes to have occurred in psychiatric departments around the world is that they abandoned organic psychiatry, they abandoned neurology, they abandoned medicine, and they only study psychiatry. So psychiatrists are becoming more of social psychiatrists than biological psychiatrists. To earn a degree to become a psychiatrist, I think you have to understand medicine, you have to understand neurology, and you have to understand psychiatry. Without the presence of these three, you'll never be a good psychiatrist. This is the only way that we can ensure that psychiatrists will not become an endangered species, if they do not change the way psychiatry is taught, the way it is being examined at the moment.

I: Is psychiatry brainless or mindless?

TO: I think it has to be brainful and mindful. Psychiatric disorders are secondary to changes in the biology of the brain; this is important as we know what an important role brain biology plays in depression, regarding the hippocampal size, the changes that occur, the neurogenesis; this is all brain pathology. But at the same time, the mind is related to how things are created, how we think, how patients hallucinate, how patients are deluded. There was a time when it was mindful and brainless, and then it became brainful and mindless. The best approach is for psychiatry to be both mindful and brainful.

I: What do you see as problems with psychiatry?

TO: As I mentioned earlier, one of the main problems I think is with training. We are training our residents more in social psychiatry. It's like tubular vision, as if you're looking through a microscope. I'm very lucky that I trained as a neuropsychiatrist until I finished my master's degree in both neurology and psychiatry. I believe without the presence of neurology in my training I would have not been a good psychiatrist and I've seen a lot of programmes where the method of treating patients proves that they have never seen organic psychiatry, never seen neurology patients. I think this is a big deficit in the training of psychiatry.

I: Mentioning training of younger doctors, how would you improve recruitment in psychiatry?

TO: Recruitment has to start with undergraduate teaching which is essential. All medical schools have to teach psychiatry at an undergraduate level and it has to be presented as a biological, not a social or psychological branch. Undergraduates have to understand about brain pathology, neurotransmitters, signs and symptoms, pharmacotherapy, and not just try to explain psychiatry from a psychoanalytical or cognitive approach; this is for postgraduates. A biological approach is essential because all medical students have entered medicine to learn the medical concept and approach and not because of the psycho-social-biological model that we promote in psychiatry, so maybe a little more influence could be placed on biological psychiatry at the undergraduate level to encourage students to take up psychiatry. Another thing is that the people teaching undergraduates should be the most experienced and senior psychiatrists, those who are charismatic and able to draw students into choosing psychiatry. As long as we're allowing people who are not as charismatic, or not very interested in teaching, to teach undergraduates, we cannot expect change as this will cause students to leave for other branches of medicine. To sum up, I think charismatic professors and taking a biological approach within undergraduate teaching are the two things that will attract more students into psychiatry.

I: What do you see as characteristics of a good psychiatrist?

TO: I think a good psychiatrist should first have some personality traits like being slightly extrovert, slightly talkative, cultured, flexible, in order to accept, deal with, and discuss different views and opinions that are not their own. They should also be able to understand different cultures as well as religion and spirituality, especially now that the world has become one village and you have to deal with patients from different countries around the world. At the same time, a psychiatrist should be persistent, knowledgeable, and reliable. Patients and, particularly in our part of the world (Africa and the Middle East), relatives and families of the patient always feel that doctors and psychiatrists are sort of their backbone when the patient is ill. The ability of a psychiatrist to convey information to the patient and to their family in a scientific manner needs good communication skills. That is why having all these traits help in making a great psychiatrist. You can be a good surgeon even with very poor supportive psychotherapy and poor doctor–patient relationship because your skills here are in your hands, but this is not the case in psychiatry.

I: What do you see as gaps in the practice of psychiatry?

TO: The most important gaps in the Middle East and Africa are the number of psychiatrists, clinical psychologists, nurses, and psychiatric social workers who make up the mental health team which is not available in most countries. Another thing is that most countries in the Middle East and Africa should try and put at least psychiatric disorders into their primary care units. Luckily in Egypt we now have the new National Insurance system that is being implemented, and this will include psychiatric disorders. As long as psychiatry is considered as psyche and other medical disorders as soma, psychiatry will be considered of less importance to the body's proper functionality. If we are able to convince the policy-makers and are able to push our colleagues to convey the message that the body and soul are connected, the mind and the brain are one and the same, and that the organ that is sick in psychiatric disorders is the brain, then we will be able to change the practice of psychiatry. Increasing the number of psychiatric clinics in general hospitals in Egypt, the Middle East, and Africa will help in destigmatizing psychiatric disorders and help increase its acceptance.

I: What do you see as gaps in training in psychiatry?

TO: The gaps in training are that psychiatrists are trained as a biological psychiatrist, a social psychiatrist, or psychotherapist. In many residential training programmes, a resident might become certified in psychiatry and have never seen or given an ECT session, a person can finish training in psychiatry without completing a psychotherapy course with a patient. You will find that in many psychiatric departments in different countries, psychiatrists are purely biological, purely social, or purely psychological. I think psychiatric training should be eclectic and they should study all of these together. The presence of cultural psychiatry and spirituality is also very important. You should learn to respect and understand other people's beliefs, whether religious or spiritual, and never make fun of such things, because for patients these are essential. If you do make fun of them, this will negatively affect the doctor–patient relationship. So understanding the patient, understanding culture and spirituality besides the cultural syndromes we have in the ICD and DSM will help people understand each other, and help psychiatrists to understand their patients beyond their textbook knowledge and studies.

I: How do you think psychiatry's social contract can be delivered?

TO: I think that society, stakeholders, and family members now expect the psychiatrist to do more than they actually can. Unfortunately, psychiatrists have accepted the responsibility of talking about and dealing with things that they're unable to manage. So everyone believes that psychiatrists have magical solutions to all medical, social, and intellectual problems; if people are bad at school, psychiatrists will help, and they will help with deviant behaviour, crime, well-being, and many other things. People should understand what the actual job of a psychiatrist is: dealing with psychiatric disorders, which is completely different from mental health and the concept of improving mental health. A psychiatrist should understand that even if a patient visits him suffering from depression or schizophrenia, there has to be a contract with the patient and his relatives about what they expect from the treatment. It is completely different if a patient is visiting for the first time after a psychotic episode, regardless of prognosis and outcome, compared to a patient who has been suffering from schizophrenia for the past 20 years, regarding the outcome and prognosis. We as psychiatrists should know our limitations, what we have to do, and the stakeholders and society should realize that we do not hold the wisdom that will solve all social and economic problems.

I: What would you tell your younger self?

TO: I would tell my younger self to take psychiatry again and that studying and working in psychiatry is a lifelong journey. There is no need to rush in order to complete anything, like finishing exams, looking for promotions, publishing; everything will come in its own time. However, never forget that as a psychiatrist, you are a doctor with responsibilities towards your patients, but at the same time, you have a family, you have friends, you have colleagues, and you have a life outside your practice. There will be a time when work can be overwhelming, and you might end up neglecting the rest. So, you have to try to compromise between work, physical activity, social interaction, and hobbies; this will make you a better person and an even better psychiatrist.

I: What would you tell trainees of today?

TO: I would tell them the same thing because most trainees today are very impulsive; they want to finish everything quickly. Unfortunately, due to the problems in economy, finances, daily living, stressors, all trainees want to make money quickly, which might make them more concerned about their social status than their educational status. Education takes time; psychiatry needs experience, it needs time with patients. Current psychiatrists are always looking for quick answers. Residents today want to fulfil the criteria of ICD-10/11 and DSM-IV/5 without actually looking at the psychopathology of the patient, the delusions, or the hallucinations; they just want to tick everything off their list and finish their paperwork. Once they finish ticking all the diagnostic boxes, they're ready to move on to the next patient, and so on. This will not help them become good psychiatrists in the long run. Also, the future of psychiatry is very promising with the introduction of pharmacogenomics in psychiatry, the work on the connectome, the possible introduction of nano-psychiatry within a few decades, and the approach towards personalized psychiatry. There is a lot waiting in the future for both psychiatry and junior psychiatrists.

I: What would you like to be remembered for?

TO: I would like to be remembered for being a good teacher and being able to transmit knowledge to my students. One day when I'm no longer here, I would like my students to remember me for the things that I have taught them, not just as psychiatrists but as professors, as a teacher, as part of a scientific community, and that they are able to help their students and help pass on knowledge to the younger generation. I would like to be remembered as someone who tried to help his patients and for being a good friend, husband, father, and hopefully grandfather.

I: Which of your achievements are you most proud of?

TO: On an academic level, I'm very proud that I was the youngest zonal representative for North Africa in the WPA and the youngest executive committee member as well, and the second WPA executive committee member one from Egypt after my father Professor Ahmed Okasha, who was President. I'm also proud that I was chosen as the chairperson of the supreme committee of higher education for promoting all professors and assistant professors in psychiatry in Egypt. I am also proud that I am the Editor-in-Chief of the highest ranked psychiatric journal in Egypt and the Middle East, the *Middle East Current Psychiatry Journal*. On a personal level, I am very proud of my daughters Salma and Nada who have both finished their university degrees, their diplomas, and their Master's degrees, and are starting their doctorate degrees.

I hope that I can accomplish more things that I will be proud of as well, and hopefully we can discuss those accomplishments in the future if there will be further editions of this book.

17
Maria A. Oquendo

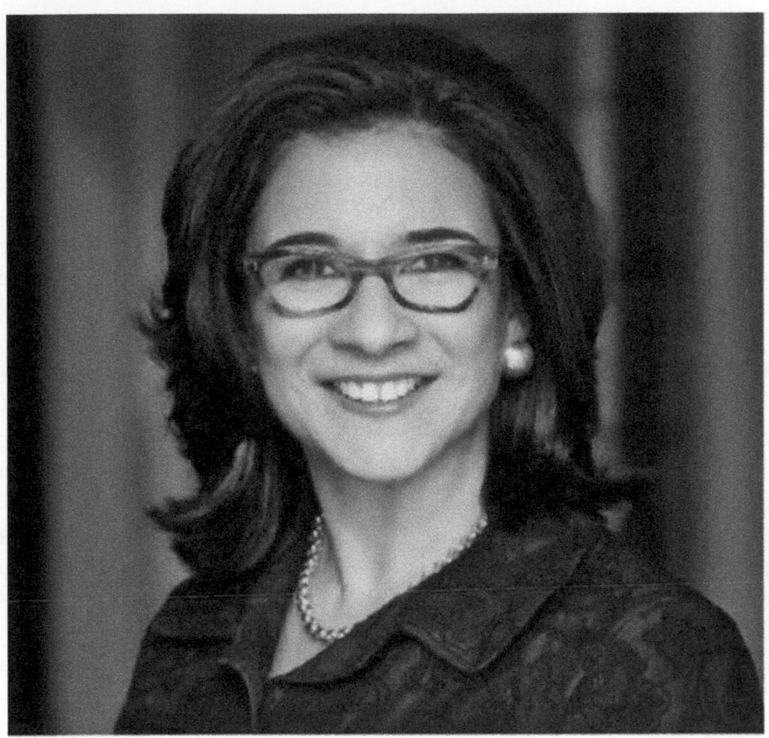

Biography

Professor Maria A. Oquendo is the Ruth Meltzer Professor and Chairman of Psychiatry at the Perelman School of Medicine at the University of Pennsylvania and Psychiatrist-in-Chief at the Hospital of the University of Pennsylvania. Dr Oquendo graduated Summa cum Laude, Phi Beta Kappa from Tufts University in 1980. She attended the Vagelos College of Physicians and Surgeons of Columbia University and completed her residency training at the Payne Whitney Clinic of New York Hospital Cornell. Until 2016, she served as Professor of Psychiatry and Vice-Chairman for Education at Columbia University and the New York State Psychiatric Institute. In 2017, she was elected to the National Academy of Medicine, one of the highest honours in the fields of health and medicine.

Her expertise is in the diagnosis, pharmacologic treatment, and neurobiology of bipolar disorder and major depression with a special emphasis on suicidal behaviour and in global mental Health. Internationally known for neurobiological studies of suicidal behaviour, Dr Oquendo has used Positron Emission Tomography and Magnetic Resonance Imaging to map brain abnormalities in mood disorders and suicidal behaviour, to disambiguate common and divergent biological contributors to each. In 2003, when issues regarding antidepressants' potential risk for inducing suicidal behaviour first arose, Dr Oquendo and colleagues were commissioned by the Federal Drug Administration (FDA) to develop a classification system to examine suicide-related events in the data. This system is endorsed by the FDA and Center for Disease Control (CDC) and now used worldwide. Dr Oquendo first proposed suicidal behaviour should be its own diagnostic category in 2008. Arguing it would facilitate tracking of high-risk patients in medical records, she succeeded in adding it to DSM-5's appendix in 2013. Critically, this conceptualization addresses the fact that suicidal behaviour occurs in conditions from schizophrenia to autism, not only as a depressive symptom. Her research to support its validity and reliability as a diagnostic entity is ongoing. She has authored or co-authored over 400 peer-reviewed publications and has an h-factor of 76 with over 17,000 citations

Dr Oquendo is a past-President of the American Psychiatric Association (APA) (2016–2017) and the International Academy of Suicide Research (2016–2017). She also served as President of the American College of Neuropsychopharmacology (ACNP) (2019–2020) and of the American Foundation for Suicide Prevention's Board of Directors (2019–2023) and has served on the National Institute of Mental Health's Advisory Council (2009–2013). She is a Fellow of the ACNP, APA, and American College of Psychiatrists (ACP). Dr Oquendo is a member of Tufts University's Board of Trustees, serves on its Executive Committee, and chairs Tufts' Academic Affairs Committee.

A recipient of multiple awards in the United States, Europe, and South America, her awards include Exemplary Psychiatrist Award from the National Alliance for the Mentally Ill (1993); Award from the National Alliance for the Mentally Ill for Commitment to Multicultural and Underserved Communities (2002); Gerald Klerman Award from the Depression and Bipolar Support Alliance (2005); National Hispanic Medical Association Hispanic Health Leadership Award (2009); Sociedad Espanola de Psiquiatria's Miembro de Honor (2009); Simon Bolivar Award, APA (2010); Rafael Tavares Award, Association of Hispanic Mental Health Providers (2010); Honorary Professor at Universidad Peruana Cayetano Heredia, Lima, Peru (2011); Stengel Award from the International Academy of Suicide Research (2013); Honorary Member of the Sociedad Colombiana de Psiquiatria Biologica (2014); Honorary Member of the Sociedad Española de Psiquiatria Biologica (2016); the Virginia Kneeland Award for Distinguished Women in Medicine from Columbia University (2016); the Award for Mood Disorders Research from the American College of Psychiatrists (2017); the Alexandra Symmonds Award (2017); the Research Award from the American Psychiatric Association (2018); the Dolores Shockley Award from the American College of Neuropsychopharmacology (2018); Gerald L. Klerman Senior Researcher Award, Depression and Bipolar Support Alliance (2020); and the Alexander H. Glassman Award, Columbia University (2021).

Interview

I: How are you? How are things where you are?

MO: I'm OK, hanging in there.

I: What's it like Philadelphia, Pennsylvania in the middle of the pandemic?

MO: It is really insane with the pandemic and then, on top of that, there is the unrest regarding racism in the United States. I do hope that there is lasting interest in making some real changes. The other thing is, and you may be experiencing this too, that as a brown person, I'm often asked to be a spokesperson. I have plenty of lived experience but this is an area of academic inquiry and I'm not an expert on race relations or racism. What I can do is tell people what it is like for me. I want to be helpful, but I also want to be honest about what I can and cannot represent and say.

I: I think that raises interesting questions about the whole experience of racism, and in whatever way you classify them, your own experiences are very personal experiences.

MO: Yes.

I: And it is, whether you call it institutional racism, structural racism, or whatever, that's just on top of everything else, so we are living through very weird times.

MO: Yes, absolutely.

I: Thank you so very much for making time. The aim of the book is to try to convey the essence of institutional memory, what it has been like coming through the ranks of the profession, as it were. The observations are for the next generation, looking at the path people have taken and what it was like getting to various leadership positions and roles. As you say, people are identifying you as a person of colour and its influence on your journey to leadership. Your path has been quite different from a lot of other people. Let's start by looking at your childhood and what it was like growing up and how you got into medicine and then psychiatry.

MO: As a child, even though I obviously was a girl, both my parents were determined that I should be a physician (my father is a paediatrician). Ever since I was little, they would say, 'When you grow up you should be a doctor'. In fact, my parents tell me that when I was about three years old, I would say things to them like, 'Don't be silly, everybody knows that girls are nurses and boys are doctors'. They would encourage me and say, 'No, no, you can be a doctor'. Then I got to college and of course, because they wanted me to be a doctor, my attitude was 'I'm not going to be a doctor, forget that'. At that time, I thought I wanted to be a maths professor. I majored in mathematics. I was very interested in logic and in abstract mathematics. I also majored in Spanish literature. But, interestingly, just in case, to be safe, I took all the pre-med requirements. When I was in my third year at the university, I went to talk to one of the senior maths professors at Tufts where I was at school. I told him that although I had met all the requirements for the pre-med, I really wanted to be a maths professor and was thinking of applying for a Ph.D. in mathematics. He looked at me and said, 'Don't be crazy. If you can go into medicine, do that. Here I am, a tenured professor, and I make no money whatsoever. Just go and be a doctor'. I was really stunned. I did not expect him to say that at all. In retrospect, I wondered whether he was thinking that I didn't have what it takes to be a math professor (laughs). Anyway, the bottom line is that I then decided to apply to medical school. At that time, I had not even heard of psychiatry. I didn't even know what it was. I thought I was going to be a surgeon and when I went through my clerkships and my rotations, I was stunned at how interesting psychiatry was. And yet I was not sure whether I wanted to do it, in particular because I found it very painful and stressful to hear about all of the suffering. That is what you hear from patients. It is about terrible, terrible suffering and even though other physicians also see suffering, it is communicated in a very different way. For a while, I thought about doing anaesthesia. I had realized that I did not want to be a surgeon; that seemed just too difficult and too beastly a lifestyle. I said to myself that I would go into anaesthesia and in fact I had a position to train in anaesthesia. As I was trying to decide, I went to talk to the director of medical student education in psychiatry. I told him that I was struggling because I really liked psychiatry but that I was worried that I would take the stuff home with me and then it would be hard to be a happy person. I remember he said, 'Don't be silly—part of our job is to teach you how to manage it so you don't take it home'. So then I thought, well, that makes sense, and that's when I decided that I would go ahead and pursue a residency in psychiatry.

I: And have you regretted it?

MO: No, not at all. I think it's a great field. I think it's really interesting. One of the things that I really love about it is, even through all of the changes in healthcare delivery, that it is still one of the few specialties where you get to know your patients really well. It is like being an old-fashioned family doctor, one who knew their patients and their families all their life. No, I don't regret it at all. I think it's a great career.

I: It is quite interesting that you said that somebody who was interested in logic would go on to do mathematics. How would you say logic works in psychiatry?

MO: It works in medicine and in psychiatry because in an ideal situation you are going through very logical deliberation about what you think the patient's problem is and what you think the right approaches are. My specialty was in psychopharmacology, so being methodical and logical was extremely important. Then, of course, when I started doing research mathematics and logic were extremely useful. They provided a strong foundation for how to reason through problems and come to conclusions that can be supported. That is extremely important in the scientific endeavour. Another thing that happened is that as I learned more mathematics, my writing prose got much better. At the time I was puzzled by this, but it makes sense because if you are writing prose and writing papers, irrespective of the topic, the more the internal logic of your arguments remains intact, the more compelling the papers are. I think it really helped me with my scientific writing.

I: What attracted you to psychopharmacology?

MO: I thought that it was really interesting that you could change people's mood, perceptions, and their lives using targeted psychopharmacology. For example, you might have a patient who was depressed and hopeless and thought that there was no point to life, and then, in response to medication, the patient could actually change and feel very differently within a relatively brief period of time.

I: And while you were doing medicine and then subsequently psychiatry, who have been your role models, heroes, heroines?

MO: I think one of the most challenging things, even when I was in school which is not all that long ago, is that there was a lack of female role models. That was a really difficult issue and so many of my role models and mentors until very recently have been men. Someone who was extremely helpful to me in my early career as a researcher and continues to mentor me and is a great sounding board is John Mann who is a professor at Columbia. He taught me everything I know about research and he has been a fantastic mentor to me. Even at times when I thought I was going to quit, that it was all too difficult, he would work with me and talk to me about the importance of sticking with it. He continues to be very important as an advisor.

I: Looking back on your clinical work, what kind of lasting impressions do you have? Who was the kind of patient that you remember the most? There are some people who leave an image on the mind.

MO: I had a very small private practice until recently. I guess I would generally say that I don't know if the patients always appreciate how attached the doctor can become to them. And because I treated chronic mood and anxiety disorders often, I would treat patients for years. I could talk about any number of them but to really give any detail, I would have to ask for their permission. It was always interesting determining how to assist people in the best way. Some people really wanted to work hard and get better. Other people were afraid of what it might be like to give up the role of being the sick person. That is not to say that they were making themselves sick on purpose or anything like that, it's just that for someone who has been depressed their entire life, it's very difficult to imagine having a different life or perspective. There are several patients with whom I worked for 10 to 15 years and finally was able to get them better. Those were really, really rewarding situations.

I: Have there been any 'Eureka' moments in research?

MO: Yes, it won't surprise you because I was very interested in maths that I loved doing the statistics myself. I particularly loved that I was the first one to find out what the answer was (laughs). But of course now I work with statisticians because they can do statistics in a much more sophisticated way than anything that I could do. I think perhaps the most surprising thing that we found was something that we published in 2013. We were working on this model of suicidal behaviour which was based on the stress-diathesis hypothesis of suicidal behaviour. The idea was that individuals who are suicidal have a diathesis, a disposition towards thinking about suicidal thoughts and acting on them. Thereafter, that predisposition, which included things like having a tendency towards aggression or irritability or having a more pessimistic outlook, would result in suicidal behaviour in the context of stressors or triggers. We were conducting a longitudinal study of 400 patients. We looked at the interaction between these various predisposing factors or the diathesis and the stressors or triggers in the subsequent years. What we found was really surprising. Certainly the predisposing factors had some influence, but we felt pretty confident that people would be at the highest risk it they had both the diathesis and had a life stressor during the follow-up period. But that's not what we found. What we found was that some individuals appeared to have suicidal behaviour in the context of one or more stressors, but for others, we couldn't identify a stressor. This latter group made suicide attempts in the context of having an active depression. We did not find that people who had both stressors and a depression were at higher risk; there was not an additive effect. Thus, it seemed like there were two different paths towards suicidal behaviour. This observation and finding led us to develop some models with subtypes of suicidal behaviour with different biological underpinnings. And in fact we published a paper about predictors of stress reactive suicidal ideation and that people who show stress reactive suicidal ideation tend to continue to exhibit it over two years, suggesting it is a trait. Our hypothesis was that people who have a lot of variability in their suicidal ideation and have large increases in suicidal ideation in the context of stressors tend to have more impulsive attempts that are less planned (we are still collecting data on this). On the other hand, we hypothesized that there is another type of individual who has a more steady-state suicidal ideation, chronic ideators for example. These are people who are much more methodical and plan carefully regarding their suicidal behaviour. Their suicidal behaviour occurs outside the context of a stressor (i.e. a stressor is not what brings it on). We often read about this type in the news, reports of suicides where everything seems to be fine, and the suicide came out of the blue, there was no particular thing that had happened to trigger it.

I: When did you go into psychiatry?

MO: I started my residency in 1984.

I: You are far too young. In your view, in the last 36 years how has psychiatry changed in that period?

MO: I think there's been a really salubrious shift towards measurement-based treatment, towards evidence-based interventions. I think we still have a lot of work to do but I believe that those are really good outcomes. I am also very excited for new developments in psychiatry. For example, here at Penn we are developing and implementing models of care that are integrated into the work that internists and surgeons are doing. In this way, we can reach the patients ideally before they are so ill that they need specialty care. Also, some people never get that ill but still are suffering a lot and deserve to be treated. So I'm very excited about those types of models and figuring out how to make them work from a financial standpoint so we can afford to deliver them.

I: What are your views on the current state of psychiatry?

MO: I have some views that I think might be unpopular. I believe that we as psychiatrists need to be realistic. There are not enough psychiatrists even in countries like the United States. For example, the Organisation for Economic Cooperation and Development estimates that ideally you want to have between 15 and 20 psychiatrists per 100,000 population. And in the United States we have 13 and it's been dropping. The last calculation which was done by a different organization, I think, found that we were down to 11 per 100,000. Hence, we need to be realistic. We cannot be the only ones prescribing psychiatric medication in specialty settings. I think that nurse practitioners and other biologically trained individuals need to be able to prescribe because we are never going to be able to see all the patients that need help.

I: In your view, is psychiatry brainless or mindless?

MO: (laughs). Well, I hope it is neither because I think of the brain as the seat of the mind. For us, as sentient beings, it is impossible to imagine that our feelings and perceptions are chemical reactions and electrical processes that are happening in our brains. Whether we like it or not, that's true. But that doesn't mean that the mind isn't real or doesn't exist, it just happens to have a biological seat.

I: In psychiatry, one of the big tensions has been the push from NIMH on RDoc criteria, that if you can't demonstrate biological underpinnings then the disease doesn't exist, that takes it to an extreme that everything is biological.

MO: Well, we do know that experience is extremely important but it does have a biological impact. Every day, we understand more about how that happens. There appear to be many pathways through which the environment impacts biology, whether it is through modifications to the genome and epigenetics or through inflammation. We now know that these types of processes can lead to changes in the hypothalamus and adrenal–pituitary axis, for example. We are understanding more and more how experience actually impacts people's well-being and mental state, but in the end it is biological. At least that's my view. I think that the RDoc initiative is a really interesting initiative but I think it is a hypothesis. We don't know that it is true. I think that we just need to be cautious and not reify the RDoc concepts, just like we shouldn't reify our psychiatric diagnoses. Although diagnoses are based on centuries of observation they nonetheless may not be precise enough.

I: What do you see as problems in psychiatry at the present time?

MO: Well, I think there are lot of problems in psychiatry and they probably vary, depending on where you are in the world. I think the problem that we have in psychiatry in the United States is the lack of parity because insurance companies tend to pay poorly for psychiatric services. This, in turn, discourages psychiatrists from accepting insurance. What results is an incredibly unfair system wherein some systems of mental healthcare are covered by the insurance companies and others are more constrained by either public or private insurance. Finally, there are also cash-based practices in which what people get may not necessarily be better but certainly they have easier access to service. That's a huge problem for psychiatry.

I: And in terms of training, do you see any gaps in psychiatry training?

MO: I think that psychiatric training probably still has gaps, in terms of training residents in the biological underpinnings of psychiatry, although again not everywhere. Also, I think that there should be more training in some of the briefer therapies that are so useful like cognitive behavioural therapy or interpersonal therapy, etc. Importantly, I think that we should really train our residents, certainly in the United States, about the financial aspects of healthcare so that we have psychiatrists who are versed enough to be able to come up with clever solutions to the problems that we face.

I: I agree that training them in therapies is important and I think it also encourages people to think about transference and countertransference issues. It was something that you mentioned earlier, that one never really understands what feelings you are generating in patients and vice versa. In the United States, is there not a sort of uniform emphasis on that?

MO: I think that many programmes still teach psychodynamic psychotherapy, and certainly at Penn, we do. At Columbia, when I was there, we did and I think it's a very important foundation. I think that the issue really is access, right? When you have protracted treatments, it means that another person is not able to get help. And yet, there are brief psychodynamically oriented psychotherapies which may improve access. In fact, Luborsky developed that approach here at Penn, back in the 1970s. There are brief ways of delivering that kind of treatment and an important body of work has demonstrated their utility. I always think that if we take five or 10 years to treat one person that means there are a lot of people who aren't getting access to that clinician.

I: You mentioned earlier about the number of psychiatrists per 100,000 population decreasing. What do you think can be done to improve recruitment into psychiatry?

MO: I think there are a couple of things. One of them goes back to the parity issue. I think it's difficult. You know that medical students, at least in the United States today, graduate with huge debts and they might owe US $250–300,000— it's a lot of money. Therefore, selecting a specialty where you know your income is not going to be high is really challenging. I think that is one thing that we need to address. I think the other thing is that the amount of time that medical students spend training in psychiatry tends to be very short, in the order of four weeks out of a total of years or a year and a half or two years of clinical work. This short duration does not allow the students enough time to really understand how beautiful a field it is.

I: Do you think that the whole Cartesian mind–body dualism plays into that somehow, so that psychiatry is out on its own and the mind is out there and the body is somewhere else?

MO: Thank you for mentioning that because you are right. I think stigma still prevents many people from choosing psychiatry as a profession. In fact when I told my parents that I was going to be a psychiatrist they were devastated. They asked why? They didn't quite say 'Why don't you want to be a real doctor?' but that was the gist of it. As I mentioned, my father is a paediatrician so he, of course, wanted me to be a paediatrician like him.

I: We did a big survey of burnout in medical students in 12 countries and one of the factors that emerged from India, for example, was that there was a lot of parental pressure on people to choose specialties their parents were in so that in due course they could take over their parents' practice.

MO: Yes, that's right. That's what my father would have loved, for me to take over his practice.

I: What would you see are the main characteristics of a good psychiatrist?

MO: Well, I think that there is space for lots of different phenotypes but clearly being able to listen well and carefully is very important. Not everybody is good at that. Not every psychiatrist is good at that.

I: And are there other gaps in training at the moment? You touched on some of psychiatric training, particularly biological underpinnings, and in some places, you could have training in some form of psychotherapy but are there any other gaps that you can think of that we ought to be focusing on?

MO: I mentioned the financial aspects, learning more about how the healthcare system works. That is a gap. I also think that in many residencies people don't have the opportunity to learn to read the literature in a critical manner, and that is a problem.

I: Coming to psychiatry's contract with society, how do you think we can deliver that? The social contract is partly about certain expectations that we as psychiatrists have from our patients and public. In return, they have certain expectations about us. For example, here in the United Kingdom, the third part of the contract is with the government because they have to fund the services. In the United States it may be the insurance companies as well as the government who are part of this contract. How do you think we ought to be looking at it and how do you think we can deliver it?

MO: I think that the path forward will be through integrated models of care. I believe that we can reach many more people this way. I find younger psychiatrists really love these models. As I mentioned earlier, in our work with internists and surgeons, we give them advice about how to manage psychopharmacology, help them to determine what the diagnosis might be. They are working hand in glove with us and I think that we can have a lot more reach if we use these types of approaches.

I: What would you tell your younger self?

MO: I think one of the things that I would have never believed if someone had told me was that my career would take very surprising turns. So for example, if somebody had told me when I was starting in medical school that I was going to be completely enamoured with research, I would have told them that they were crazy. I think that the idea of keeping an open mind about opportunities that come one's way is incredibly important. A lot of times, people ask me, 'How did you plan your career, how did you think about it?' My response is, 'I didn't plan it, it just happened', but it did have to do it with a certain openness to try new things. For example, I mentioned my mentor John Mann. When he came to Columbia back in 1996, he essentially offered me a job. He had known me when I was a resident at Cornell. I tease him that he was smart because he already knew that I was a workaholic (laughs). When he offered me a job, I was in a situation where I needed a change. I had been on a teaching unit, teaching residents for a while, taking care of really sick patients. I had been doing it for eight years and it was getting a little tired. In fact, if you look at the trajectory of my career, I seem to change things about every eight years (laughs). I accepted John Mann's offer and I went into the research, not knowing if I would like it and I just loved it. Then eight years later, I was approached to take on the position of Vice-Chair for Education at Columbia and again I didn't know if I would like it but I took the job. It was really interesting and I learned a lot. And then people around the country and my Chair (Jeff Lieberman) started telling me that I should run for APA President. My response was to tell them to go away as I had a child to get into college. I kept saying that I did not have time for that, but they kept insisting. Under all that pressure, I finally agreed. It was really life changing to do that. In a very surprising way, I found that it gave me much more of a voice. And what I learned is that I love advocacy. It's one of the things that I liked the most, other than travelling and meeting people all over the world; I loved getting to know you and all that that was really fun. I was travelling regularly to Washington DC to meet politicians, to explain to them why it was important that they fund research and to keep parity. Also, why it was important that we get rid of stigma. When the opioid epidemic broke out in this country, I had the opportunity to talk to politicians about how we needed to really focus on it because it could get out of hand, which it did. That was important and those experiences were really life changing.

I: What was it like being President of the APA? It is the largest membership organization of psychiatrists in the world. The WPA is different because it has organizations as members and not individuals, whereas APA has individual members. What was it like? You said that you loved advocacy and meeting politicians but as a leader, what were your challenges and what were the skills that you brought to it?

MO: One of the things that Saul (Levin CEO and Medical Director of the APA, Chapter 9) and I still joke about is my data-driven approach and my measurement-obsessed attitude. Because the APA spends a lot of money on committees and work groups and things like that, I wanted to make sure that the money was well spent. I also wanted to be certain that we had robust products that were the result of the work of these committees. I didn't want people just meeting to talk. I wanted to see serious output. I also was very focused on making sure that decisions were based on data. In fact, Saul still says it today. 'Show me the data. If you think that's what we should do, then show me the data to prove it.' I think that was something that was very useful. The other thing that I brought was people skills. There were some minority and under-represented groups which were really struggling and not feeling connected to the APA. I really felt strongly that my job was to engage with them and spend time listening to them, and also figuring out how the APA can serve them better so that they would feel embraced by the organization. I did a lot of work on that.

I: What would you like to be remembered for?

MO: I think that I pride myself in being very fair and predictable and that's very important to me, even though my children used to say that I was boring because I was so predictable (laughs).

I: That shows reliability.

MO: Exactly. I said to them that predictable mothers and boring mothers are really good, trust me (laughs).

I: And what would you advise to the trainees of today?

MO: To keep an open mind about opportunities and to remember the reason we go into medicine for the most part is because we care about people and we want to be helpful. That is the kind of altruism that can sometimes get lost but it is an incredibly important part of being a physician. Not only because it's good for the society but it is also good for the physician. We know that altruism actually helps people be more resilient.

I: And the last question is: which of your achievements are you most proud of?

MO: I was certainly very honoured to be inducted into the National Academy of Medicine because that speaks for the integrity of my work and my scientific accomplishments. I also care very deeply about the work I do around suicide, which is not only research but also a lot of advocacy, working to change systems and things like diagnostic approaches and coding. The goal is to improve the tracking of individuals at risk.

I: Thanks very much, look after yourself and keep safe.

MO: You too, take care.

18
Michael Rutter

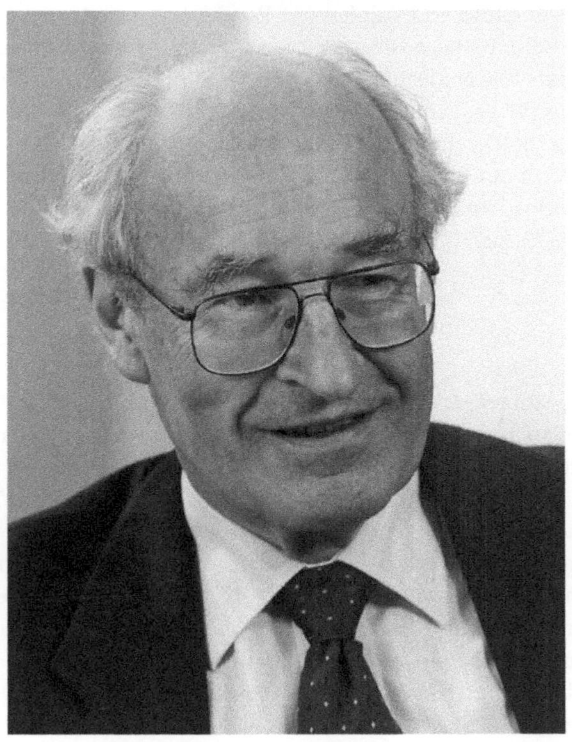

Biography

Sir Michael Rutter was true pioneer in establishing field of child psychiatry in the United Kingdom for which he was awarded CBE in 1985 and a knighthood in 1992 for his contributions to child and adolescent psychiatry. He was born in Lebanon and was evacuated to the United States along with his younger sister in his early childhood due to the Second World War. He spent four years of his childhood in the United States and saw the family he stayed with as his other family and maintained regular contact with them. After his return from the United States, initially he studied at the local grammar school and then went to a Quaker school in York. He came from a family of doctors and studied medicine at Birmingham Medical School in the UK. As a medical student he worked with Willie Mayer-Gross, which was of particular influence in shaping his interest towards psychiatry. After arrival at the Maudsley

Hospital and the Institute of Psychiatry for his training in psychiatry, he was strongly influenced by Sir Aubrey Lewis. He worked in the MRC Social Psychiatry Unit and developed further interest in child development and the epidemiology of childhood disorders. He was encouraged to spend time in the United States and returned to the Institute of Psychiatry in 1973. He was the first Chair of Child Psychiatry in the United Kingdom and directed the MRC Unit of child psychiatry. He then directed the Social Genetic and Development centre for its first five years. He edited the first major Textbook of Child and Adolescent Psychiatry with Lionel Herzov which is now in its sixth edition and has become a classic. His studies on children in Isle of Wight have become the gold standard for research in the field. His subsequent work in Romania on orphans, genetic twin studies, and maternal deprivation paved the way for bringing social genetic and epidemiological factors together. He was a prolific writer and led a number of initiatives and unique studies. He was a true pioneer in the field and helped establish child psychiatry as a discipline worldwide. He passed away on October 23, 2021.

Interview

I: Shall we start with your childhood and growing up and what was it like?

MR: Well, I had an innocent childhood. I was born in Lebanon, where my father was running a community and hospital medical service focusing particularly on obstetrics and eventually we returned. During the Second World War, I was evacuated to the United States. I spent four years away from my parents with a wonderful American family whom my parents never met but they had friends in common. Although they had never met my parents, they somehow managed to keep them alive in my mind through discussions over the dinner table, but not in any formal way. We simply talked. It was a very happy time, people assume that it was very stressful to be away from my family but it wasn't. I simply had two families, both of which were wonderful. I came back towards the end of the war, just before the doodlebugs started. I got used to the drones of the doodlebugs coming in.

I went to Wolverhampton Grammar School where I was very happy. I was admitted to the Grammar school under the so-called 10% quota rule whereby 90% of the children were selected on the basis of exam score. The headmaster had the right to choose the 10% and I was selected because I had none of the schooling that was relevant. I came in at the bottom of the fifth stream and I was near the top of the third stream at the end of the first term, this was a tremendously morale-boosting experience. I moved from there because they didn't do biology which seemed quite extraordinary. So I had to go to another school. I went to Woodhams, a Quaker boarding school that my father had gone to. There I jumped streams twice which was very good and again, a boost to my morale. I was younger than everybody else. I loved sports but was not good enough at them because of my age. It was basically a happy time.

I learnt to cope in a very different setting and it worked out. Then I had to consider what to do when I left school. I guess I had two sorts of main interests; medicine was one, my father was in medicine, my grandfather was in medicine, my uncle was in medicine, so it was very much part of the family. I was aware that they were very successful but also that they enjoyed medicine enormously. Curiously, law was the other alternative but in Britain we have two types of lawyers: solicitors and barristers. We don't have lawyers in the US style, and the life of a solicitor was likely to be rather boring. I didn't have the dramatic skills to be good as a barrister. So I didn't follow that path. I went on to study medicine in Birmingham, where my father had been earlier on.

Why did I choose psychiatry? Well, I would pick out one or two decisive moments, which is a little odd but I believe in decisive moments. There was Mayer-Gross who was professor but he worked away in a mental hospital there. One thing he did was to give you a patient to examine for an hour. I had to interview them and then tell him about it but I could not make head or tail of the patient. When I came to the end, I decided that I had to confess to total failure so I said, 'I'm awfully sorry. I have tried making heads and tails of the patient but it's a total waste of time and I'm sorry to waste your time too.' He asked me to go through my observations. I went through what I had observed and the patient had hebephrenic schizophrenia in the terminology of the day. He showed me that I had made all the necessary observations to come up with the diagnosis. Of course, I had not appreciated the significance of it but he converted a total failure into a pseudo-success. It was a wonderful experience, teaching at its very best. That made such a difference and meant that I paid a lot of attention to his advice. He advised me not at that interview but subsequently that I should do medicine and then to go on to psychiatry. I needed training in internal medicine, paediatrics, and neurology first, which I did. It was very good advice. One of the regrets at the present situation is that one cannot do that today. I think we have lost something by not training that way. The knowledge and the skills that I gained doing paediatrics, neurology, and neurosurgery were tremendously handy both in my clinical work and in my research. I think that has been a real loss. Can we ever reverse that? I don't know if the system will allow that to happen.

I: My understanding is that the system has become so rigid that it expects you to make decisions in your foundation year two and stick to them with loss of flexibility. In particular, the Maudsley had the expectation that you would do your MRCP before you came to train, so you had a much broader and longer period of training than you do now.

MR: Well, the longer period of training is not a bad thing at all and it's not that long. I do think that is a move in the wrong direction. It's not of course necessary that everybody had that sort of background and among the cohort of people that came with me to the Maudsley at the same time I did, some did and some didn't. We were not divided according to different experiences. The teaching at that time at the Maudsley had a number of qualities, which were very important, I think. The key teaching was done by senior people. For example, the teaching on psychology was done by Hans Eysenck. Although I disagreed with most of Hans' views, he was a spectacularly good teacher and he interested me in psychology. I ended up with a very different view in psychology to the one he would like me to have, but that didn't matter. We have now moved to a situation in which most of the teaching is done by younger people. I think that's based on a view of teaching which is mostly involved with the transmission of dry statistics. When I spent a year later at Stanford in California, I was very struck that the introductory courses were all led by international stars and they were not teaching facts but answering questions about exciting subjects and the messages to learn from these. We should be doing that but we don't. The teaching by the young people after Hans gave up was much worse. His view was biased but it aroused interest and Maudsley trainees, being the rebellious bunch they usually are, didn't feel that they had to agree with all the teachers they interacted with. Aubrey Lewis who was, of course, head of the place encouraged debate and argument. You did so at your peril but Aubrey loved nothing better than somebody who said that he (Aubrey) was wrong. You argued your case, he was pleased, and he never tried to put you down. He too was a wonderful teacher but not in the same style as the others. He established interest in multiple disciplines.

I: At what point did you choose child psychiatry? You are a pioneer in child psychiatry. You did paediatrics and neurology. Were the seeds sown then?

MR: Yes and no. If they were then I didn't recognize at that time. When Aubrey said that I should do (child) psychiatry, I did not take that very well. He was the boss and he actually knew better than I did what I was good at. One of the other lessons that I did learn from that is you don't always know what's the best (for yourself). He said that he wanted me to be an academic child psychiatrist and made two conditions. One was that I never be trained in child psychiatry. I thought that was a bit surprising but he said, 'Well, of course training is very important', but at that time the training was of a bit different quality. It did not encourage creative thinking. He emphasised 'If you are going to be a researcher, creative thinking is the *sine qua non*'.

The second was that I received training in child development in the States and I welcomed that. Of course, I learned a lot from mentors and others, so it wasn't that I lacked learning about child psychiatry, but I didn't undergo the formal training available at that time. Training now is of course much better but at that time his perspective was correct. I welcomed going to the States to study child development. Aubrey made various suggestions as to who I should work with, including Skinner which did not appeal to me particularly, and then that was put on hold until Herzberg gave an invited lecture here. He was riveting and after the lecture I went to Aubrey and said, 'That's the man I want to be trained by'. So Aubrey agreed that Herzberg was very good. He was very bright; he had trained initially in psychology and did his medical training on the side. Aubrey recognized that I had picked the right man and so the next thing of course was to get funding to do this. I had to apply for fellowships, which I did. I went and worked with him and his colleagues Alexander Thomas and Stella Chess at Bellevue Hospital in New York. Those were exciting days. It was the time of the New York Longitudinal Study on Temperament, but Herb (Herbert Birch-one of the researchers on the study) knew everything. Well, his colleagues and students warned me that he was right 95% of the time, the challenge was to spot the 5% when he was not (laughs). It was a great year and they were very generous to me, I have to say, not just Herb but Stella and Alexander as well. They were an interesting trio, nothing much in common, but they complemented each other. He was a researcher, Alex and Stella clinicians—Alex in general psychiatry, Stella in child psychiatry. But they recognized each other's different skills and each could contribute in their own way. I think it was a wonderful model and one that is good to follow. One of the things about Alex and Stella and Herb was that they knew everybody who was anybody so they put me in touch with Lee Robins, for example. They also put me in touch with Leon Eisenberg, who I see as the only child psychiatry mentor I had. Lee Robins certainly was a mentor and of course a personal friend later on; she is a sociologist. And Jerry Kane, a psychologist was also a mentor.

Mentors are different from supervisors. Mentors are there to help you develop your own ideas and creativity in a way which they should be critical and challenging but on the other hand they should not be controlling and entirely directive. I was very fortunate during that year to be working with some of the best brains in the field. The two that I have not mentioned yet are Ben Pasamanick and Hilda Nablock, who were very, very bright and challenging people. They were a great group. In addition to Lee Robins, I got to know Eli Robins, her husband, who ruled Washington University (in Seattle) with a rod of iron; he was a great challenger. Eli was fearsome, Lee was much gentler. She was a Southern lady in style and rather undervalued initially at Washington University; she was not a psychiatrist and there, psychiatry dominated. But then local people recognized her as one of the outstanding brains in the field as well as one of the nicest people in the field. She ran the study 'Deviant children growing up'. She told me that she saw smoke coming out of the chimney across the road and on asking what it was, she was told that they were burning their records. She said was, 'Hold off, I might find them interesting'. That is relevant to our situation here now because we are destroying records without any recognition that it is important to hold on to them.

I: A lot of old Bethlem case notes would have disappeared if they had not been kept. We would not have accurate historical accounts but also not been aware of evolution of symptoms and diseases and relationship to social changes.

MR: D.R. Davies gave seminars on this. One of the things he used to do in his teaching was to show a case and ask if you knew what would happen. He would ask you to predict along the line, a very interesting style of teaching. Of course, you quickly learn that you couldn't predict very easily. He was a much better at it then we were but even he found it quite difficult because unexpected things happen, the social context of the patient changes and the like.

I: You came back and went into epidemiology of childhood disorders.

MR: Well, I joined the Social Psychiatry Unit, of which Aubrey was the director, and that's when my interest and skills in social psychiatry started. Aubrey had a creative imagination. In typical fashion at that time, although I was the consultant, I was paid as a senior registrar (laughs). Well, did it matter? But obviously it didn't. I raised this with Aubrey, who said, 'Well I take your point, but do well and jobs will be found', and of course they were. He had power and clout that modern professors don't have. He recognised what he needed to do, and as I said he was a great teacher. He was also an anthropologist; he trained in anthropology before he trained in psychiatry.

I: I didn't know that, but that would explain a lot in terms kind of thinking outside the box.

MR: Yes, he did think outside the box and when you presented cases to him, he wanted you to think outside of the box too, not in a totally open-ended fashion. He, of course, had an encyclopaedic knowledge about psychiatry but also about music, the arts, and he brought this broad range of interests into his thinking.

I: How did you think he would have responded to the current fad of algorithmic diagnostics?

MR: He wouldn't have liked it (laughs) at all. No, that wasn't a bit of his style. Others might have responded positively to that I suppose, but not Aubrey.

I: When you started your Isle of Wight studies, they were through the Social Psychiatry Unit?

MR: Indirectly, yes. The leader there was Jack Tizard who, like most of my mentors, became a close personal friend. He was a very generous in letting me lead the study, together with others. We used to go down to the Isle of Wight on a Sunday evening and come back on a Thursday evening. We worked very hard, all day, all evening, sometimes into the night. But we had to get back and do our regular jobs, and so it was very hard work but it was exciting and we were learning about all sort of things. We had to interview children and their parents for half an hour to derive a lot of information. That taught me a lot about interviewing. I learned about different types of interviewing and it became an interest of mine. The later studies derived from all this, where we had to study comparing different interviewing styles in terms of what they could give you. One of the things is clear that what you need to do in order to gain facts and what you need to do in order to gain feelings are really not the same things, and there are a lot of alternatives. You need both to explore those, so we compared interviewing styles, which in itself was an interesting experience.

I: Would you say that the style for interviewing for research purposes and for clinical purposes have to be different?

MR: No, they have to be the same. In research as well as clinical work you must be open to the unexpected. If you are not, you are missing something really important and so what you need is an interviewing style which is vigorous and systematic. It has to be done in a way in which if something unexpected comes up which is likely to be important, you pick it up.

I: Do you think the use of structured questionnaires is problematic?

MR: Structured questionnaires are different. They are used for other purposes but that's not the same as the interview.

I: I see some research questionnaires get bogged down in very simple Yes/No answers which is not always straightforward.

The Isle of Wight studies became the gold standard in epidemiology. Following on from these and your work in Social Psychiatry Unit, what was the most exciting research that you did?

MR: Many psychologists, psychiatrists, and researchers want to prove that they were right about something or the other which seems to me as a foolish misguided way of thinking about things. Because if you've been right all along then all your career has been a waste of time. The research that excited me the most is where I was learning about the unexpected. The Romanian adoptee study would be an example of that. Yes, we had our expectations of what we would find, which were all proved wrong, but this didn't mean that it was unsystematic but instead that one learnt new things. For example, what was unexpected was that although there were quite serious deficits found, if the children left the relevant institution under the age of six months, we could not detect those deficits, and that was a surprise. This could be interpreted in terms of a critical sensitive period. Another thing we found was not just an increase in anxiety, depression, and conduct disturbances but what we came to call deprivation-specific patterns—things like quasi-autism, disinhibited attachment, etc. It was a style of research I think which I've always enjoyed. I would pick that as one of the most interesting studies I engaged in. The Isle of Wight study would have to be another one. It was my pattern those days to give feedback to the people who had helped us in our research. I had been giving feedback to the teachers who helped us and there was a lady in the fifth row of the class who grilled me very hard. I felt that I had a hostile critic but I was utterly wrong. What she ended up saying was that this study was very important; did we influence the children in this particular way, or were they like that before they came? She was a teacher and became a tremendous supporter of the study, comparing Isle of Wight and London when looking at schools. While we were doing the study and teachers went on strike, she persuaded her colleagues to support the strike throughout except to do the work required for our study, which they did. Therefore, the research was all the better for being a partnership, which is the way she described it. We tried to live up to that in planning future research and again that influenced me in terms of recognizing the importance of the collaborative style.

I: You said that you went to do child development in the United States. Were you tempted at any time to take up psychoanalysis?

MR: No, never.

I: Why not? Did you see it as unscientific? Did it take up too much time, time away from getting where you wanted to be?

MR: No. First it demanded an acceptance in advance of things, and so a questioning approach was frowned upon. Of course, I have been influenced a lot by Leon Eisenberg who was a wonderful man and his writings on how psychiatry had gone from being brainless to being mindless. He had the gift of the gab, but he was right and it's not just brainlessness and mindlessness that is dangerous. Psychoanalysis is a style of psychiatry which is determined in a very particular kind of way, and that's not a good thing.

I: I find one of the most exciting things about psychiatry is you can be as nosy as you want to be.

MR: Exactly.

I: At that time, did the Maudsley have a lot of psychoanalytic influence?

MR: Aubrey had chosen some of the world's best psychoanalysts for his staff and he was always up for the challenge from any one who would question him. He did not like being told that people were just coming along to say to him and others that this is the truth, the whole truth nothing but the truth. Stengel, for example, was very much a psychoanalyst but he was also a questioner, as was Heinz Wolff, so Aubrey appointed a lot of people like these (who questioned him) which was the right thing to do.

I: It sounds as though as a leader, he did not surround himself with people who were exactly like him.

MR: No. To the contrary, he wanted people who would question him, challenge him, and, as I said a while ago, you did so at your peril. But on the other hand, if you succeeded in challenging him, it would please him more than anything.

I: It is a sign of a true leader to have people around you who can challenge you, who can disagree with you rather than saying yes to everything.

MR: Absolutely.

I: From the time you worked with him and then went out to set up your own research network and research groups, how did that come about and what are the lessons for next generation? When I used to teach trainees quite often, they didn't know who Aubrey was, and I used to get quite irritated that they were not remotely curious about the people after whom these wards and buildings are named.

MR: When we were talking about naming the building here, I suggested Aubrey Lewis. Someone said, 'Nobody knows anything about him. You say that he was a great man, I will take your word for it but nobody else thinks that.' Aubrey was not somebody who pushed himself forward, but he was no shrinking violet.

I: I would guess Aubrey was one of these people who generates strong feelings.

MR: Yes, yes, he did.

I: Both of loyalty and of anger and frustration.

MR: This would be true. No, there were some trainees in my own group who were frightened of him. He would be shocked to hear that because he said he never intended to scare people, but he challenged them. I enjoyed it, I have to say, and we got on well, I suppose partly because of that.

I: You have touched a couple of times on how psychiatry has changed. Has it changed for the better or worse?

MR: Well, that's a good question but I think a complex one. We have tools at our disposal now that would have been unheard of when I first came here and that is definitely for the good. On the other hand, there is sometimes a danger that these tools are seen as an end in their own right; they are not, they are tools. So, at the time when we didn't have any of these tools, we were certainly worse off in most ways, but we were forced to think.

I: Are you referring to scans and the like?

MR: Yes, yes.

I: Biology?

MR: Biology or genetics. I make use of both of them for my research but tools should not drive research just because they are handy.

I: There are two training-related questions: one is what do we do to attract people like you into psychiatry, who may be walking away from psychiatry because it is seen as wishy-washy, unscientific, touchy-feely, and all that; and the second is about training itself—what do we need to change?

MR: Well, we have some intakes of really outstanding people here but they are largely from abroad and International Medical Graduates, so from the College's (The Royal College of Psychiatrists) point of view I think I need to be concerned. Why do we get really excellent foreigners and yet so few people from our own medical schools coming into psychiatry? I think this is because teaching of psychiatry to undergraduates is often pretty boring. It shouldn't be because there are really interesting questions and really interesting findings. Two people who were most successful in recruiting into psychiatry when I came here were William Sargent and Heinz Wolff. It would deeply shock both of them to be put in the same group, but they had an enthusiasm which was very infectious.

I: This confirms what you were saying earlier which is that nowadays, quite often teaching is done by junior people which is focused on disgorging facts only. We need to change teaching. We did a survey in 22 countries looking at why medical students do not choose psychiatry and two factors emerged consistently: one was poor teaching and the other one was a lack of exposure to clinical work. For example, some places allocate patients to medical students for six months or a year for ongoing psychotherapy which is supported and supervised by psychotherapists which appeared to improve their interest in psychiatry. Somewhere along the line, we have got lost.

MR: Yes, we have. I agree with that. Many of the brightest people choose not to take part in teaching and training. We all learn through our own experience as well as that of others. You've got to be able to make mistakes, one hopes safe mistakes, but nevertheless to avoid making any mistakes is not a good situation.

I: One of the things particularly at the Maudsley was that people came here because there were big names and they wanted to learn from them and work with them. Currently there appears to be a tension because there is an expectation that you would do x amount of clinical work and bring y amount of research grants and yet do teaching on top of that. So how do we resolve the tension?

MR: Well, it is true that you can't be expert at everything—none of us is and it is also true that the amount of time you have to spend these days on administration is too much, in my view. When I first got my Chair, it would be a dull week if I had to spend more than 10 minutes or so in the week on actual administration. That's not true today. The most skilled people have a lot to do and I think as a clinical academic you do have to work harder than most. I don't see a way around that but I think we need to try and make it possible.

I: And going back to what you were saying earlier, do you think psychiatry is mindless or brainless or both?

MR: Well, it's in danger of being both, but it shouldn't be.

I: How do we change that and what's your vision? What do we need to convey to the younger generation?

MR: The excitement of it, whether we're talking about treatments or research methods. Let's talk treatments for a moment. Methods like Cognitive Behaviour Therapy (CBT) didn't exist at all when I started here and people like Alan Kazdin and books like John Weisz's *Evidence Based Psychotherapy* were very good. They both take a stance of wanting to excite people in the potential of psychiatry, not pretending that even with CBT we have got all the answers but that we have got something good going for this. Let us make use of that but let us also be aware that there are further things which need to be done. Of course, in terms of medications it is the same sort of thing. We know that prescribing medications is better than doing nothing at all but we know very little about one medication compared with another, and I think that is a problem.

I: And your textbook which is I can say is the Bible as far as child psychiatry is concerned, how did that come about? It must have been a lot of work at that time.

MR: Oh yes, it was. The idea of it came from Lionel Herzov, I think. I don't remember it, but he was approached by a publisher to do a book on the subject and he said he would have to do it in conjunction with me. So we developed a very harmonious and productive partnership and in each edition, he introduced a way of asking questions in an enquiring way. I think each edition is somewhat better than its predecessor. The one which I had nothing to do with was the last one which was edited by Anita Thapar and Danny Pine together with a broader team, and they did it even better still. Now, the contributors to the first edition were largely from the Maudsley and the Institute of Psychiatry and that was not a bad way to start. But by the time of the second edition, it was clear that we were narrowing the field too much. It is true, in the early days that anybody who was anybody came through the Maudsley.

I: You have touched upon some of the issues and problems in psychiatry and recruitment.

What do you see as the characteristics of a good psychiatrist? What should we be inculcating in the next generation?

MR: Well, I don't know if there is such a thing as a good psychiatrist or if there's a model. I feel bad about the way that Peter Medawar felt about science. He talked about the importance of gathering facts and the importance of telling stories about what those facts might mean. If I think of the psychiatrists who I worked with or seen around the place I admire most, they all have a quality of excitement about what they do although they do very different sorts of things. I do see that the excitement is something one loses at one's peril.

I: I guess that's true of medicine as a whole. For me, something that you said earlier was incredibly important: that we should be pushing to engage our curiosity, that's what makes it fun. Patients come to us and share the most intimate, innermost things; sometimes you think you have seen it all and somebody comes along and shatters your preconceptions. It is communicating that excitement, which is important. If you were to write a letter to your younger self now, what would you say?

MR: I would say that the mentors have been hugely important in my life and I think that's not specific to me. Mentors play a huge role. Leon Eisenberg is the only psychiatrist who has been a mentor to me, but also Ernie Gruber, though not in the close way that Leon was. I don't believe one has just one mentor. I had Leon and Herb and Alex and Stella and Lee Robins, each playing a different role, that kind of broad input, I think, is important in almost everything. I once wrote a paper about the importance of being wrong. None of my friends without exception liked it. They thought that was ridiculous, a shameful thing to say but it comes back to what I was saying: if you're going to be right all along, your career is a waste of time. So, what is different about being wrong, which is good and being wrong which is bad. I would say there are very few examples where my factual findings were proved wrong. On the other hand, there are certainly set of examples were my interpretations were mistaken and I felt the need to put that right and, if I was in a competitive frame of mind, I would say you want to see the error before your competitors do and put it in right.

I: What is it that you wish that you had done but didn't get a chance or opportunity to do it?

MR: I wish I had gained skills in the things that I was not good at. I think the learning lies in the breadth of training; it is really important and that was certainly one of the things that was important at the Maudsley when I came here.

I: Looking back, and looking ahead, what are you most proud of?

MR: Well, I think like most researchers I would like to be remembered for particular discoveries I have made in the course of my career. I think actually we will be remembered for who we have trained at least as much as a particular discovery. Is it a bad thing? No, I think it's quite a good thing. Thus it is important to see that the training has an important part of what we do. I have no place in my mind for the pure researcher who does no teaching.

I: That's a very important point, who we train in a way, that is a living legacy.

MR: Yes, that's right.

I: Thank you so very much for your time and sharing your life story and thoughts. Really appreciate it.

19
Norman Sartorius

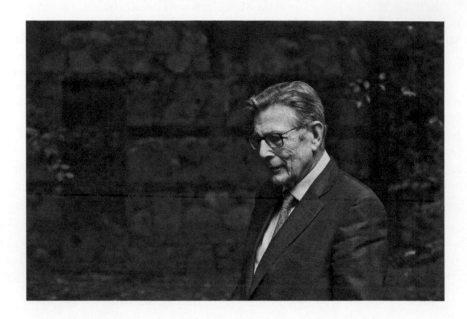

Biography

Professor Norman Sartorius, MD, MA, DPM, PhD, FRCPsych, was the first Director of the Division of Mental Health of the World Health Organization (WHO), a position which he held until mid-1993. In June 1993, he was elected President of the World Psychiatric Association (WPA) and served as its President until August 1999. Subsequently he became President of the Association of European Psychiatrists (EAP), a position held until December 2001. He is the President of the Association for the Improvement of Mental Health Programmes and a member of the Geneva Prize Foundation, having been its President 2004–2008. Dr Sartorius holds professorial appointments at the Universities of London, Prague, and Zagreb and at several other universities in the United States and China.

Professor Sartorius has published more than 500 articles in peer-reviewed scientific journals, authored, co-authored, or edited more than 120 books.

He received honorary doctorates from universities in the Czech Republic, Denmark, Romania, Sweden, and the United Kingdom, and is an honorary fellow of the Royal College of Psychiatrists of the United Kingdom and of the Royal Australian and New Zealand College of Psychiatrists, and Distinguished Fellow of the American

Psychiatric Association. He is an honorary member of many other professional organizations including Medical Academies in Mexico, Peru, and Croatia, and a corresponding member of the Croatian Academy of Arts and Sciences and of the Spanish Royal Medical Academy.

Interview

I: Thanks very much for sparing the time for this interview. In previous interviews and conversations, you have talked a bit about your childhood and upbringing which was during the Second World War. That will be a good point to start. Your childhood was quite a rough time, wasn't it?

NS: I was born and spent the first three years of my life in Germany where my mother, a specialist in paediatrics, worked at the time. As Nazism took hold, life there became unbearable and she returned to Croatia, her motherland, in 1937. She continued to work there as a paediatrician and then when the war started she joined the resistance movement and took me with her. So, as a small boy, I spent about two and a half years, from 1943 to 1945, in the forest with the partisans. I wasn't an active fighter but I was helping my mother who worked as a doctor. When the war ended, we came back to Zagreb where we experienced all the consequences of the war, shortages and uncertainties and the like. The memories of the war remained very clear for many years: one of the things that stayed with me until today is the conviction that the only way to build or develop things is to base them on friendships and trusted relationships with people. During the war it mattered tremendously whether you had somebody you could rely on. Some other memories also stayed with me for many years. For example, during the war when the enemy launched offensives the partisan troops had to withdraw and hide. When this happened, the partisans would take their wounded and ill persons (and, whenever possible, also a nurse or a doctor) into underground bunkers whose entrances were covered with earth so that you could not see them. Those in the bunkers then spent as long as was necessary—it could be weeks—waiting and hoping that the things above them would get better and that the enemy troops will leave the territory, allowing you to return to the surface. I stayed in those bunkers several times, and the memories of the time spent there remain with me. There was no light, at most there was half a potato with a little oil, and a wick that which served as a source of some light. As time went by, some of the wounded died and were covered. There was not much to eat; usually there was a barrel of water, a barrel for garbage of all types, a block of marmalade or some other food. Whenever you heard some movement on top of the bunker above your head your anxiety rose; you could not be sure whether it was an animal, a friend, or an enemy who could dig you out and kill you, as usually happened when a bunker was discovered. It was a frightening time. But it was also a time when you really learnt how important it is to have friends and have people on whom you can rely.

I: How old were you when you were in the forest?

NS: I was there from the ages of eight to ten years.

I: I recall that once you had said that perhaps it was because you were passing messages on between various groups during the war that you became very good at identifying names and faces. This has been incredibly important because you are absolutely astonishing in terms of remembering names, and not only remembering but also pronouncing names correctly and linking the name and face together.

NS: Well, I learned very early that remembering a person's name and knowing how to pronounce it was very important because sometimes if you didn't this could have bad consequences. People get very offended when you call them by a wrong name or when you pronounce their name in a funny way (laughs). People stop trying to become friends with you if you pronounce their name wrongly. Paying particular attention to names was also encouraged by my family who for many years moved from place to place because of my grandfather's occupation (he was an engineer who constructed plants in various locations in the Austro-Hungarian empire and elsewhere) and from meeting people from different backgrounds, with different occupations, and in different countries.

I: At what point did you decide that you wanted to do medicine? Was your father a doctor as well?

NS: Both my father and mother were doctors, as well as my grandfather's brother. Before them, the family always had some members who were medical doctors since I was the oldest boy, there wasn't much choice. It was to do medicine or to disappoint the family. I decided to do medicine and I think that all family members were very proud that I followed their advice and did medicine, but it was preordained by tradition that this would happen.

I: How did they respond to you becoming a psychiatrist?

NS: Before she became a paediatrician, my mother worked in the clinic of Professor Oswald Bumke who was one of the great leaders of German psychiatry at that time. Working with him, she became interested in mental illness and developed a positive attitude to psychiatry. My becoming a psychiatrist was partly a matter of choice and partly a matter of necessity. I was interested in ophthalmology but I could not get a position because they were all taken by people who were politically better connected than I was. Some of the other specialty trainings were not open at all to new graduates, others were not of interest to me, such as dermatology. The department of psychiatry was offering postgraduate training to those who were ready to work without being paid, as volunteers. So I took psychiatry. My mother was very supportive. She felt that it was a respectable discipline and never discouraged me in any way.

I: And this was in Zagreb?

NS: Yes. At that time, neurology and psychiatry were together and it was a university clinic. It was an interesting time in many ways.

I: And after that, obviously at some point you would have learnt English because without that further movement would have been very difficult. Was that in Zagreb or somewhere else? What about other languages?

NS: My grandmother as well as my mother often spoke to me in German, so German became the first foreign language I learnt. During my secondary education in the gymnasium (school), Russian and Latin were obligatory, and in addition we had to take another language. I took English and continued with it until the graduation from the gymnasium. After I had finished medical school, I started a four-year course for an MA in psychology. In those days, in order to study psychology, you had to take another set of courses for what they called a subject B. I took French as the B subject and passed the necessary exams. After that I went to conversation evenings. These were organized by the French Consulate and were events in which a small group of people spent time together in conversation with a teacher present to help if needed. That is where I met Vera, my future wife. She was fluent in French and her family wanted her to attend this conversation evenings to maintain her fluency. She was not keen to attend these sessions, in which she had to converse with old ladies, but promised that she would attend for one more year and that is where we met. Thus foreign language education can be useful, sometimes.

I: How many languages do you speak?

NS: I am fluent in French, English, German, and Croatian. I can understand Bulgarian although I don't speak it. I can also understand Italian. I used to be fluent in Russian and Spanish but I have got out of practice as I use them rarely now. More recently when Serbian, Bosnian and Montenegrinian gained independence from the serbo-croatian language I suddenly became fluent in three more languages without any effort.

I: You went into psychiatry because there was a lower level of competition. You did the first-year unpaid internship and then you obviously decided to stay on. What attracted you to stay on in psychiatry?

NS: Well, I'll first tell you what frightened me about psychiatry. In those days as students we went to a psychiatric hospital. And at that time it was like going to a museum to watch 'the crazy people'. I felt that something should be done for them. The treatments offered at that time were not very attractive. I remember my first day of my postgraduate training. I went to see my supervisor in the morning. The patients were just being woken up from insulin coma, at that time a popular treatment for schizophrenia. Often when they woke up, they would cry and shout out loud. The atmosphere did not appear to be therapeutic at all. I almost stopped going on to see the supervisor to start my training in psychiatry.

I soon discovered that listening to patients carefully and being interested in what they had to say was a powerful way of helping them. I also soon learned that the likelihood that patients will follow advice depended to a large degree on the way in which advice was given—the emotional envelope of the advice, the wish to help on which the advice is based.

I: Obviously it is very important and helpful to have good non-verbal skills too.

NS: Exactly.

I: This is what makes psychiatry really fascinating. Over the years, you have gone from strength to strength. Have there been any times when you regretted choosing psychiatry?

NS: No, I don't think I regretted that I went into psychiatry; I regretted that psychiatry wasn't what it should have or could have been. Also, when I started psychiatry, it had entered an era of hope caused by the discovery of medications. Medications seem to promise that many of the biological treatments—such as insulin coma treatment—would cease to be applied and that it would be possible to help many patients quickly, without long-lasting and complicated psychotherapy. We felt that psychiatry will become a medical discipline and that patients will, like in other medical disciplines, come to meet a psychiatrist who will be a person who would listen to them and give them some medication and reasonable advice. I think that my teachers at that time have also contributed to my optimism about the future of psychiatry. Several of them were immensely good teachers but also very good doctors with a lot of heart and a lot of knowledge.

I: Who have been your heroes and heroines in psychiatry? Who influenced you?

NS: Well, I think all of my teachers have contributed to my education. I had great admiration for Sir Aubrey (Lewis), whom I met when I came to England. I admired his encyclopaedic knowledge but even more his insatiable curiosity about and interest in people. He really wanted to know you and he really listened to you, willing to hear what you had to say. Professor Kielholz from Basel was an outstandingly good clinician with an amazing capacity to understand human problems and find solutions for them as well as being a charming and generous teacher; he was another person whom I held in high esteem and from I have learned a lot. Professor Stromgren was another person whom I highly respected; he was one of the leading people in genetic epidemiology. Many people were role models for me but these three stand out over the others, as does also my first teacher, Professor Bohacek who later became my best man at our marriage.

I: Earlier you alluded to your view that there's something wrong with psychiatry. Your regret was not that you went into psychiatry but there was something missing in psychiatry. What was that about and when did that occur?

NS: I was referring to the conditions in some of the mental hospitals and to the use of force which was a characteristic of psychiatry at that time. I saw patients who were punished if they did not behave as the staff wanted. I was struck by the fact that most of the patients were amenable to reasonable proposals yet they were considered to be out of control. We had only male nurses at that time because it was felt that you needed force to deal with patients. The nurses, and some of the doctors, saw all the patients as being dangerous. There were of course also nurses and doctors providing humane treatment and respecting their patients, but the notion of needing to protect society from patients was very prevalent and made the use of force a general strategy.

I: Over the years, how do you think psychiatry has changed? You mentioned that when you started, it was in an era of hope with the introduction of medications. Over the last five or six decades, how has psychiatry changed?

NS: When I started my training in psychiatry, psychotherapy was not very much practised nor accepted in Croatia. It was considered as an invention which in capitalist countries allowed some of the rich people—not necessarily people with mental illness—to ventilate their personal problems with a psychiatrist. As time went by, the value of psychotherapy as a treatment method became accepted. The availability of medications was also big step forward. It was not only that medications were helpful but also that prescribing them was something which was in the realm of medicine, and that led to a tremendous change of spirit within psychiatry. The question was no longer where the person with mental illness should be placed to lessen any threat they posed but what treatment would be reasonable at that point. Despite these changes, psychiatry was still at the bottom of the pile in every possible way. Mental illness and all that was linked to it was stigmatized—patients, doctors, institutions, treatments. There was less money for psychiatry than for any other medical discipline. The department of psychiatry, which was also the place where students were taught psychiatry, was in the cellar of the general hospital in Zagreb. Gradually, however, psychiatry became recognized as a medical discipline rather than a form of imprisonment.

I: One of the things that strikes me is the regular swing from social psychiatry to biological psychiatry and now to epigenetics to socio-biological psychiatry. How do you feel about these regular swings in fashion?

NS: I think that the problem is that over time, for a variety of reasons, psychiatrists have split into different subgroups. There is no common spirit in psychiatry. The psychotherapists believe in psychotherapy and those who deal with psychopharmacotherapy believe in psychopharmacotherapy even within psychotherapy there are divisions into various schools and subgroups. The discipline as such doesn't have an ethos that inspires everyone who practises it. Instead of being one discipline which allows the use of different methods of treatment, we have a group of disciplines defined by the method of treatment rather than by the type of illness which is at the focus of its attention. This tremendous variety of subdisciplines of psychiatry is an enemy that we have to remove because it does not allow us to speak with one voice.

I: How do we bring it together? One of the challenges for me in the Royal College was precisely that. Any report to the College Council, when discussed, would lead to somebody saying there is not enough neuropsychiatry or perinatal or eating disorders or whatever, so often that there was always that tension. I had the same difficulty as to who speaks for the whole profession.

NS: Many years ago, Henry Walton wrote a wonderful paper that described the loss of interest and engagement in social matters during medical education. He noted that students come to medical school with ideals and ideas about ways to help people and to be with them, to accompany them on the road to health. However, as they progress in their studies they become less and less interested in these matters—the education makes them medical doctors who know the facts but have much less empathy, less interest in people whom they treat, less feeling about their profession. I think that earlier exposure to psychiatry and emphasis on the psychological and social issues arising in medical practice would prevent this development. The problem with psychiatry and the behavioral sciences teaching during the medical studies is that students are taught these late in the curriculum and often in a bad way. By the time they come to psychiatry, students are already conditioned in a certain way. Often those who finish their medical training have a solid set of prejudices about psychiatry and do not really understand what psychiatry is about. Starting with some training in psychiatry during the first years of medical school education would make a difference. Early instruction in psychiatry is becoming even more important now that the comorbidity of mental and physical disorders is becoming more and more frequent. In the present system students learn how to recognize the physical illness and how to treat it, but not having any training in psychiatry disregarding the presence of the mental illness in the patient whom they see. The organization of medical education allows this to happen in many countries.

I: Do you feel psychiatry is brainless or mindless?

NS: Your question reminds me of another person whom I forgot to tell you that I admired: Leon Eisenberg. He wrote a paper under that title drawing attention to the fact that psychiatrists are unfortunately split into a group that believes in and practises brainless psychiatry and the other who disregard the mind aspect of their profession. I believe that this division of the discipline is harmful to its progress and makes it less useful to the people who have mental illness and less useful to society.

I: You have mentioned that there are some people who are quite interested in psychiatry from an early stage and others do their medical school and then decide to take it up. What do you think we can do to improve recruitment overall?

NS: I think that it is important to postpone the decision about the choice of a specialty and make arrangements which will ensure that medical students become physicians with knowledge about all subjects before they are allowed to become specialists. An early decision about one's specialty will lead to the neglect of many subjects which are a necessary part of knowledge and skills of a well-qualified physician.

I: And what would you see as the characteristics of a good psychiatrist?

NS: (laughs) Above all I think that it should be a person who is reasonable. A person who knows and can think rationally about the world and who can formulate options in any situation. Being reasonable is not enough: a good doctor should have empathy for other people and should be willing to understand them. It is empathy and common sense which I would put as two basic needs for a good psychiatrist. After that I would put knowledge and the mastery of the use of simple treatment methods, the simpler the better. Problem-solving techniques and the rational use of psychotropic medications could be taken as examples of treatments in that category. Skills and knowledge of this type should be sufficient to help a vast majority of patients who will be seen. If there is sufficient time and interest, the 'general psychiatrist' could learn more sophisticated methods of treatment and restrict his field of action to helping a particular group of patients.

Another area of knowledge which psychiatrists should cover is that of primary prevention of mental disorders. I think psychiatry is in part considered as less valuable because it is not doing enough about the primary prevention of mental disorders. Much of the primary prevention of mental disorders will depend on the action of people other than psychiatrists. Take the example of iodine supplementation for women in child-bearing age: if iodine supplementation were to be regularly taken by these women it would prevent severe mental deficiency in several million children every year. Iodine is readily available and pregnant women would surely not refuse to take supplements if they were advised that taking them prevents the birth of a child with an intellectual impairment. The task of psychiatrists should be to inform decision-makers about possibilities of primary prevention and in this case, insist that iodine supplementation should be a normal part of perinatal care: To be successful in convincing all those involved—government officials, perinatal care providers, and pregnant women—psychiatrists have to know about methods of primary prevention and should have the communication skills which will permit them to convince those who need to act to do so.

I: In the past you have spoken about varying durations of training necessary to qualify in psychiatry. You had mentioned that in Mongolia, one is called a psychiatrist if one works in a psychiatric hospital, even for a short time. In the United Kingdom it is seven years. What's different in the training? What should we be doing to standardize training? What do you see as gaps in training and how do we respond to that?

NS: I think that a significant part of training in psychiatry during medical school and onwards should focus on helping people who have comorbid mental and physical disorders. I would give one-third of curriculum time to learning about the recognition and management of comorbid disorders. Another third of the training should focus on public health issues. This should include training in communication skills, the epidemiology of mental disorders, and management techniques, including those of team leadership. The remaining third should be spent learning about the recognition and management of mental disorders which at present takes up most of the training time of specialists.

I: How do you think psychiatry's social contract can be delivered? Psychiatry has a contract with society, including patients and their carers and families, and it has the power in many countries to lock people up and take away their liberty. It also has a contract with the government or funders of services and has expectations from both. How do you think we ought to be dealing with this tripartite contract and delivering it?

NS: When speaking about training I mentioned that psychiatrists should acquire communication skills—to know how to speak to people. At present, very few psychiatrists know how to communicate with patients, politicians, community leaders, nurses, and colleagues although they have to speak to all these people and convince them to take part in mental healthcare programmes. When psychiatrists meet a politician or a community leader, they should be able to use that opportunity to convey clearly what they need in order to improve services. When invited to speak on television they should know how to use this opportunity to convey these needs to the audience and explain what should be done. At present, most psychiatrists do not know how to behave in such situations, how to use them for the betterment of the position of their discipline and the improvement of care for people with mental disorders.

I: Looking back on your life, what would you tell your younger self?

NS: I probably didn't spend enough time with my family: today I know that spending more time with them would have been the right thing to do. Second, I have travelled to many countries and seen many people and today I regret that I did not keep a systematic record of these travels and experiences. I should have listened to one of my uncles who told me that he has a little block of notes for each of the countries which he had visited. If he went to the same country again, he continued adding notes and so had reminders of what he saw, what he did, and whom he met. That would be also advice that I would give to my younger self. I should have also spent more time keeping in contact with the many people whom I met and whose company I enjoyed.

I: Looking back, what would you have done differently, if anything?

NS: **Apart from what I just said** I don't think I would have done things differently.

I: You started your career as a clinical psychiatrist but did not treat any patients after you joined the World Health Organization. Did you miss clinical practice?

NS: The answer is yes and no. During the years working as a psychiatrist I found work with people who came to be treated or sought information about their health and care or care for others inspiring and rich in emotion. It was wonderful when the treatment which we prescribed worked and the people got better; but even when the illness was resistant to treatment helping people who had the disease to fight it was giving me a sense that I am engaged in a profoundly humane and useful profession.

Recently I received a letter from a lady whom I have seen and whom I have looked after, in the Bethlem Royal Hospital in London when she was 18, some 50 years ago. She had seen an article in the press mentioning my name and location and wrote to thank me for being very careful about her diagnosis (most of the other doctors thought that she had schizophrenia and I had disagreed). She fully recovered and led an interesting and full life. Her letter made me very happy—she was my patient who was doing well—and reminded me of other people whom I have seen as a doctor in the early years of my career. It also made me think about the impact that a diagnosis which carries stigma can have on one's life and somehow confirmed that the fight against stigma—which was an important part of my work over many years was a wise decision.

When I joined WHO I sometimes had people come and ask for advice about their problems, but this did not replace the clinical practice which was the main occupation I had previously: but soon I found that being actively engaged in advising others how to build and develop services for mental illness (and seeing some of that advice used) gave me a feeling of being useful to people with problems and in many ways replaced clinical practice. In most parts of world the services provided to mentally ill people left much to be improved: this was true in poor countries but also for a large proportion of people with mental illness in countries which had high incomes. Advice which came from me—being a speaker from WHO—was often followed particularly also because I kept thinking and listing interventions which could be used even if there is no additional money or other support to the services. Seeing things improved was a major source of satisfaction.

I: In the WHO, you led on cross-cultural research comparing rates of various psychiatric disorders. Looking back at the reports and papers, it feels as if everything went very smoothly. I'm sure that wasn't necessarily the case. What was it like coordinating so many academics in so many countries?

NS: As I mentioned, earlier during the war years, as a child, I learnt to rely on people. Most of the programmes we undertook at the WHO were based on friendships. Having good relationships with people was both important and helpful. Recently we did a study on diabetes in which we got 14 centres in different countries to work together without being paid a penny. Now, as well as during my time in the WHO the main challenge in the development of programmes is to find people whose interests coincide, who can understand each other and who are willing to work with others. It was keeping this in mind that made it possible to run programmes and to help collaborative research grow although we had a very modest budget. Many of the programmes which we did are remembered with pleasure because they were built on friendships and on mutual respect. In our programme we almost never paid for the work which people were doing in collaborative studies and other projects. I believe that the most useful activity in my life was to bring people together and to keep them together. Keeping them together was not always easy because it was often impossible to avoid negative or misunderstood comments, dislike of a particular gesture or action, or misunderstandings. Strengthening the cohesion among all involved required constant attention. It was important to have meals together, to know and care about everyone's families, to spend good times together, to reward achievements by praise, and to listen to each other. We had the pleasure of seeing most of those with whom I worked at our home and visiting their homes as well. Programmes stayed alive because of good human relations.

I: I guess one of the big challenges is when you bring a group of researchers from different countries and different cultures who have different expectations. There is also likely to be some academic rivalry and jealousy. How do you suggest that these issues can be dealt with, particularly if you are a youngster coming through the system and you want to take part in joint thinking and joint work?

NS: Well, you have first to listen to people to understand what they really want. To get a group of five people who will do a project together, you have to speak to 50 and select those who have a similarity of interest, personality, and position features which will match. Some projects cannot be done because you cannot find enough people who are interested in participating and who are suitable for inclusion in a joint project. In those instances it is better to abandon the idea or postpone its realization. If you speak to a sufficiently large number of people, you will usually discover those who, due to their personal chemistry and their interest and enthusiasm, are willing and able to do things together. Once you have identified these people you will have to invest time and effort to create a community which will usually last far longer than the project. Some of the grandchildren of the original investigator who participated in some of our projects are still spending college holidays together. What began as a research project became a well-connected group who know one another, are willing to help each other, and like and respect the other participants.

I: What would you advise trainees of today?

NS: My advice is that they should invest time in creating strong social networks. They should join networks and try to meet people, speak to them, listen to them, help them, possibly make them part of one of their own networks. I think that developing their social networks should be their top priority. They should not be worried about what may happen tomorrow because the social networks in many ways will help them to survive. The second advice I would give them is to try to have harmony between their personal and professional life and to learn how to lead and how to follow. I would also ask them to become aware of what really drives them. They should know what is it that they really want to do and discover themselves. In addition, I would like them to acquire communication skills and of course acquire the skills and knowledge of theirtheir profession.

I: What would you like to be remembered for?

NS: (laughs) Mainly for having brought people together. I think it is a wonderful achievement when you bring people together and when they do something that is bigger than anything that any individual alone could have done.

I: You have an incredible number of achievements under your belt. Which of them are you most proud of?

NS: I would still stick to the notion that it is the number of people whom I have made work together, be together, like each other, and stay together. They have done miraculous things. One could list the results of projects which have been a resounding success, but togetherness was the real thing to be proud of. It is not that we have discovered the Moon but what we achieved we did together, we made people of different religions, different life philosophies, different experiences, and different tasks in life friends.

I: Thanks very much again for sparing the time and taking me through your life.

20
Alan F. Schatzberg

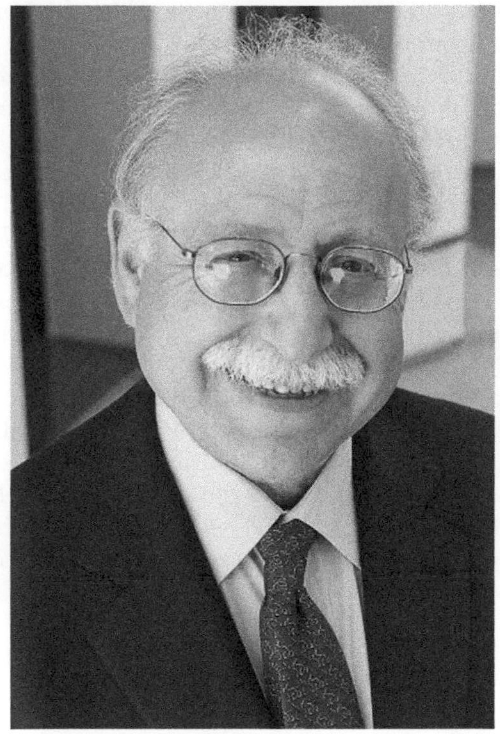

Biography

Alan F. Schatzberg received his MD from New York University in 1968. He did his psychiatric residency at the Massachusetts Mental Health Center from 1969 to 1972 and was Chief Resident, Southard Clinic in 1971–1972.

After serving in the United States Air Force, he joined the staff at McLean Hospital and the faculty of Harvard Medical School in 1974. At McLean Hospital, he held a number of important positions including Service Chief, Interim Psychiatrist in Chief, Co-Director of the Affective Disorders Program (with Dr J. Cole) and Director of the Depression Research Facility. In 1988, he became Clinical Director of the Massachusetts Mental Health Center and Professor of Psychiatry at Harvard Medical School. In 1991, Dr Schatzberg moved to Stanford University to become the Kenneth T. Norris Jr, Professor and Chairman of the Department of Psychiatry and Behavioral

Sciences. He served as Chair of the Department there until 2010 and directs the Stanford Mood Disorders Center.

Dr Schatzberg has been an active investigator in the biology and psychopharmacology of depressive disorders. He has authored over 700 publications and abstracts, including Schatzberg's *Manual of Clinical Psychopharmacology*, whose ninth edition appeared in 2019 and which is co-authored by Dr Charles DeBattista. He also co-edited with Dr Charles B. Nemeroff the *Textbook of Psychopharmacology* whose fifth edition appeared in 2017. He was Co-Editor-in-Chief of the *Journal of Psychiatric Research* and sits on many other Editorial Boards, including the *Journal of Clinical Psychopharmacology*, *Psychoneuroendocrinology*, *Biological Psychiatry*, and others. He is a past-President of the American Psychiatric Association, the American College of Neuropsychopharmacology (ACNP), and the Society of Biological Psychiatry, and was also the Secretary-General of the International Society of Psychoneuroendocrinology. He has received numerous awards, including; the 1998 Gerald L. Klerman, MD Lifetime Research Award from the NDMDA; the 2001 Gerald L. Klerman, MD Award from Cornell University Medical College; the 2001 Edward A. Strecker, MD Award from the University of Pennsylvania; the 2002 Mood Disorders Research Award from the American College of Psychiatrists; the 2002 American Psychiatric Association Award for Research; the 2005 Distinguished Service in Psychiatry Award from the American College of Psychiatrists; the 2005 Falcone Award from NARSAD; the 2013 Anna Monika Award; the 2014 Kraepelin Gold Medal from the Max Planck Institute of Psychiatry; the 2015 Gold Medal from the Society of Biological Psychiatry; the 2015 Lifetime Achievement Award of the ISPNE; 2017 Julius Axelrod Mentorship Award from the ACNP, among others. In 2003, he was elected to the Institute of Medicine of the National Academy of Sciences (National Academy of Medicine). He has received three honorary doctorate degrees.

Interview

I: Shall we start by talking about was your childhood was like, what was it like growing up?

FS: I was born in 1944 and so I grew up in a part of New York called the Bronx, which at the time was kind of a middle class and mostly had a large Jewish population. My folks fled Vienna from Hitler in Christmas of 1939 and came to the United States in January 1940. My father had been a dentist in Vienna. Dentistry was then a medical specialty and a fair number of the Jews then did dentistry because there was a lot of anti-Semitism in aspects of medicine. Anyways, he came to the United States, and he came with nothing. He had to brush up on his English and took almost three years to do this. He had graduated in 1925 from the Medical School of the University of Vienna. He did a year of internship and sat for his New York licensure exams and he became a General Practitioner in the Bronx. At first our entire family, my sister and I and our mother and my father, were all sharing an apartment that connected to the office. When I was about four or five, we moved to a more residential area but the office stayed where it was. He passed away at the age of 68 in August 1969. My sister was 10 years older than me and she was a psychiatrist too. There were very few women when she went to medical school. She was a classmate of Helen Singer Kaplan at New York Medical College at New York. Because women tended to be scarcely represented, they ended up being the smartest and at the top of the class. She did her training at Columbia at the NYS-PI. She married a man who was nine years older than she was and who was a psychiatrist. He had been on the clinical faculty at Cornell as a psychoanalyst—more of an eclectic kind of psychoanalyst rather than a neo-Freudian one. He was a member of the American Academy of Psychoanalysis. So medicine has sort of been a family trade. My father had two older brothers and both of them were physicians. My maternal uncle went from Poland to study medicine in France and then studied in Italy. He graduated from Naples and eventually went to Canada. He was a GP too. There are other doctors in the family. My sister and my brother-in-law have two daughters, one of whom is a psychiatrist, also training at Cornell. I remember, I talked to my dad about going into psychiatry, he said, 'You know, 65% of my primary care practice is really psychiatry'. That's how it was. He was fine with us becoming psychiatrists.

I: What attracted you to medicine? Was it simply because it ran in the family or was there a kind of a turning point?

FS: In medicine, I'm always struck by how many colleagues of mine who are physicians had parents who were physicians too. In those days, it was common to follow a parent's profession but beyond that, if you grow up in the context of a parent who is a physician, you become imbued by the calling. You become imbued by the sense of dedication. My father worked six-and-a-half days a week in the office. He practised on Sunday mornings too. So it just became a calling which you did. You took care of sick people and the calling to help others becomes important. I think that the combination of doing what's in the family but also the calling and trying to help people all contribute. Intelligence has a big say in the matter but I think it's really the calling, it becomes imbued in you.

I: And why did you choose psychiatry?

FS: I liked it. Well, first of all I had a sister who was a psychiatrist and my brother-in-law who was a psychiatrist, so that was one reason. The reason I chose psychiatry was that psychiatry had the intellectual curiosity of psychoanalysis, with the relationship to the arts particularly. There were the beginnings of biological psychiatry with initially a pharmacologic perspective with new drugs, antidepressants, and lithium. That really spread on to the development of neurosciences, the neurosciences of the brain in relationship to behaviour, and the behavioural sciences. So, psychiatry was not only interesting to me in terms of psychopathology but also in terms of a budding intellectual arena where impact could be great not only for developing new treatments but also for understanding a very important part of life, namely how does the brain work. These were the attractions. I went to NYU Medical School which had a very strong psychiatry programme. It had Arnie Friedhoff in schizophrenia. It had Sam Gershon in bipolar and lithium. It had Barbara Fish who was one of the leaders of paediatric psychopharmacology, and it had a tradition of psychology with Wexler and those folks in terms of intelligence testing, and the psychoanalyst Binder was there as well. So it had a tremendous tradition and that, coupled with a fair amount of New York Jews as students at

NYU at that time, led to NYU developing a fair number of psychiatrists and a fair number of academic psychiatrists. Gerald Klerman went to NYU Medical School. Richard Schader went to NYU Medical School. Eric Kandel went to NYU. There are a number of well-known academic psychiatrists who came out of NYU.

I: Do you have any regrets?

FS: About becoming a psychiatrist?

I: Yes.

FS: No, you know I think my mother thought maybe I would become an ophthalmologist as it paid better and you had an easier lifestyle. I always found surgery intriguing. I tend to think that my temperament is closer to a surgeon than a psychiatrist. But do you know why I couldn't become a surgeon. In those days you go into the operating room and you'd prep and you'd wash and then come in and you'd stick your hands in your gloves and the nurse would hold the gloves out and you do that, so the attending will go in and quickly he's ready to go. By the time I got the gloves on the team was ready to close, so I knew I couldn't be a surgeon (laughs). The other problem was that my glasses would fog up like crazy with the masks (laughs). I would be standing there and I'd start to breathe and all of a sudden, I couldn't see the operating field. All in all, surgery wasn't going to work out for me even though I've always thought of surgery as interesting. I have no regrets in becoming a psychiatrist. I think it still remains one of the great areas of medicine for various reasons.

I: You mentioned quite a few names. Who were your heroes when you were training in psychiatry?

FS: Well, I trained at the Massachusetts Mental Health Center at Harvard and there were a number of folks who were extremely helpful: Carl Salzman, who remains a very good friend, from Mass Mental Health Center is a leader of geriatric psychiatry and was among the first people to teach psychopharmacology. Dick Shader was a great teacher of psychopharmacology. Joe Schildkraut was a mentor when I became a young faculty person at Mclean in the Harvard system. We started collaborating very strongly in 1974 and we worked together for couple of decades or more, so Schildkraut was a big mentor. I knew him a bit when I was a resident and I started working with him after that. The last person who was a tremendous mentor to me was Jonathan Cole at Mclean. Jonathan and I wrote the *Manual of Psychopharmacology*, now in its ninth edition. He taught me a great deal about psychopharmacology, about writing, about taking care of patients in terms of how to prescribe and how to think about psychopharmacology in practice.

I: You said that it was an interesting time for psychiatry, particularly with psychoanalysis and biology included, and yet you veered towards psychopharmacology. How did that come about?

FS: I always had a strong interest in research. Even when I was a resident, when I started doing projects and publishing papers, I think that it was clear to me that the impact of psychopharmacology, particularly in the early period, was so phenomenal in terms of helping people to get better much faster than it using a psychoanalytic approach. That to me was extremely attractive, in terms of pursuing an area of investigation. You can actually do experiments and studies and control trials, things like that, all of which are difficult, you know.

I: Were there any kind of occasions that stick out in your mind and as really memorable?

FS: The first peer-reviewed paper that I published was in 1972 and it had to do with psychoanalysis indirectly, interestingly. It was a single-author publication in the *Archives of General Psychiatry*, published a couple of months after I finished my residency. It was a study of the trial and appeal of Wilhelm Reich. Reich was the only person to be thrown out of the International Psychoanalytical Society and the German Communist Party within a year as both institutions felt that the ideas of each were incompatible with the other. He was a cantankerous, somewhat crazy guy who wrote some really brilliant books. The first half of his book on character analysis is spectacular. It really explains the theory about how you form character structure; however, the second part gets a little wiggy. He had developed this idea about cosmic energy and he had a thing called an orgone box, a cube that he claimed could concentrate, out of the air, orgasmic energy that could be used to help patients. He immigrated from Europe, he was Jewish, and he moved to the United States. He had a retreat area in Rangely, Maine, in his 50s he was trying to sell his orgone boxes and the FDA said, 'Look, you're selling these across state lines and there's no evidence that any of this stuff works. You need to stop selling them.' He continued to sell them so they prosecuted him. He was convicted and imprisoned and he died in prison. When I was a medical student, I knew somebody who had an orgone box, a young woman and she was into Reich. I was curious about it and some of my supervisors at the Massachusetts Mental Health Center at Harvard knew a little bit about it. Then I started reading about Reich in prison and thought it was a pretty interesting story. I thought it was probably worth looking into. Because I used to do Boston Municipal Court work I could go down to Federal Court to review the papers of the case. He was tried at the Federal Court in Boston because that is the jurisdiction for Maine. I got a hold of his transcripts from the trial and his appeal. What is important is that in the middle of his trial Reich fired his lawyer, James D. St Clair. He was a very famous Boston lawyer who was Nixon's lawyer during Watergate and he was fired by Nixon because he told Nixon that what he was doing was illegal. Reich fires St. Clair and he represents himself. Then he goes to prison and writes his own appeal, it was the last thing he wrote. I studied his trial and appeal. I was a young guy. I sent the paper to the *Archives of General Psychiatry* which made some very good comments about it. They thought I was a little too negative about him and should be a little more critical about society so it ended up being called 'Wilhelm Reich: Self-Destined Victim and Social Casualty' and they published it. It was the first paper I ever published, single author in the *Archives*. My career has gone downhill ever since (laughs) for the past 48 years. I want to tell you that in the days of H factors and citations, it was one of my least cited papers but I think that is the best paper that I ever wrote. It was really good. I had a chance to reread it lately because one of our folks wrote something about Wilhelm Reich, and it was a pretty damn good paper.

I: That takes me neatly to the next question about how psychiatry has changed in your lifetime. Obviously it is much more biological with focus on publications with the highest impact factors and the influence of Altmetrics. You went into psychiatry almost on the cusp when things were beginning to shift. From a psychodynamic to biological perspective. How do you think it has changed? And do you think it has changed for the better or have we lost something?

FS: It has changed because in that it has become more scientific. We have a better sense of rigour and scientific method, we have controlled trials, we have developed all sorts of medications, we don't have enough medications, we need better medications, but we have done a lot. The field has progressed with developing new and different classes of medications with unique mechanisms of action. I think it has progressed pretty well in terms of biological psychiatry. In the context of trying to develop some rigour to diagnosis and classification, we have come a long way since DSM-III. In the United States, now we are up to DSM5. We have refined the criteria for making a diagnosis, which we didn't have before. We have a better classification system. Things used to be very vague. We have become a little too checklist-oriented and that to me is a real problem. When we used to work up patients as a resident, we would have to write an anamnesis, a 10 to 12 page report, single spaced, on that patient's history, not on just to where they were at the school and where they were born but a really understanding of the dynamic life of the patient, from their relationships with their parents, and onwards to adulthood. That helped guide a therapy or treatment plan, that was mostly psychodynamically oriented. We have largely lost that perspective. Now we have the checklist to make a diagnosis that's easy, that's good, but I wouldn't say it's uniformly optimal in reliability. It does not have much validity and thus we have a real problem. People confuse the reliability with the questions about validity and that's important. It is not just the matrix but we've become too reliant on the language that we can agree on, namely, does the patient meet five out of the nine criteria to make criteria for a major depressive disorder episode, but we've forgotten the life of the patient. It is the life of the patient that often gives you the roadmap to describe the reasons for their depression, which is usually because of social stressors. We have lost that particularly in training now. Training frequently is mindless, particularly inpatient training where patient's stays are incredibly short. Before patients used to stay a couple of months, so as a resident you really got to know them. Now, the patients stay a few days to get checked, you give them SSRIs or SNRIs, then they go on their way and you haven't made an impact on the causes for this person becoming depressed. That could be the loss of a spouse, divorce, loss of a job, a history of child abuse. Those are the things that really sculpt people's lives. We used to capture these routinely. As far as the abuse is concerned, that's a whole other issue, because I think that becomes somewhat of a male sexist approach for large number of female patients. We have lost the soul of psychiatry in some ways in the training and that is highly disturbing to me. I try to get the residents to find out something about the patients, to tell me about their life. When I do rounds, asking about the criteria and SSRIs and side effects is fine but there are little data on where are patients from, whether they have a job; I've lost count of the number of times trainees don't tell me whether a person has been working or not, when they worked last, were they successful at work, did they have any problems with their boss, what happened to them at work; that whole aspect of understanding the life of the patient is gone. We just don't have it right now, at least we don't in training. In private practice where individuals do therapy and get meds, you see it more but most psychiatrists in the

United States are pharmacologically oriented. A lot of psychiatrists do not really participate in non-pharmacological interventions and that to me is the big loss for psychiatry today in the Western world.

I: Do you think psychiatry has become mindless or brainless?

FS: It's not brainless. I mean we know a lot about the brain, but it has become mindless but I am concerned that it has become soulless. We talk about the mind but it's the sense of the person in terms, it's not just the mind, it's really the persona of the individual that they have sculpted that. We have given up talking about the mind in psychiatry.

I: I don't know what it's like in the United States regarding recruitment into psychiatry. Is that a problem?

FS: Yes, for a long time, we had about 600 people per year out of 17,000 medical graduates enter psychiatry. That's about 3.5%. About six or seven years ago this increased so there are more people today getting a grounding in psychiatry. The first reason is that the APA has worked on changing the billing codes and things for psychiatry to conform with medical practice and to have the years in Medicare. Psychiatrists could not build what's called Evaluation and Management (E&M) codes that are used by interns; we could only build the psychotherapy codes with a little bit of management. That changed, so we couldn't build E&M codes as well as in psychotherapy codes, so what that did was that it pushed up the earnings of psychiatry even when psychiatrists accept insurance which, in the United States, is not common. It pushed that up 30% automatically. There was 30% more money coming out of Medicare (which is the senior healthcare paid for by the government that affects the billing) as well as for private insurance. So that was one reason why recruitment into psychiatry increased. Two, the economy being good means a lot of people finished their residency and got into private practice which they can build at a much higher level than academics can and so private practice became lucrative. And the third reason is that medicine has become much more female oriented, in terms of producing many more women psychiatrists. Psychiatry is a good choice for women in terms of them being able to call their own working hours. So all three reasons have led to a big spurring of people coming into psychiatry. We used to fill less than half of the spots with international medical graduates in the United States. Nowadays, it is very hard for an international medical graduate to get a spot because there are just so many US graduates who want to do psychiatry.

I: Although you have alluded to it earlier, what would you see as the characteristics of a good psychiatrist?

FS: To my mind, if you're not a good listener you are not going to be a good psychiatrist. So you have to have, psychiatrists have to have patience, I mean if they have the patience to wait for patients to give you clues to their problem and to give you the answers. Be a good listener. Then you must have a sense of compassion. It takes a lot of patience to be compassionate. It is a lot easier to make sure of the sense of people and situations. Beyond that, intelligence is important, but most medical graduates are highly intelligent. That is the one thing that I think that medicine does very well, it screens for intelligence and for people who are highly educated—maybe not highly intellectual or highly creative—but they have the native intelligence to do it and the society demands that. Society wants to look up to the physician, it wants to believe that the physician knows more, has better judgement than other people. We usually don't screen for patience, compassion, the ability to listen. People who are strong in these suits exist, there is no question about this. Academic work requires a different set of skills.

I: What do you see as gaps in psychiatry and gaps in psychiatric training?

FS: Well, I think we need to spend more time on application of devices. We need to make sure that everybody coming out of training understands the mechanics of TMS (Trans Magnetic Stimulation), understands what people are doing with VNS and DBS. We need to have rotations in brain stimulation beyond ECT. A lot of places don't even require rotations in ECT in the United States but they require some exposure. When I was a resident, we were on the unit. Two residents per month did a rotation every morning for ECT so you learned how to do ECT. We don't do that much anymore. We need to teach folks about brain imaging, not just structural imaging, looking for masses and things but they need to understand functional imaging, like functional MRI, because these are not getting used more to screen for drugs efficacy and the like. We need to make sure folks are better educated about genetics and pharmacogenetics. We teach psychotherapy, still often dynamically oriented. Some programmes teach other manual-based therapies like the DBTs and the CBTs which tend to be more commonly taught now and they continue to be taught widely. We still require residents to have long-term cases on supervision or they tend to be taught dynamically oriented treatments. I think there are things in biology where things have changed for us that we need to keep up with if we are going to have a very modern, trained workforce in psychiatry.

I: How do you think psychiatry's social contract can be delivered?

FS: Social contract in terms of taking care of the patients?

I: The social contract is kind of an informal contract between funders, patients, the public, and psychiatrists, so what is it that we expect from funders and what do we expect from the patients and what do they expect from us in return?

FS: We haven't figured out how psychiatrists have to fit into the overall mental healthcare of the society. There is way too much psychopathology on a prevalence basis, and way too few psychiatrists, and that's not going to change even though we have more psychiatrists coming into the field, more people coming into psychiatry then we had before. American trend, you know, we don't really have the system set up to get beyond the guild to kind of have an effective approach, you know, to taking care of the mentally ill. Now that may change by setting, may vary by setting. Some of the problems lie in the tension between the various professions, some of it lies in the philosophical basis of treatment. You will see this in the United Kingdom where everyone reporting major depression is offered CBT, and patients who don't get CBT are offered pharmacology. You know we need something that's a little bit more logical rather than just carving out things by one group or another. The big issue for psychiatry is that there just aren't going to be enough psychiatrists to cover psychiatry. And so then the question is whom do we train? Is it the primary care physicians? They write most of the scripts for antidepressants. Do we need to train the nurse practitioners? I think that would be a natural alliance for us. The problem is that there aren't many of them compared to the number of psychiatrists. We produce many more psychiatrists than we have access to nurse practitioners so that's not our solution on a local basis. We need to figure out how to take care of everyone who has psychiatric issues. There are things that we could do that may be more or less popular. When we started in psychiatry there were two groups of patients. One group was a severely ill person with depression who was agitated, psychotic, or showing other symptoms, whom we hospitalized. We took care of him well, unusually well with tricyclics or ECT. And then there were others—the walking worried—who were largely taken care of by psychoanalysts and some psychotherapists. So the field was defined as a very different field. We also had patients with schizophrenia, we had bipolar disorders. There is a problem with DSM by its having criteria for a disorder such as major depression that can be met by a certain percentage of people. Thus, we have had a lot of depressed people because they meet the DSM criteria. Maybe those are people who don't need the treatment. Maybe on a society-wide basis, we need to have greater acceptance of varying degrees of psychopathology that can be targeted by social reforms. We never talk about that. We talk about the shortages of caregivers so maybe we need a social kind of solution to help people. We see this now with the riots that are going on in the United States that are not just about police brutality. The riots are really about people who are truly being disadvantaged. They don't have jobs, they don't have their education, they don't have healthcare. Fifty per cent of some groups of people under the age of 30 in the United States are people of colour. They are not necessarily Black, they're Latinos, they're Asians, they are people of colour. I'm not talking about the Italians, Jews or whatever, they are Caucasians now. The disadvantaged grow up in a very different environment, they expect diversity, they don't see any reason for why there should be White privilege. We need a social system that supports performance and people feeling better, so then in fact there is less burden placed on the psychiatrist. Then we need to do something about child abuse. We need to think through our substance abuse policies. These are largely social issues and they often lead to a diagnosis of depression. Maybe if we had taken care of the social issue, if a person had a job or wasn't going to be destitute, maybe they wouldn't be so depressed.

I: What would you tell your younger self?

FS: Here is what I tell the residents, when they are starting out: psychiatry is very different from any other specialty. You are handed a privilege, and that privilege is to hear about a person's life, the things that are good, the things that are bad, the things that ail them, their disappointments, their stress. That is a privilege and that privilege needs not only to be respected but you need to do something with that privilege. It doesn't have to be psychotherapy, but it has to be an understanding of that person. When I see a patient, I want to know what's happening with them, I want to know where they went to school, I want to know what's happening with their families, what's happening with their kids. I want to be able to say, 'That's good' or 'That's difficult. Is there anything I could do to help?' I may be too chatty but it's a privilege for somebody to open themselves up to you and that always needs to be respected. It also needs to be a motivation for people so they understand the pain the person has. They can hopefully do something to help that person eventually; it could be pharmacologic or psychosocial. The psychiatrist could do things where they might avoid hurting the person by saying something without thinking that somebody might feel as hurtful or insensitive. I think that getting a sense of people is crucial. This moves us on to being a good listener, being patient, and being non-judgmental. Those are difficult things for people to develop. So I would emphasize trying to understand patients. We spend a lot of time, historically, in psychiatry on countertransference which is if somebody's acting like a jerk with a patient—you might better understand your countertransference, I agree with that but a lot of countertransference is that people being impatient with trying to understand what's eating into the patients. It's not just not understanding oneself, it's being more respectful of the other person.

I: What would you like to be remembered for?

FS: I think first for being a good person, for being a decent person. In terms of academic work I think I've done a lot of good things: I ran Stanford Psychiatry and built it up again after it had been decimated to become a world-class research and clinical unit. *The Manual of Clinical Psychopharmacology* has been through nine editions. At the APA we named it *Schatzberg's Manual of Clinical Psychopharmacology*, which was very kind. That book gets used by people who practice every day, here and around the world. Every edition has been translated multiple times. The *Textbook of Psychopharmacology* has been through five editions; I co-edited it with Charles Nemeroff. I've been fortunate to be the President of the American Psychiatric Association, the American College of Neuropsychopharmacology, and the Society of Biological Psychiatry. Those were very great honours for me, as was being elected to the National Academy of Medicine. Overall, being a contributor to understanding the biology and treatment of depression.

In the end you want to be remembered as being a decent person. That's always a good legacy to strive for.

I: Which of your achievements are you most proud of?

FS: I'm probably most proud of building Stanford Psychiatry. It was almost a 19-year effort and we produced some of the top investigators in the world, Karl Deisseroth and other people, so that I think is probably the thing that gives me the most pride and I think *The Manual of Clinical Psychopharmacology* gives me great pride. We published it with the APA Press with Jon Cole. We wrote it and wasn't edited. Donald Klein had done a great book with John Davis where they reviewed all the studies in tricyclics and phenothiazines—a wonderful and remarkable book, encyclopaedic. So (we thought) the thing was to tell people how to practise. In 1986, people were just getting into psychopharmacology. How does psychopharmacology work in practice. You can read about its side effects and you know is it severe. Do you need to worry or not worry? So we set out to write that book and it came out in 1986. Jon passed away a few years ago. Before Jon died, Charles DeBattista joined us as an author. He also runs the Depression Clinic here and now we are up to the ninth edition. It's still used by people every day and that gives me great pride. The impact of that book is huge. I still get people coming up and talking to me about it at the APA. Chuck DeBattista and I run a course based on the book and sometimes Charles Nemeroff will join us. We may get 300 people who come to that course. That gives us, gives me great pride, in terms of professionalism.

I: That's all the questions I have. Is there any kind of parting observation advice?

FS: Well I'm honoured to be asked to participate in this, Dinesh. It's great to have international friends. It's really very important. Psychiatry is not exclusively a US specialty. Psychiatrists differ around the world but you know, we are in an international brotherhood.

21
Nada L. Stotland

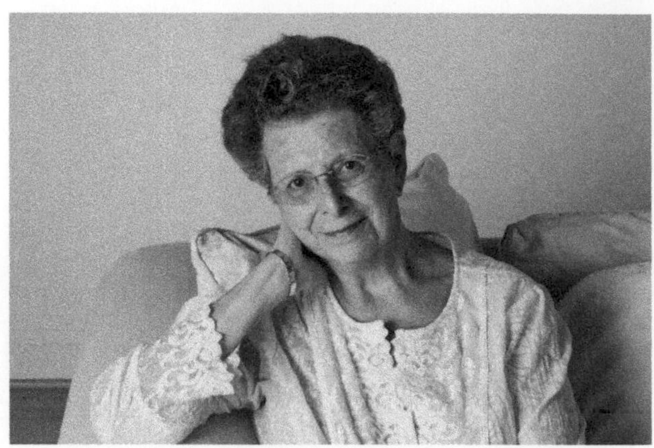

Biography

Dr Nada L. Stotland, MD, MPH, completed her undergraduate and medical education and psychiatric residency at the University of Chicago. She has served as a Director of Consultation/Liaison Psychiatry, Director of Psychiatric Education, Medical Coordinator for the State of Illinois Department of Mental Health, and Chair of Psychiatry at the Illinois Masonic Medical Center, all while maintaining a clinical practice. She is a graduate of the Chicago Institute of Psychoanalysis and earned a Master's degree in Public Health from the University of Illinois. The author of over 80 articles and author or editor of seven books, she has had an abiding interest in women's mental and reproductive health. In furtherance of those issues, she has testified against anti-abortion laws in state courts and the United States Congress. She has appeared on major television shows and for articles in the *New York Times* and other national publications. Dr Stotland has been President of the North American Society for Psychosocial Obstetrics and Gynecology; the Association of Women Psychiatrists; the Senior Psychiatrists of America; and the American Psychiatric Association. She has been invited to speak at meetings all over the world, and has led psychiatric delegations to Australia, China, Japan, Iceland, Russia, Rwanda, South Africa, Myanmar, Botswana, Taiwan, Hong Kong, and India. She and Harold Stotland met as undergraduates and married 57 years ago, shortly before she started medical school and he graduated from law school. They have four daughters and four grandchildren. Throughout countless professional meetings, and travel to and from them, she knitted sweaters for all of them. Now largely retired from practice and confined to Chicago by in unconscious conflict, and that mothers were to blame for children's pathology. When the World Psychiatric Association met in Berlin, where the country was apologizing for Nazi atrocities, I thought we needed to apologize to the mothers of all the children with autism and children with schizophrenia. I believe and hope that the era of mother-blaming is just about over now.

I: One of the things that I found when I was in therapy as part of our training was that it taught me about transference and counter-transference which were incredibly helpful. They get you to think why a particular patient is irritating you.

LS: Of course, I don't know the history of training in the British Commonwealth, but when I visited the United Kingdom, I learnt that things are much more segmented than they were when I trained in the United States; trainees choose psychotherapy or some other modality. We trained in everything supposedly, but psychoanalysis certainly informed psychotherapy. I did the whole thing, on the couch four days a week and listening to yourself, which is mostly what you do, without censoring. I still remember—and use for myself—the 'ding!' I would have when my free association had led me to something significant that I hadn't realized. As I say, it did me an enormous amount of good and has helped my own patients as well. I think in that sense it's a shame that we have lost it, but it took itself down for a number of reasons.

I: Do you have any regrets about doing psychiatry?

LS: No. I love psychiatry. I love the intellectual challenge, I love the work, and I love the nature of my colleagues.

I: When you were in medical school or training, who were your role models? Who were the people who left a lasting impression on you?

LS: It was strange. We had a larger-than-life training director and he was often considered a bully. Psychoanalysis very unfortunately conferred arrogance on practitioners. You could never have a negative or a critical thought because that was deemed to be resistance. It was a defence. So we worshipped all our teachers because they obviously could see through our souls. Our training director did teach us a number of very useful things. In our three years (we had a year of internship before we started psychiatry) there was one other woman altogether. Women were an oddity (in training) and we were there in a way on sufferance. The rest of the faculty were at a stratospheric level and we were merely peons. And then both of us had babies during training; not a day of training did we miss, there was no maternity leave, no such thing. We both had babies on purpose. It was going to be three years since my first baby and I didn't want to wait any longer. So we had babies and that made us weirder and it was talked about for years after. There were men who missed much more training than we did. I had to time my pregnancy so I could have my two weeks of vacation from one year and two weeks from the next year together. There were trainees who were too high up and academic and too analytic to be role models. I can't say they were role models.

I: Have there been other people who made you think things differently?

LS: Well, a couple of people. I got involved in organized psychiatry at the state level in Illinois. I organized two things: a committee of residents, the first one there was, I think, in the country and a committee on women.

I: That is incredible!

LS: And during that time, there was a woman President of the Illinois Psychiatric Society. There had been another one but that was a distant memory. This woman was a very solid, together, not mushy but supportive woman and she said to me, 'I'm going to put you on the finance committee. I want you to chair the finance committee.' I said, "I have no interest in finance." She said, 'You be quiet. You'll become the Chair of the finance committee and then you'll become the treasurer and then you'll become the President.' And I was blown away. The notion that I would ever be in an elected position in the Illinois Psychiatric Society was a complete revelation. It happened as she said. Meanwhile, I got to know Carol Nadelson (see Chapter 14) a little bit. Just the very idea that there was a woman running first for Vice-President and then President of the APA and at the same time as we had the first woman candidate for Vice-President of the United States was wonderful. It provoked feelings somewhat similar if by no means as strong as Black people felt about Barack Obama. I mean, the very idea that women would be in the leadership positions. When Carol ran, I was working. I had finished my training and I was able to arrange for her to come and give grand rounds. That was how those campaigns worked in those days. I had her come to Chicago and I met her. I took her to dinner. Our grand rounds were in the evenings at that hospital. After dinner, she made a call home. I'll never forget. Ted, her husband was annoyed because he had to take their son for a prep school interview and his suit hadn't been taken to the cleaners and son and father were fighting with each other, you know, arguing during the phone call. She started to quieten them down, Ted eventually realized that he was capable of taking a suit to the cleaners. Then she came out and did her grand rounds as though nothing had happened. It took me decades to get anywhere near that level of confidence. There was nothing more she could do for Ted. She had done what she could. She knew everybody would be fine at home. I would have agonized; I would have sat saying to myself, 'How can I give a grand rounds when they are fighting at home? Why do I have to handle these things?' She did not do that. After being elected, she put me on the Committee on Women of the APA, and that began my involvement at the national level. Also, she and Malkah Notman had edited a series of books about women which I immediately bought and read. That was awesome to me, to edit a book. Then, not so many years later she was asked to write a book. She told the publisher she didn't have time and she referred them to me.

I: That was really kind of her.

LS: And they came to me. I don't know if more than five copies of the books ever sold, but I wrote a book and that was something you didn't even aspire to, it didn't even occur to you in my family. A different class of people wrote books. Carol did an enormous amount for me. Her campaign for Presidency of the APA was much better than mine. At one point I became chair of a major council of the APA, so I sat on the side-lines of Board meetings for years. I watched how Boards work, and I watched each President confer something on himself. Carol became the editor of (American Psychiatric Association) Press, and she moved the press from being a sort of little in-house thing to a huge operation.

I: Yes, that is true.

LS: Time after time she did things which were very impressive to me. At the time a set of publications for young professionals: the *Young Engineer*, the *Young Lawyer*, the *Young Doctor*. They interviewed her for the *Young Doctor*. I learned how little sleep she got. I had never needed a lot of sleep either. I don't think there's any other way I would have known that. She went to bed and then she got up at 4 a.m. or 4:30 a.m. in the morning and did her writing and research until it was time for her children to wake up.

I: In your clinical practice, what's your lasting impression about patients?

LS: I like patients. I have had only one patient who was hard to like. Now, I just have three patients. Mostly, if you try to understand people, they are interesting and they are likeable and you look forward to seeing them.

I: Do you see patients now?

LS: Yes, I have three patients. They are stable on medication, but I won't do just medication; I still do psychotherapy with them. I think they will all tell you the psychotherapy has been a great benefit to them. I'll turn 77 in August and for now I'll keep seeing them.

I: Excellent.

LS: There are a couple of patients who bounced off. One moved away; whenever she comes back to Chicago to visit, she usually sees me. Another one lives in Chicago but only pops up when she gets into trouble of some kind or other. There are others who are not off the books yet; I still see them now and again.

I: In your opinion how has psychiatry changed in your practice time?

LS: Well, it's awful. I still love psychiatry but the takeover of American psychiatry by med-checks, and 15-minute visits is an abomination, very sad. I won't do it. but I have that luxury. I don't have anybody to support. I can't take insurance because to take insurance in the United States you need to have staff because it's so complicated. It's just not worth it. I lost the opportunity to treat quite a few people because they insisted on having somebody who would take their insurance which means they are not going to get psychotherapy. And I think as I said, I don't think classical psychoanalysis is a very useful modality, but to do psychotherapy and understand it is important. We psychiatrists were the repository of how to talk to people and how to listen to people for the whole profession of medicine. And now we are taught very little about that, as far as I can tell. I was a training director many years ago but I don't know a single resident now. I have written a couple of chapters with a lovely young woman who just finished her fellowship about a year ago; that's the closest I have got to the younger generation. I don't really know what the rules are, I don't know what they do in residency anymore. I can't see that anyone is really being prepared to do psychotherapy. I think psychotherapy is life-saving, wonderful when done properly. It's been left to other professionals. Often it is important to have medical as well as psychotherapy training. Positive developments take a long time to replace outmoded practices. The 'recovered memory' thing hung on years after a lot of innocent pre-school teachers were prosecuted and many people needlessly alienated from their parents. It trickles down to people who are not as intensely trained. Physiology affects behaviour and emotions. All the same, I think the field of psychiatry remains fascinating.

I: Do you think psychiatry is brainless or mindless?

LS: Neither. I think it has both. Philosophers have spent millennia considering what the mind is but I don't think we will ever know how one translates physiology of the brain into behaviours, feelings, thoughts, etc. I think they are in different domains.

I: You suggested that psychiatry without psychotherapy is not acceptable. Keeping American psychiatry to one side, in your view are there other issues or problems for psychiatry?

LS: Well, reimbursement and discrimination are huge problems. I just read in the news that again a healthcare insurance company has been fined by a court because they systematically deny mental healthcare to increase their profits. There is worldwide discrimination against people with psychiatric illnesses. What bothers me as much in terms of discrimination is the self-abnegation of psychiatrists. The Scientologists didn't have trouble finding someone to interview unwittingly. When I gave my Presidential address, I talked about a recent article in the *New England Journal of Medicine* saying that regarding cardiovascular care, something like 10% of the interventions have empirical evidence. Nobody in medicine knows anything.

I: Are they better at pretending, you think?

LS: Exactly. But, at the same time, doctors won't leave anything alone. Nobody knows anything in medicine, but we certainly don't know how to leave anything alone. When I was in medical school, the canon was that if there is one malignant cell in the breast, the patient must have a radical mastectomy. I said, 'How do you know some malignant cells don't just go away?' It took 50 years before they started looking into that. Of course. It's nice to remember the things that you are prescient about.

I: Yes.

LS: In my Presidential address, I asked, 'We know what causes diabetes, right?' Well, it's caused by not having insulin and that's caused by an autoimmune response, but what causes that? But when it comes to much more complicated ailments that have to do with the brain, which is a much more complicated organ and very difficult to study then suddenly we blame ourselves for not knowing what causes things.

I: You were talking about your Presidential lecture, what was the most challenging thing about your Presidency?

LS: Honestly, the most challenging thing about my presidency was dealing with the staff. And the Board, although I remained on very good terms with the Board, as far as I know. I didn't remain on good terms with some of the staff. I had been on the Board of the National Mental Health Association, the Board of my kids' Montessori school, and several professional organizations. I have sat at Board meetings for many years. It is the Board's responsibility to oversee the management of the organization. But I couldn't get my Board to question some things and staff, even though I tried to prepare them and built in time on the agenda. So I had clashes and I had frustrations. The other challenge that arose during my presidency was the big scandal over pharmaceutical relationships with the APA.

I: I remember that.

LS: During my first Board meeting as President, the *New York Times* published a story on the front page accusing psychiatry of being in thrall to the pharmaceutical industry. I was drafting an op-ed piece while chairing the meeting.

And then I met with the two authors of the article, one of whom still gets in touch with me now and then when he wants to run something past someone. I and the medical director met with these guys in Starbucks. We were not defensive and it was not contentious. I said, 'I don't know that psychiatry gets more money from the pharmaceutical industry than any other specialty.' They said, 'It seems like psychiatry fights harder for the new and more expensive medications.' So I said, 'I can't tell you about other specialties, but I can tell you one thing: our patients get less social support than people with other diseases; we have to fight harder for them to get the latest thing than anybody else.' There was never another article on the front page about this; I think I succeeded. I was just very honest and straightforward. But that issue ran through my whole Presidency. There's a US senator who liked to do these kinds of investigations.

I: From Iowa, wasn't he?

LS: Yes; he demanded every piece of paper, every record of every interaction that the APA had had with the pharmaceutical industry for the previous five years, and he wanted it almost immediately. Of course, most of those records were in storehouses. We succeeded in getting an extension on the delivery deadline because it was a big job for the staff. Eventually he was given what he wanted. I don't think anything came of it because there was nothing horrible in all those documents, but that ran through my Presidential year. Another challenge was the DSM 5. One colleague and I fought with the leadership and staff to institute a rule that people in the leadership of the development of the DSM 5 couldn't get more than $10,000 a year from pharma. Prominent psychiatrists asked me how those leaders were supposed to live and send their children to college if we mandated that restriction. They doubted whether the DSM 5 process could have leaders with any credibility if we excluded all the people getting hundreds of thousands of dollars from pharma. But we did it. Of course, when you do the right thing, there are people who think that is still not enough. That same $10,000 sounded like a lot of money to most people, but it was a fraction of what these people had been getting. Of course, it didn't mean they couldn't go back to getting large sums when they finished with DSM 5. You asking me these questions reminds me of useful things I did as President. I'm much more likely to be thinking about what I didn't do and should have done.

I: Don't you think that is always the case? One looks back and thinks I wish I had done A, B, and C rather than X, Y, and Z.

LS: Exactly.

I: I guess from your perspective, one year is not long enough. By the time you get your feet under the table, it's time to move.

LS: We have the year of being the President elect. In fact one of the things that helped was that Carolyn Robinowitz was the President before me. When I announced at her Board meeting that when I became President, I was going to appoint an ad hoc committee about our relationships with pharma, Carolyn said, 'Go ahead and set it up now', which was very good of her and it also worked very much to our benefit with the *New York Times* because we already had a functioning committee looking at the issue by the time they wrote the article.

I: I don't know what it's like in the United States but certainly here in the United Kingdom there have been periods when we have had major problems in recruiting into psychiatry. In your experience and view, how do you think we can improve that?

LS: Well, my database, as we speak, is very old. My latest skirmishes with this issue were when things were more in the process of changing than they are now. My observation was that senior people in the field were so upset by changes in insurance coverage that all the students heard from them was complaints. As I said earlier, I think we have too much internalized self-doubt. The joy of making somebody better or relieving their pain, which we can do in spades, is not sufficiently on display. It is harder to demonstrate our work than demonstrate successful surgery. Surgeons think they have the solution. They remove something and then sew the patient up. Actually Stuart Yudofsky, whom you probably didn't know, was the chair of our department when I came back to the university where I had trained, now as an attending psychiatrist. He used to do interviews with patients for the students practically on the first day of medical school. He used to tell them that he started out in surgery and found that it was too easy and that that's why he switched to psychiatry. He would do an interview that blew them away; in one empathic interview, he could reveal such important things and such beneficial things. That was awesome; I don't think we do that anymore. I don't know how it is elsewhere in the world. I understand that recruitment is up, I see young people writing wonderful articles in the APA's *Psychiatric News* and the publications of the Royal College that show we're attracting very bright, thoughtful, dedicated young people, but I don't know what the numbers are. It's also a matter of status and reimbursement. We certainly don't get a lot of respect from hospitals; what they want is orthopaedic patients and cardiac surgeons to fill the beds and do expensive procedures.

I: About 10 years ago in the UK, we were getting about 1.2 applications per vacancy and now it's gone up to 1.7

LS: Oh! That's very good.

I: And the trainees in some settings, certainly at the Maudsley were expected to interview a patient and record it and bring the tapes for the group and a senior consultant to look at. The teacher then would take you through the presentation frame by frame, pointing out what you did right and what you could have done better, including body language and the words used. About 20 years ago there was an expectation that trainees would undergo psychoanalysis and that's all gone.

LS: Right.

I: What do you see as characteristics of a good psychiatrist?

LS: The characteristics sound very trite; you need to be humble but not subservient, you need to have self-respect. You need to listen, you need to hear, you need to respond, you need to not get ahead of the data. We have to be both honest and optimistic, supportive with patients and their families. We have to tell the patient, 'You are going to feel better'. That has a beneficent value beyond measure. You have to take that responsibility. When you do nothing but give people statistics about treatment outcomes, so that you won't be responsible for the decisions they make, the worried patients and families always ask, 'What would you do?' Because that's what they want to know. I think that's sad. I had an attending pediatrician during my internship who was from Sweden. I remember that he said, 'Let's say a child has a terrible heart lesion and the surgery is dangerous but the child won't live to adulthood without it and the parents ask you, what would you do? It's your obligation to say what would you do, so that when there's a bad outcome, the parents know that the doctor would have done the same thing, so that they don't feel alone.' You have to be willing to do that.

I: There is psychiatry's contract with society; how do you think that can be delivered?

LS: I think we need more teams because we can't do it all. There will never in the foreseeable future be enough psychiatrists to see all the people who desperately need psychiatrists. When I was a resident, insurance would pay to keep psychiatric patients in the hospital for six months, and then they reduced it to three months. We had an inpatient unit where the patient was seen by the attending and resident psychiatrist, mostly the resident, but also the psychologist and the social worker and maybe an occupational therapist, and then you all would meet. We all respected each other because we each were experts in that aspect of care. I think we gave much better care. We have to keep pushing for appropriate reimbursement and appropriate respect. The *New York Times* reporter once called me a psychologist; that has happened to me many times, coming from otherwise very sophisticated writers, so I think part of our contract is to explain what we are, who we are, why we are there, and why that makes a difference. I think the incoming President of the APA, Jeffery Geller, is going to be in that sense great. He concentrates on the least empowered people and the people who suffer the most.

You know, this conversation has made me realize the good things I did. When I was the President of the Illinois Psychiatric Society, I convened a meeting with the President of the Psychology Association, the social workers' organization. They were very wary to even meet with me. There was so much interdisciplinary rivalry and distrust. We started an umbrella organization to address the needs of the public system. At that time, there was no interest by the Psychiatric Association in anything but private practice, really. We had very little and very bad exposure to the public sector in medical school and residency. That organization is still going and effective 25 years later. In terms of our contract with society, much of society doesn't care either. Society doesn't even have a very good contract with itself, but we need to pay more attention to what our relationship and contacts are with the society. When I chaired the psychiatry department in a large community hospital, I started a service especially for African-American patients. I hired two Black women psychiatrists and boy oh boy, did we get patients! Because you have got a whole population of people who are afraid to go to White doctors.

I: Yes, we had something similar here in the United Kingdom.

LS: Apropos of what's going on in the world right now, even then we didn't pay attention to the needs of other underserved populations.

I: I think the attention to the underserved populations varies according to a number of factors. Looking back, what would you tell your younger self?

LS: It's hard to say. I might warn myself that painful and unfair and destructive things can happen to you during your career, but that might not have helped me prepare. I guess I might have been able to forestall one or the other, but probably not. I couldn't have imagined it. I lost three positions, over the decades, when the leadership or other external circumstances changed, despite having done a demonstrably very good job. Possibly, in one situation, the problem was my insistence on telling the truth, but I wouldn't want to change that, really. I have lived without a job for the last 20 years. I set up a private practice in my home. I really threw myself into successive elected and appointed positions in the APA. As President, I spent at least eight hours a day on APA business both at home and while travelling on APA business. I did not see any desirable job in Chicago and my husband, as an attorney, was not moveable.

I: What would your advice be to trainees of today?

LS: It's tough partly because I don't know what they already do so I'll repeat some of what I have said. Don't let anybody put you down, don't ever think psychiatry isn't as good as the specialties where they poison (chemotherapy), burn (radiation), and cut sick people and call that cutting-edge science, while we mostly talk to people and give them medication which is much more humane—and interesting—and our research is fascinating. I would say be in touch with trainees from other programs, be involved in organized psychiatry. Otherwise you are isolated in your own cocoon and you don't realize all the ways people can be trained or what wonderful things they are learning somewhere else—or maybe you are very lucky and they are not learning things that you are. Get involved. Don't tell yourself you don't have enough time no matter how busy you are because it's worth it, and of course nowadays you know you can do everything electronically. Now you don't have to travel very much. Seeing psychiatry around the country and the world is wonderful. I love travelling, so I didn't mind doing it. When my children were young, I took one of them with me to each meeting, in rotation; all four of them as adults are very comfortable speaking at meetings. I would advise young trainees to keep an open mind and be prepared for change. It's still a sacred tradition.

Since I was in training and practice they have made residents' lives less punitive, but they have also taken some professionalism and self-esteem and joy out of medicine. I think that young people have to be prepared to deal with the fact that the electronic medical record is a great idea in theory and a mess in practice. They should struggle to improve it.

I: What would you like to be remembered for?

LS: For being honest, for caring. I managed to be a good enough mother and a good enough doctor. I did some things that were hard and not popular like becoming the psychiatric expert on abortion. I got thrown into that. I chaired the APA Committee on Women. I was very interested in preparation for childbirth and postpartum. Ronald Reagan was elected President of the United States, he appointed a Surgeon General who was anti-abortion, and ordered him to produce a report about abortion. The Surgeon General held hearings about abortion. The then President of the APA detailed me against my will to represent the APA to talk about abortion to this fearsome guy in a military uniform. The APA staff helped me put together and review the literature, and I went and gave evidence. I was in psychoanalysis at the time. I was a nervous wreck over the prospect of testifying before this man in Washington DC, and my psychoanalyst all of a sudden says it'll be OK. This is not an analytic thing to say. I turned around and asked him, 'What did you say?' He said, 'I went to college with him, he is an honest man'. After hearing all the evidence from all perspectives and interested parties, that anti-abortion Surgeon General refused to do what Ronald Reagan wanted. He wouldn't write the report. He sent a letter to Congress saying, 'The public health effect of abortion on women in America is miniscule', but I became the abortion expert. I gave professional talks, and testimony against anti-abortion laws. Giving the testimony was extremely painful because it entailed listening to anti-abortion witnesses who lied. That took a lot of courage. I decided to mention my advocacy in my Presidential address. One of my daughters said she cried with pride on hearing that. I'll never forget that; I'm proud of that.

LS: When you finish your term as APA President, you stay on the Board for two years, and you will know more about what's happening than any other member. I have a happy mostly retired life, a husband, and four grandchildren, and a rapidly diminishing, though not absent, awareness of what is happening in the field and in the APA.

I: Thanks very much for your time and sharing your memories and thoughts.

22
Paul Summergrad

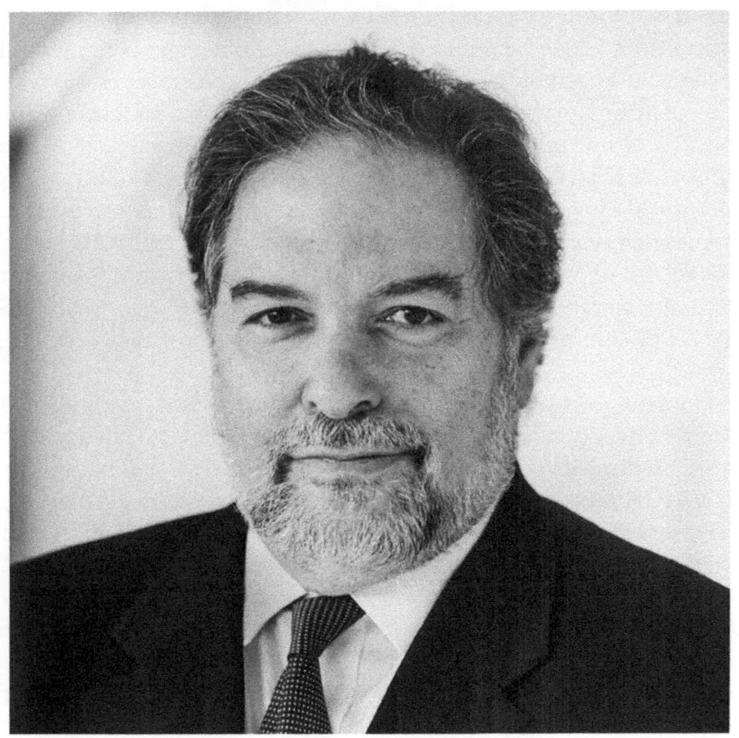

Biography

Professor Paul Summergrad, MD, is the Dr Frances S. Arkin professor and chairman of the Department of Psychiatry and professor of psychiatry and medicine at Tufts University School of Medicine and psychiatrist-in-chief at Tufts Medical Center. In 2014–15, Dr Summergrad served as the 141st President of the American Psychiatric Association, and he is a past-President of the American Association of Chairs of Departments of Psychiatry. He serves as Secretary for Finances of the World Psychiatric. Association.

An international leader in medical psychiatric disorders and care, Dr Summergrad's research focuses on mood disorders, medical-psychiatric comorbidity, and health system design. He has published extensively with over 150 peer review publications, book chapters, and other communications. He has edited three books: *The Textbook of Medical Psychiatry*, *Integrated Care in Psychiatry*, and *Primary Care Psychiatry*.

He currently serves on the Editorial Boards of *Current Psychiatry* and *Personalized Medicine in Psychiatry* and guest edited a special issue of *Academic Psychiatry* on strategic planning in academic departments of psychiatry. A sought-after speaker, educator, and consultant, he has served as a visiting professor and has given invited lectures throughout the United States and internationally. He was a member of the Diagnostic and Statistical Manual (DSM) 5 Steering Committee of the American Psychiatric Association and the Standing Committee on Nominations of the World Psychiatric Association where he currently serves on the Standing Committee on Finances and from which he received Honorary Membership. He chaired the work group of the APA Board of the role of psychiatry in healthcare reform which commissioned the Milliman report on the total healthcare costs associated with psychiatric illness. He is a distinguished fellow of the American Psychiatric Association, a fellow of the American College of Psychiatrists, the American College of Physicians, and of the Royal College of Physicians—Edinburgh, and has received numerous other awards and honours. He received the Distinguished Faculty Award from Tufts University School of Medicine in 2015 and the Leadership award of the American Association of Chairs of Departments of Psychiatry in 2018. He was elected to the Honorary Fellowship of the Royal College of Psychiatrists, their highest honour, in 2020.

After completing his training in internal medicine at Boston City Hospital and Boston University and in psychiatry at the Massachusetts General Hospital (MGH) and Harvard Medical School, Dr Summergrad served as chief of Inpatient Psychiatric Services at MGH from 1987 to 1998 and as associate professor of psychiatry at Harvard. He served as staff to the Partners Now MassGeneral Brigham) Mental Health Strategic Planning Committee of the Partners Board of Trustees in 1996–97 and as network director of the Partners Psychiatry & Mental Health System from 1997–2004. From 2000–2002 he served as the Executive Vice-President for medical affairs and chief medical officer of the North Shore Medical Center where he oversaw quality, physician integration, and the physician group while also serving as chief of psychiatry. He was a member of the Partners Healthcare System Executive Committee from 2000–2004. He served in 2013–14 as the chair of the American Hospital Association Governing Council for psychiatric and substance abuse services. In 1999, Dr Summergrad chaired the Harvard University Provost's Committee on Student Mental Services and he currently co-chairs the Tufts University Mental Health Task Force with the President of Tufts University. Dr Summergrad served from 2005 to 2019 as the founding chairman of the Tufts Medical Center Physicians Organization, a multispecialty faculty medical group for which he also served as interim President and chief executive officer from 2014 to 2016. He chaired the search for the Chair of the Tufts Medicine Board of Trustees in 2020 and is a former Board member of Tufts Medicine. He is a member of the Tufts Medical Center Board of Trustees.

Dr Summergrad earned his medical degree from the School of Medicine at the State University of New York at Buffalo in 1978 where he was elected to Alpha Omega Alpha in his junior year. He served as chief resident in psychiatry at MGH. He completed psychoanalytic training at the Boston Psychoanalytic Society and Institute. He is board-certified in psychiatry, internal medicine, and psychosomatic medicine.

Interview

I: Shall we start off with your childhood and growing up and what was it like and where was it?.

PS: I grew up in New York City, in an area called the Bronx which is north of Manhattan. New York City is divided into five boroughs and Manhattan is obviously the part that everybody knows because it's where all the big buildings are and the United Nation and the Empire State building, you know where Wall Street and all of that is, but people live primarily in the surrounding, outer boroughs. So the Bronx, where I lived was between lower class to working to middle class, there's one small upper class area but we didn't live in the upper class area. And initially I lived with my grandparents and my cousins and really it was almost like a classic extended family, which was wonderful actually. My parents lived in an apartment building that was next to one of the complexes and it was a very interesting building and complex which actually had an article written about it in the New Yorker by Calvin Trillin in probably the year 2000 or so. The article starts out by saying that there was a time you could live in the Bronx in a building based upon your political ideology. This building was actually run by people who were, I don't know if they were communist but they were very left-wing Jewish people to the extent that in the 1930s when the depression hit and they were running out of money, people couldn't pay their bills, they said, "are we going force people to pay their bills or evict them?" They said, "we can't evict them, we are not going to behave like capitalists" and then they went bankrupt. (laughs) So that was the context in which I grew up and so it was a very non—religious Jewish background, so intensely Jewish culturally and ethnically but my parents were not at all religious. They came from left wing political not so much anti-Zionist but maybe neutral, but certainly not particularly focused on Zionism. They really came much more out of a left wing political background, so my mother and my father—used to march in May Day parades for black and white reconciliation. There was a parade where they would march to free the Scottsboro Boys—that's how they were described—who were a group of black youth who had been incarcerated somewhere in the South. So I was really brought up with my maternal grandparents. My mother's cousin, her first cousin moved and her family lived around the corner and then there were a lot of other people that we lived with. In the summers we would spend time going up towards what was called the mountains, which is the small area in the north of New York called the Catskill Mountains but it wasn't in the mountains, it's not like you know the Himalayas or the Alps or something. It is like foothills and worn-down mountains. So we spent a lot of time there. I would spend summers there probably until I was about 8 to 10 before starting summer camp. I was surrounded by my entire family, my extended family. I grew up in an environment where I was the eldest child, so I grew up at the centre of attention to some degree and within a very warm rich environment that was very much in extended family. When I was about four (this is traumatic) we moved about three miles away. My parents got their own apartment, their own kind of area and then I went to elementary school just down the block although that was great. So I grew up in the Bronx where kids would play in the street, we'd go out on our bikes and we would play various kinds of urban baseball games, stoop ball or what was called in our neighbourhood "slug" or stick ball or punch ball. Things we used were a small kind of rubber ball to play in a concrete setting and there were two parks nearby and then we lived there until about I was 11 in 6th grade and then we really did get a traumatic move and which was we moved to the suburbs as my father wanted to have his own house and we went to north to Westchester county and that was really hard for me because up until I was 11, I lived in an entirely Jewish area and I thought everyone in the world was Jewish till I was about 11. My parents had not suffered in the Holocaust as they were born in the United States. My dad had fought in World War II as had my uncle. My dad was a sergeant and a medic and been and done a whole range of things. I was so American but I very much remember living there and moving to a place where my friends were not next door so I was much more socially isolated. In that geographical area, Jews were a significant minority. It was the first place where I ever really began to encounter anti-Semitism to the point where I remember when I was in high school there was one guy who called me dirty Jew or filthy kike or whatever. I remember fighting and shoving him when he was a senior in high school and I was a junior in high school in the locker room. I think I acquitted myself okay but I don't remember exactly so that was where I grew up and the other piece where I very much wanted to be in New York and stay in New York, I thought in New York kind of felt like the centre of the world at that point—it really was. It is a very exciting place to be. There were exam courses that you could do in New York and then you could be accelerated. It looked like that was the track I was on but I never got a chance to take the exams, go to one of these exam schools because we moved to the suburbs and it wasn't an equally good environment to do my secondary education as it would have been if I had stayed in New York but it ended up, so that was kind of where I grew up. There were a lot of other advantages not to ignore such as the summer camps which were really important until I went off to college really in the New York City area.

I: At what point did you decide that you wanted to do medicine and what attracted you to it?

PS: So when I was in high school, I think there were two influences. One is that I worked in the summers for a camp which was a Jewish social agency camp called Camp Willoway which was run by the by the YMHA which was basically like the YMCA the Young Men's Christian Association, this was Young Men's Hebrew Association and there was a co-ed camp and the camp was run by social workers and there was always a subset of kids there, who had some form of emotional or medical difficulties usually more emotional difficulties or they came from difficult family situations or environments that were more challenging and so I remember when I became what was called the counsellor-in-training and then a counsellor and then have my own bunk of kids that they would instruct me about how to manage to deal with kids who were having emotional difficulties and I enjoyed doing that and I just liked learning about that. The other thing was in high school, we read Freud and I think it was more of his social writings and may have been about Moses and Monotheism or something like that or the future of an illusion,

We began to do more reading in social psychology and II was taking what was called Honors History, I remember writing a paper about the role of propaganda in Nazi Germany and how propaganda was utilized by Goebbels and others. So I was very interested in the interface between politics and psychology and social psychology. I began to think when I was about 15 that I wanted to be a psychiatrist. Now that's not the youngest—one of the people in my department who said that he wanted to be a psychiatrist from the age of nine. I thought that was very precocious. So I was very interested and there was something about being a psychiatrist, it was something about being a master of hidden knowledge to some degree, I think it was also about being respected medical professional although being a doctor per se I'm not sure was, my younger brother who passed away, he at one point wanted to be a surgeon, great hands for being a surgeon. I don't have good hands for being a surgeon but I would not say that my primary way of thinking was scientific. In other words, I'm not somebody who you would say was a biologist or a chemist. Interestingly my father was a junior high school/high school science teacher and when I was a little kid when I had days off, he would take me to his classes with him and I remember going to his classes and he taught me a lot of science. I remember him teaching about experiments which disprove spontaneous generation of insects and so I saw the scientific methods that was very important but I would say frankly, probably my more natural inclinations are towards history, philosophy, law, politics, that kind of way of thinking. I tend to be more of a synthetic thinker than an analytic one. I don't tend to discover through scientific experiments, I tend to discover more through introspection and experience. But psychiatry somehow was kind of a calling-it called me and then things got completely derailed in the 1960s—derailed completely.

I: Why did they get derailed? What happened?

PS: In some ways it's the most foundational or one of the most foundational experiences of my life. What happened was, I was smart enough to be able to get away with most things without working too hard and there was a part of me that wasn't disciplined enough. I believed that if I was really intuitively into something or gifted, I should be able to do it without a lot of hard work and I was smart enough to get away with that for a long time but then eventually I actually needed to do some reparative work. I wasn't strong in maths, I could have done more probably, I did okay in geometry when I got to calculus and stuff, it was okay in college but before college geometry was great. I had major difficulties with French, primarily because I was out of sequence. I had been kind of slotted into taking French and when I moved to the town I was in, kids were very familiar with it, so I never really learned it from the ground up and it just never quite stuck for me so I did not do very well. I had a couple of blemishes on my record and I ended up not getting into the college which I wanted to get into. I ended up getting waitlisted at the University of Chicago, which is where I wanted to go because it's a very intellectual environment. I probably could have gone to other places that were almost as good but I wasn't knowledgeable about them, my parents didn't know about that, they weren't familiar so I ended up going to a safety school which was the State University of New York at Buffalo, it is actually a very good school but it wasn't distinguished as the same way as other places were. I felt very wounded by that, but it was really hard for me to acknowledge that I was wounded. I was 18 years old, most 18 years old guys don't do well with narcissistic injury and I was no exception to that rule and when it intersected in a way which was very powerful with the 1960s. It was 1967. The war was burgeoning, the country was beginning to fall apart, it felt like it was a period like now, normal things were very difficult in 1968, the spring of '68 where there was worldwide you know the French Student Riots in Paris in 1968 and it I also intersected with other things. I got exposed to marijuana and started smoking a lot of weed at that point which I have never gone back to. It was just that one year but it was enough and I hated being in Buffalo. It was cold, it was snowy because it sits east of a large lake, the clouds roll in September and they don't leave till May. It snows every day. They put all the freshmen in overflow housing, no women there at all, you have to walk or take a bus to campus, it was just not a good scene and it felt like it was nothing redeeming about it. I'd walk on this campus and the snow would be ripping around and would be cold and I felt like I was in the scene from the movie "Doctor Zhivago" you know Zhivago was walking across the tundra to come back to Moscow whatever and it just was awful. So that combined with the war, combined with my own personal sense of injury threw me into. I don't believe that I was clinically depressed, my parents sent me off to see a psychiatrist who had been recommended to them. I think he was the chair of the department of psychiatry in Buffalo, he thought I was depressed, I didn't think I was depressed, I didn't see him again that was not particularly helpful. But I paid very little attention to school. I did take a course in the Dhammapada which is one of the foundational Buddhist texts. It is very accessible among the Buddhist texts. I'm not aware—it's early—where it fits in the kind of sequence of Buddhist texts but I really liked it and enjoyed it and in the spring of '68 when I was still a freshmen, I had my one and only LSD experience and I took LSD and I have written about this and I have talked about this but it actually came out when I did interview with Ram Dass in 2014. We talked about something and I had written for a book when I was a resident training in psychiatry at Harvard about resident experience you know, things have transformed them. I wrote about taking LSD. I had a profoundly religious experience, it was like being dropped into the middle of what is known in Sanskrit as the "Prajnaparamita Sutra" The Heart of Perfect Wisdom Sutra which I later studied when I did Zen training "Form is no other than emptiness, emptiness is no other than form, feeling thought and consciousness is the is the same as this". It was as if you could see where we always stand is "Nirvana". Nirvana is no different than samsara, it's just seeing it from a different perspective and with self/object differentiation dropping away not in a scary way but in a good way and in a sense of mystery the world—everything was perfect that when seen under the aspect of eternity there was only compassion and caring and love and absolute order and perfection and that the universe was filled with compassion and order and love. And I was perfect and had always been perfect but I didn't become perfect, I was intrinsically perfect, everything was intrinsically perfect and there was nothing to strive after, it was the cessation of striving because there was nothing to strive after to complete myself. And I sort of went "wow!" It completely blew me away and I became really interested in returning to that state and figuring out how to get there but without drugs, and through some circuitous path about a year and a half later I ended up in Rochester, New York which was just down the road from Buffalo at the Rochester Zen Center which was run by an American named Philip Kapleau. Kapleau had been the court reporter whose company had served as the court reporting company for the Nuremberg war crimes trial and the Tokyo war crimes trial after World War II. He had been so disturbed by what he experienced that he ended up eventually moving to Japan to get into Zen training to get some peace back in his life. I ended up studying with Kapleau and spent the next year training intensively with him. When I got there, I was able to do independent study, this is where I was great actually when I was in Buffalo, I ended up graduating with many credits of independent study for doing Zen meditation, so I ended up getting my degree. I actually did take courses in American studies and got my Bachelor's degree but a piece of it was based on the work I had done basically by doing Zen meditation. I spent a year doing Zen meditation five hours a day, two hours in the morning, an hour at lunch time and two hours in the evening. Working at the Zen centre doing manual labour, physical projects, eating a vegetarian diet, losing a lot of weight and getting very focused, what would be called in Hinduism or Sanskrit "Dhyana"—one pointed concentration which gets translated into Chinese as "Chan Buddhism" and then gets translated from Chinese into Japanese as "Zen Buddhism" so it's a kind of very much, you would think about it more as samadhi, intensely focused concentration work as opposed to vipasana meditation or loving kindness meditation or chanting or the kinds of things you see in some parts of Hinduism, chanting a mantra or something like that, it was less based on that. It was based on really intensive meditative practice and I did that very intensely for about four years and in the second year of that I realised that I was not going to be a Zen Buddhist monk. I realised that was probably not my path and I really was stuck, I had no idea how to get, what was I going to do in the world that incorporated all of these, that incorporated these wishes and urges, what was I going to do that was actually practical in the world and I could not for the life of me figure out the solution to this and I ended up spending a year, actually I wasn't lonely but I ended up spending a year living alone. I cut myself off. I was in touch with my family and friends. I still was meditating but I cut myself off from all kinds of extraneous social contact; no newspapers, no television, radio, music, and I lived by myself. I would go to my meditation. I was doing some substitute teaching just to make money and working in a couple of other stores to make money but I didn't have a lot of expenses and I was still getting my independent study credit or maybe actually I was done with that at that point, I don't remember. But mainly I think I spent about a year doing walking meditation through the streets of Rochester, so I would just go out for very long walks and you know I learned how to keep my concentration while walking and you know you plant your attention at the bottom of your feet and you walk and that's what I did. And through it I was reading a lot of Zen Buddhism and I was also reading a lot about Jung and one of his disciples Eric Neumann who was a German Jewish Psychiatrist. He was initially a psychologist and so I think he went to medical school then I think he moved to Israel but he wrote a lot. It was very hard to read him, He is not a great writer actually but he wrote a bunch of books, it somehow seemed relevant and I read those and then I read some Jung and towards the end of this period I had a couple of very powerful dreams and it was the second one which really ended up resolving the crisis and it was one of these great dreams that presents a solution to your life. It reconnected me to being Jewish and it reconnected me to psychiatry, It was like I went to sleep one night I was still in crisis the next morning I woke up and the crisis was abated and it was absolutely clear to me that I had a way forward that I was going to become a psychiatrist. I saw a way of integrating psychiatry which was always linked in some ways to me to be the depth psychology with integrating that with a religious trajectory that somehow would incorporate being Jewish and at the same time would incorporate Buddhism. And it all was put together around the metaphor of travelling to the other shore which was both a metaphor in Buddhism and a metaphor in Judaism and at that point the crisis was over, it was absolutely crystal clear to me that I should go to medical school and become a psychiatrist and that's what I did—I never looked back—it was a transformation which occurred in the very depths of my soul and in some ways has never left me—the annealing of these various parts of myself was so complete. I went and got my pre-med courses and I went to the university of Rochester for two years, I did about three years' worth of the course working for two years, I did a bunch of backup work in history, I did a bunch of stuff in Chinese history and European history just in case medical school didn't work out. If I couldn't get in, I figured out I could go to law school. My fallback positions were medical school, law school, maybe rabbinical school, I actually had an exploratory interview at one of the rabbinical schools but then decided that really wasn't for me and psychiatry was, and I loved the idea of being rooted in something that was very medical and very scientific, it fit with my relationship with my father and what I had grown up with. From that point on it's never been really unclear in my mind, I never looked back, I never had doubt about the idea to go to medical school but once I got to medical school, I did really well in medical school because I had really learnt how to study, I had all these concentration skills that I had gotten from been trained in Zen. The Zen teachers had taught me how to sit for 14 hours a day staring at a wall, reading a textbook was easy after that, you know this is not hard work and I did really well. I graduated at the top of my class in medical school and I decided that, you know, they said "No, don't waste your time being a psychiatrist, you should do internal medicine." I actually wasn't quite ready psychologically to do psychiatry, I thought it would be too internal and I wasn't quite ready to go back into the depths, so I went off to Boston and did my internal medicine training and then in the middle of my internal training, they asked me to stay on to be Chief Resident in medicine, this was at Boston City Hospital which was a legendary kind of place to train in Boston. Midway through that realised that I had to really train in psychiatry and I finished my internal medicine training but I then I got accepted to train in psychiatry at Massachusetts General Hospital and Harvard. Mass General was the most medically oriented psychiatry training programs, the most prestigious hospital really in the US and I had just gone through two and a half years of seeing all these people with all sorts of medical disorders who were presenting with psychiatric illness. At Boston City Hospital so many patients had an abnormal mental status due to their medical illnesses and it was like enormously complex and interesting patient population and a place to train and I was still in and was doing medical kind of mode and MGH had the most kind of connection to that in its history and I ended up then going on Faculty at Harvard and for the next 20 plus years staying at Mass General until I came to Tufts so all of that really derived from that early interest and that transformative crisis.

I: Do you have regrets doing psychiatry?

PS: No, no, I haven't regretted doing Psychiatry for a minute. I mean there are times when I thought it would be fun to be a constitutional lawyer or something or might have been interesting to be a rabbi but in terms of being a doctor, in terms of being a psychiatrist I never doubted that was the right choice for me, I never doubt that. When I was a junior medical resident, I had just been asked to be chief resident in medicine which is a high honour in this program. They only selected two people out of 30 people to be chief resident, it was being tapped for academic growth and development. One of the people who did that before me became Chair of neurology at Brigham and one of the neurology chairs at Harvard. The guy who was just a year ahead of me did that and ended up becoming the neurology chair at Cornell. It was a group of people who did very well. One of the guys who I was supposed to do it with eventually became the assistant secretary for health for the department of health and human services for the United States, which was equivalent to being a four-star Admiral—A flag officer. The idea of doing psychiatry never ever felt like it was a mistake, but I struggled against it. I was in the middle of my junior residency in medicine, I resisted the idea of doing psychiatry mightily. I fought against it for probably about a year and I finally realized that I could no longer resist the call of psychiatry and then I had to come out and tell people that I was going to be a psychiatrist and it was uncomfortable, it was painful but once I did it I felt like it was absolutely the right thing to do. I felt completely at home in myself and so I tell people that this the closest I had to a coming out experience but there's never been a hints worth of a doubt after that.

I: I mean you mentioned a couple of names, who have been your role models, heroes, heroines?

PS: Besides you? (laughs) I always liked Freud a lot. I think Freud is misunderstood, I don't particularly like his views on religion and obviously some of his theorising, but I do have a sense of understanding some of what he was struggling with. I liked the idea of his self-analysis. So he has always been a touchstone. Jung in his own way but he has a really interesting perspective. Buddha is an important figure (for me). Moses to some degree, I mean those are people and in the greater world. But I think in psychiatry itself there were two people in training who had the most influence on me. One was Tom Hackett who was my chief of psychiatry at Mass General who helped me publish and pointed me in a direction to study medical psychiatry. So that I would be able to publish my first really serious academic paper with him as the co-author. He died extraordinarily young; he was chief in his early 50s I think and he died at 58 riding his horse. He literally died on the saddle and my first major paper was co-authored by him—it was his last academic paper. For me he was a very powerful figure, he was a polymath, he was the director of herpetology at the Cincinnati Natural History Museum when he was 13 years old.

He was one of these kids who was just a prodigy, but he also was a raconteur. He was a great storyteller and he was a late night person which I am too and so he wouldn't come in until about 10 o'clock in the morning except when we had our early morning meetings which I thought was a great job and I said that's the job I want. But he'd get tired and if you get to bed at like 2 o'clock in the morning, he worked very late so, if you weren't able to keep him interested, he would fall asleep during meetings. You had to learn how to be pithy and entertaining to engage with him. He was certainly an influence. And then there was Gerry Klerman, who had been the head of the research at Massachusetts General in Psychiatry and had been the head of (what was then called) ADAMHA, which was the mental health-related National Institutes put together. He was a brilliant teacher and a really significant influence. I would say those two, more than anybody in my analytic training, had a significant impact on me and some of my colleagues as well.

I: You mentioned analysis; did you undergo psychoanalysis yourself?

PS: Yes, I did. I did analytic training at the Boston Psychoanalytic for a long time. I hadn't graduated. You are supposed to write up your cases when you do the control cases and the first time, I wrote them up, they said, 'There is not enough process. Rewrite them.' So I rewrote them and then they said, 'Too much process', so I said, 'Screw this. I'm just not going do it.' I just slid the whole thing to the side. It was kind of irrelevant at that point. Eventually I decided that I needed either to finish it or become an affiliate member and give up or rewrite the cases in a way that could be acceptable. So I finally got those cases rewritten and I graduated; I certainly use those skills to some degree and I liked the intellectual piece of analytic training and certainly learnt a lot from the training. It's actually easier to do psychoanalysis than it is to do psychotherapy in some ways because you're not sure what to say today you will see them again tomorrow, you're not looking at them, they are not looking at you. You're taking notes, it's a very different feel but I did the whole training and the training analysis. My own experiences have been my own self-analytic experiences both when I was in my early 20s and then in my late 20s or early 30s when I decided to leave medicine and go into psychiatry and these years were much more powerful for me than anything I went through in analysis in part because my soul was on fire at those moments. I imagine if I had been in analysis at a moment when I was going through crisis, it would have been much more useful and meaningful but to do a training analysis just because that's when you have to do it from the sequence standpoint feels a little like you're eating a meal and you're not hungry and so that had a more limited impact on me. It had a beneficial impact in other ways personally but in terms of the depth of it, it wasn't that impactful.

I: How has psychiatry changed in your time?

PS: I started doing psychiatry just as psychiatry was emerging from its analytic focus on the US and it was moving towards a more biological, scientific, and randomized controlled perspective. I trained in a place that also included a lot of psychotherapy training as well as the medical psychiatry focus on being a physician. I think that psychiatry has changed in a couple of ways. One is that I think that there has been a decrease in the stigmatization of both mental illness and psychiatry as a profession by the general public. People are more open to talking about these things. I think psychiatry in part continues to suffer from feeling as if it's not quite scientific enough; this was true when I was in training and growing up in early years in my career and even still now to some degree. It feels a little bit like a piece of the struggle for biomarkers and biological mechanisms and neurologic mechanisms is in part to legitimate psychiatry, to put it on a better scientific footing, but it's also to say, 'You see? We really do have disorders, we really do have diseases, we are real doctors too.' And on the one hand, doctoring is much broader than simply diagnostic and aetiological certainty; on the other hand, I think psychiatry that's why I conceived of and edited a textbook on medical psychiatry because I think that there's actually a huge number of general medical and neurologic disorders that affect the way in which people feel and think in a pretty pronounced way. If psychiatrists became familiar with that or knew that and felt comfortable with that, they would understand that they already are all sorts of things that require the medical skills in the training and the background that they have, syphilis being the great nineteenth-century example. I don't know if COVID will be the great twenty-first-century example, I hope not but yes, certainly there are many conditions, for example various forms of thyroid illness. I think that one thing about being a psychiatrist that sometimes gets lost is the need to be centred in the body as well as centred in the brain, psyche, and the soul. All of those things are necessary to acknowledge, of course and I think that to be extent that you know we can obviously find genetics and other mechanisms that tell us about what would otherwise be idiopathic illnesses I think that would be extraordinarily good. However I think there are times in which biomedicine feels overweighted a little bit in a way in which research dollars are distributed or some other way the field talks and thinks about itself. Probably the biggest change is that psychiatry as a field is also becoming more popular again with medical students in the United States. The numbers of medical students going into psychiatry here have doubled on an absolute basis from about 3% to 6% of graduating classes in the last seven or eight years. That's a reflection of a number of things including the fact that it's hard to have the kind of in-depth relationships you can have with patients outside of psychiatry. I think that there is more flexibility about how long you can practice and there's greater public acceptance of psychiatry. As a field it has become more heterogeneous, which is good. From my standpoint you have to use the tools that work for particular conditions or situations; you shouldn't be bound by a theory and have to force conditions or people into those theories. There's a recognition that not everything that looks or smells like an emotional difficulty is necessarily psychiatric illness. Sometimes it's just a developmental growth, experience, or crisis. Not everything needs to be pathologized. We have enough business and work to do; we don't need to take on everything.

I: Do you think the current state of psychiatry is brainless or mindless?

PS: (laughs) Leon Eisenberg gave a lecture called Mindlessness and Brainlessness Psychiatry in 1985 or 1986 to the Royal college of Psychiatrists and it's one of my favourite lectures which he then published in the *British Journal of Psychiatry* in 1986.

I: Yes, it was and I think it Bob Kendell responded to it.

PS: Leon was a teacher of mine and another person I consider as an important mentor at Harvard. He was really very brilliant and had an excellent sense of humour. You meet certain people where they clearly have twenty IQ points on everyone else in the room. I have met about half a dozen people like this where they are just scary smart and Leon was like that. He came from a fairly left-wing Jewish background but he was a little too hostile to psychoanalysis per se. He grew up at a time when psychoanalytic orthodoxy ruled the roost in US psychiatry. He was fighting against that. I think that while it's true that psychiatry was brainless, probably in the 1930s, 1940s, 1950s, or 1960s to some degree, and it became increasingly less focused on the mind, I'm not sure if it's either brainless or mindless right now. My impression is that it is a little bit more in equipoise. I don't know that we have a set of overarching principles that help us understand the ways in which the brain produces the mind, if that's the way it happens, or whether mind and brain are what I think Freud called dependent concomitants, something he got from Hughlings Jackson. I always thought that Leon underestimated the degree to which Freud was actually linked to neurobiology, even when you get to, for example, Freud's 1923 paper, 'The Ego and the Id'. In that paper, he describes the speech apparatus and he draws a little brain cartoon in the middle of the book which shows the acoustic area on the left side of the brain and he says in the text that the ego is a drawing of the human figure that's hanging upside down on the left side of the brain, with overly large lips and thumbs and hands, identifying the ego with the speech apparatus and a homunculus. The ego is more concerned with the discrete, particular, time-bound verbal components of mental operations as opposed to dreaming, which occurs in a different form of organization of the brain which is more visual than verbal, less time-bound, and more fluid in its operation. That part of psychoanalysis got suppressed to some degree in part because it wasn't until 1950 that the Project for Scientific Psychology was published and people understood some of what Freud was struggling with in the early 1890s (when it was written), even though he had the wrong solutions for these very fundamental problems. He was struggling with these fundamental questions which are still very cogent: how did these things—the brain and mind—relate to one another. I think one of the places where you see both a brain-focused and a mind-focused psychology in psychiatry is in some of the focus and interest that young people have in psychedelic research where you find very small doses of 5HT2A agonists in the form of classic psychedelics having profound effects on neural organization, both acutely and potentially longer term, and at the same time having profound impacts on the mental state and mental well-being. I'm not arguing that these are necessarily anything other than interesting compounds that are worth studying. I don't know yet what their real efficacy is, if any, and there are risks associated with taking them, but I do think that there is an interest in both right now, particularly among the younger generation of psychiatrists.

I: What do you see as the problems in the current state of psychiatry?

PS: I think one problem is that people are still too self-conscious about being a psychiatrist. A huge problem in every country that I'm aware of is that there is enough stigma still that surrounds psychiatric illness that the payment systems for psychiatry (and this is not so much from psychiatrists standpoint because I'm yet to meet a lot of starving psychiatrists) but the care for patients tends to be very discriminatory. Because psychiatry touches on and so often then impairs mental functioning and behaviour. Look at what is happening in the United States right now with COVID. Hospitals have been intensely busy so they have to restructure what they do to provide COVID care; but because of the way in which medical care is paid for in the United States, the most profitable care is elective surgery which can't be done if all the beds are taken up with folks with COVID. We therefore have hospitals throughout the United States that are losing money because they are providing necessary medical care but they are not providing the care that generates a lot of profitability, all of which is artificial. This doesn't effect psychiatry alone but it puts psychiatry clearly at the bottom of that heap and understanding this is a major issue. There is still a lot of stigma surrounding psychiatry but let me go back to my comparison with the gay and lesbian communities. My struggle to become a psychiatrist is a little bit like a coming-out experiences, my sense that I had to fight resistance, internal resistance because I was afraid of how I would be viewed and I was also afraid of how I internally viewed myself. I think those elements remain very powerful, more so in some cultures than in others. I don't want to assume that all bad behaviour is related to psychiatric illness and all good behaviours are unrelated to psychiatry. I think that the stigma around psychiatry prevents an adequate basis of investment in both research and the clinical services which people need. Even in the UK National Health Service (NHS), which has a lot to commend it, I have been aware of the need for a parity of esteem, equity around funding for services. That needs to be challenged and it's certainly a challenge in the United States as well in many other places of the world. I think the second great challenge is whether or not the focus on neuroimaging and neurocircuitry in genetics will eventually yield the kind of results that we think will emerge from very large genome-wide association studies and other concept studies. The President of Tufts University, Tony Monaco, who has an MD, PhD, and who was at Oxford for many years as a geneticist, was looking at some of the data on heritability compared to what allelic variation is. He has raised a really important issue about the degree to which epigenetics modifications have not been fully taken into account as having a role in heritability. If you begin to add that in, you know the role of social factors and other factors needed to be considered as number two and I think the third thing is that part of it because psychiatry deals with the most intimate parts of human experience in oneself and one's sense of self makes psychiatry a complex and interesting field. Elyn Saks, who is a famous constitutional lawyer at the University of Southern California, had schizophrenia, became ill when she was in college, and then again when she was at Oxford. She got lots of really good care in the NHS then came back into law school at Yale and continued to be ill. I've heard her speak and she said at one point that it was only when she finally got treated with Clozaril that she got better and she realized that having a psychiatric illness didn't define who she was. For people who live with conditions like this there's a sense of saying your intrinsic being is somehow ill or defective in some way; that's what others hear us saying when we talk about having a brain disease or genetic disease. Part of what generates some (not all) of the anti-psychiatry feeling is this prejudice that someone who suffers from mental illness is defective. And this prejudice seems to me more prevalent in the United Kingdom than it is in the United States.

I: What would you see as characteristics of a good psychiatrist?

PS: I think characteristics of a good psychiatrist are partly the characteristics of a good physician: an interest in people, wide and excellent training, and knowledge of illness and disease, medicine, neurology, other conditions in general. I think deep experience taking care of people over long periods of time is essential. I don't think there's any substitute for a lot of clinical experience because without it you don't have a mental model, you don't have an internal bell curve to know if something is unusual or not. Interest in people and a willingness to listen, an ability to tolerate uncertainty and silence, being able to engage with people, and humility; all these are really important. I think avoiding making definitive pronouncements about people is also a requirement. What makes a bad psychiatrist is the absence of those things or someone who has the need to control other people; that can create a lot of difficulties.

I: If we look at psychiatry's social contract, how would you say that can be delivered? It is a tripartite contract between psychiatry, the public, and the funders, whether they are the government or insurers. How can that be delivered?

PS: I think quite a lot depends on what gets put into the bucket of psychiatry. Psychiatry needs to be careful not to create new diagnostic categories for every potential illness. That doesn't mean there aren't things that should be separated or reorganized in different ways; diagnostic categories are limited in medicine and they are limited in psychiatry. The second thing is to think about what is most needed then, to the extent that we can, define that. It ought to be where we put the greatest amount of effort and energy. I think that becomes hard for funders if we're so focused on things that are necessarily important but maybe out of the traditional realm of healthcare. The funders get confused about what psychiatry is. For people with serious mental illness who are sleeping under bridges or whose lives have been blown apart by severe mental illness or people who have catatonia or they have got very severe life threatening illnesses; we owe a special obligation to those individuals. I think defining what psychiatry is and there's a piece of us that always has to define ourselves. On the one hand, we are embedded in the earth, embedded in biology, embedded in general medicine, in human medicine. And then there's another part of us that is in the stars. It's a difficult balance to maintain. We have asked all our hospitals and health systems right now, during this COVID crisis, to be public utilities, public goods. We have said to them, 'You may not have the resources, you may not have the money, you may actually end up losing money, may spend on things that are not in your budgets, but we need you to do this work because this is an overarching social obligation.' So I think that the sense of overarching obligation towards people with serious mental illness in particular gets lost. It is unconscionable that people with serious mental illness are dying 10 to 15 years earlier mostly due to untreated medical disorders. There are now a number of studies that suggest that targeted interventions exist to help people with mental illness, we can do better. I think that's part of our obligation because we may be on this position seeing people who have serious mental illness and medical conditions and if we are not attentive to those and we are not advocating for that, you know that's a terrible outcome. The way we think about hospital-based care also worries me. There is a tendency to see hospital-based care as negative and to try to limit the length of patient stay. At the same time, we know that the greatest risk for suicide is probably in the week to a month after discharge and that either means we are doing something wrong or it's a reflection of the patients we are admitting that are at high risk. But it also suggests the possibility that we are not keeping people in hospital long enough or not creating the protective steps for them that are needed after discharge, and the kind of outreach to stabilize them through the transition and re-entry into their daily lives is not sufficient. I worry about those who are most at risk.

I: What would you tell your younger self?

PS: First, that you will be fine most of the time. Not all the time. Secondly, that you should have compassion for yourself; don't beat yourself up too much. Thirdly, be more attentive and kinder about other people and listen to them better, spend more time with them; you'll never know how much time you actually going to have with them. Don't get too wrapped up in yourself. This is still a problem that I have. I'm too wrapped up in my own career and in my own evolution. At the end of the day, that's important but the other stuff is very important as well. In particular, and I probably would tell my younger self that you really should have studied a little bit harder in high school (laughs). Even Mozart worked hard!

I: What would you advise the trainees of today? Exactly what you have just said or something else, or something in addition, perhaps?

PS: I think the trainees that we have at Tufts are wonderful. All the trainees in other programmes that I have met are wonderful. We are getting fantastic young people into psychiatry. I would advise them of a few things: one would be that they must be sure that they want to do psychiatry because it's a hard field. One of the things that I look for most when I interview applicants is their passion for psychiatry in a sense that although it doesn't formally require a 'calling', it would be better if the trainee in the United States and the registrars in the Unites Kingdom had a sense of calling because it's not the easiest field to enter, for all of the reasons we have been talking about. Secondly, I would strongly encourage them to get a strong foundation in medicine or neurology, and if they were interested in child psychiatry, then paediatrics, perhaps a little bit of surgery, but certainly medicine and neurology. I think experiences in other medical specialties are very important for practising psychiatry. Thirdly, some form of personal growth and development is helpful, not that they must have been through psychotherapy or analytic training but something where they have the experience of calling on deeper parts of themselves or deeper resources is essential. These, I think, are all really important because they'll need them and their patients will need them. The fourth thing is the value of good science, not to be pulled into every trend or fad that comes along, to learn about other things that will help them a lot such as getting good training in statistics. For me, learning statistics was really valuable. The last thing is humility and also the ability to act when things are uncertain and not assume that because somebody else told you that this person doesn't have a medical, neurologic disorder that they don't. If you think something is not quite right with the patient, no-one has more experience than you do with what psychiatric illness looks like. You have to learn to trust your gut.

I: What would you like to be remembered for?

PS: I would like to be remembered for some of my focus on medical psychiatry. I think I would certainly like to be remembered for the fact that I hope I was an open-hearted and a generous advocate for both the field and for patients with psychiatric illness. The opportunity to lead an organization, be President of the American Psychiatric Association (APA), was certainly very important. I certainly would like to be remembered as a good parent and husband and family member and friend. Somehow maybe clarifying some of the tension points between what psychiatry on the one hand is and kind of normative human development on the other hand but might fall under the traditional rubric of more religious or existential experience, I think that one's the hardest and least likely to occur. I would like be remembered for being kind, for being a good friend to trainees. Ultimately, I want to be remembered as somebody who ran a good department, who focused a lot on residency training, who made sure that trainees that felt good about their training, did advocacy work and worked on medical psychiatry. I think those three are probably the most important.

I: Looking back at your Presidency of the APA, what was that like?

PS: It was great, I loved it. My wife Randy said it fitted me like a glove. I think I'm the only person that's ever had their spouse introduce them in the final Presidential address. Partly that's because she's a much more talented public speaker than I am. Partly because she had done a lot of this type of stuff when she was very young. After she gave the introduction to her Presidential address, Carol Nadelson President of the APA came to Randy and said that she really ought to do more leadership in psychiatry. Carol and Randy are good friends; they have known each other from their Brigham and Women's Hospital days and Carol had been at Tufts early in her career when she was President of the APA. Randy had been the international girls President of B'nai Brith, representing Jewish girls at the age of seventeen throughout the United States and in the world. She met Lady Bird Johnson and Robert F. Kennedy. Randy told Carol that she had gotten all her needs for leadership out of her system at age 17. But I think the things that I cared about most coming out of that were really three things. One was that we made a decision through a lot of planning to decide where the APA headquarters were going to be. We made a decision and went through a good process to buy the building that we now have and I'm glad that we did that. And the second one was people often ask the APA President what the theme of each year is going to be and I have always replied that it is not my Bar Mitzvah. I said this is not about me, it's about the long-term benefit for the organization. We are putting a strategic plan in place. We did branding work during that year 2014. All of this has continued and has helped to inform the organization. I'm very glad of having the opportunity to speak on behalf of patients and families and the profession in a way that wasn't primarily focused on how much we are going get paid. If you are not speaking up on behalf of people, patients, and their families, nobody else is really going do it. And the secondary obligation is to make sure that doctors are well treated and hospitals are adequately funded. But the primary obligation is one of speaking on behalf of others, many of whom can speak for themselves, some of whom are in conditions where it's harder for them to speak for themselves, and to speak for them not just nationally but internationally. I think that to me is the most important part of it.

I: Which of your achievements are you most proud of?

PS: Of course, my wife and family—that transcends all of this. From a professional standpoint, probably my Presidential year when I was President of APA. I think the second was being chair at Tufts, probably the third one is the textbook that has just been published, medical psychiatry textbook. I have a generation of young psychiatrists who have trained with me and in my department and to accept that we created an environment where people feel like that they get good training and they have gone on to things that have both benefitted themselves and others and they have been successful, all this feels like a gift to the future. You know, your trainees are your professional progeny, they are your professional offspring and so they are very important.

I: Thanks very much, Paul.

23
Thara Rangaswamy

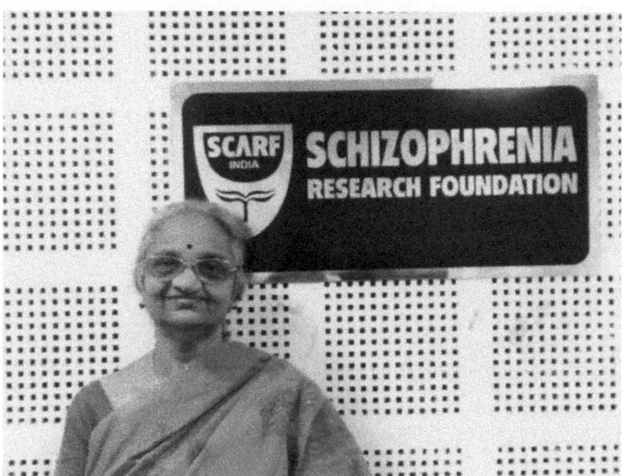

Biography

Dr Thara Rangaswamy is a trained psychiatrist and the co-Founder and Vice Chairman, of a non-governmental organization, the Schizophrenia Research Foundation (SCARF), based in Chennai in Tamil Nadu which provides care for outpatients, inpatients, rehabilitation services, and care homes. As an internationally reputed research centre, SCARF also provides extensive community outreach programmes. After having led SCARF as its Director for over 23 years, she stepped down to become the Chair of Research and Vice Chairman.

With her PhD on the subject of disability, Thara lobbied hard for the inclusion of mental disability in the Disabilities Act in India. She was also responsible for the development of a tool called IDEAS which is officially used to measure disability in schizophrenia. Dr Thara has pioneered the use of mobile tele psychiatry which is now serving more than 1,500 patients in Tamil Nadu.

She has collaborated with premier institutions around the world such as the Johns Hopkins in the United States, the Institute of Psychiatry in the United Kingdom, and others in Australia, Canada, etc. She has served on the many task forces of the World Health Organization (WHO) and the National Institute for Mental Health (NIMH) and has over 180 peer reviewed publications.

She is on the Advisory Committee to the Director General of the WHO and is on the editorial Board of several reputed journals including the *Schizophrenia Bulletin*.

the pandemic, she continues to write, and she substitutes edifying broadcast concerts and cinema to occupy her mind while knitting.

Interview

I: Could we start by talking about your childhood and growing up?

LS: I'm the oldest of three, I have two younger brothers. My parents were rebels against orthodox Judaism. They couldn't have enough Christmas trees, shrimp, bacon, etc. But we still had relatives who were observant, so I'm quite familiar with all the rules. After having three children, my parents began to fight. Eventually they were in a process of divorce, a very contentious mess during which my father died. I was eight. I was told that he had had a heart attack. Many years later, the head of the Psychoanalytic Institute of Chicago hearing the story said, 'Obviously he suicided.' It had never occurred to me. I gather that the cause of death had been falsified because of the stigma of suicide. My mother was a lot of fun, bright, had a lot of educational aspirations and admiration, but she was also in a state of rage for the rest of her life. Apparently, my father had angrily threatened to leave her with three children to support. One of the reasons I was interested in becoming a doctor was that I was determined to be able to earn enough money to support my own children because my father didn't leave money to support his. My mother went back to school and became a teacher. She was very fascinated by psychoanalysis, which was of course the rage then. We lived in the neighbourhood of the University of Chicago. She was very jealous of all the faculty wives and of everybody with more money, education, status, or marital success. She had a little bit of free college, as she came from a very poor family, but hadn't finished her degree. Both single mothers and working mothers were very uncommon in the 1950s. She had two best friends, both divorced and bitter. One of them was the assistant to the head of the Institute for Psychoanalysis. My mother fancied herself as a bit of a psychoanalytic interpreter, generally to unfortunate effect. I was fascinated by how psychoanalysis could explain everything. I wanted to do something hard. I wanted to do something interesting. I wanted to do something psychological. Being a psychiatrist was the hardest and the most comprehensive way to learn how to be a psychotherapist, which is what I wanted to be. I went to medical school in order to be a psychiatrist.

I: Did you undergo psychoanalysis yourself?

LS: I did eventually. When I was training, all the leading lights in psychiatry were psychoanalysts. But I was very eager to have children. I married at age 19, just after graduating from college. As soon as my husband finished law school and had a good income, though I was still in medical school, I decided to have a baby. I chose to have another during my residency. That kept me busy. So I didn't actually start my psychoanalysis until some years later. I graduated from the Chicago Institute for Psychoanalysis. Psychoanalysis and classical psychoanalytic theory seem to have virtually disappeared from psychiatry today. My treatment did me an enormous amount of good. I think psychodynamic psychotherapy can be a great help to people, but much of the theory is not valid. Some did a lot of harm to a lot of people, particularly the idea that every psychiatric symptom had a basis

She initiated two major programmes, an international conference, ICONS, and a film festival, Frame of Mind, which have been successfully held on eight occasions.

She has won several awards including, some from the state government. She was awarded the Honorary Fellowship of the Royal College of Psychiatrists in 2014 and also the President's Gold Medal from the Royal College in 2012. She is also an Honorary Member of the World Psychiatry Association. In 2020, she was the recipient of the outstanding award for Outstanding Clinical and Community Research from the Schizophrenia International Research Society.

Interview

I: We can start by talking about how it was like growing up in Chennai. What was your childhood like?

TR: I had a pretty uneventful childhood in Chennai. I grew up in a fairly large family where I had grandparents, great-grandparents, and of course my parents as well. I went to a normal English medium convent school where we had to go and pray in the chapel every week. I was really interested in sports and I was a table tennis player, I represented the University in table tennis. I am a great lover of animals; we had three dogs at home. Being born into a conservative Brahmin family, there were some restrictions. I was not allowed to learn swimming since it was not acceptable for young women to wear swimsuits. My grandmother, who was very orthodox, was totally against the fact that I brought dogs into the house, and she even threatened to leave home. So, it was an environment where there were a lot of restrictions but perhaps that made me feel the need to be more independent and strong-willed; I had to fight all these restrictions that my grandmother threatened to impose on me. To be fair, though, I should say that my life has not been really affected by all this. I just look upon these restrictions as experiences and issues that one has to deal with while one grows up.

I: I'm really interested to know about your orthodox Brahmin childhood and particularly your grandmother and her response to animals. How did you deal with it?

TR: Our home was large and I made it clear to my grandmother that the dogs would not bother her. She was losing her eyesight due to diabetes and was also apprehensive that she might tread on them. I think after a couple of months, she got used to the idea and then things became fine and in fact I remember when the female dog delivered puppies, she was very anxious, and she kept asking me whether the puppies were OK, whether the mother was OK. In those days, we had no dining table and our food was spread onto banana leaves on the floor. After we ate, the whole floor was swept with cow dung in order to sanitize it!

I: Were there other youngsters in the household? how many brothers and sisters were there?

TR: I have only one brother and he was absorbed with his friends and games.

I: And any cousins in the household?

TR: Cousins would come and go but did not live with us.

I: Was your need to be independent what attracted you to medicine?

TR: Probably, yes. I was thinking of law as well, at some point in time. But in those days, medicine was considered to be a more secure profession for a lady. But it was my choice, not my parents' choice or my family's choice. I chose to get into medicine and to be honest, it was not to help suffering humanity. It was because I wanted to make sure I had a profession and I was financially independent. Although my father was a rich man, I felt strongly about this.

I: Were there any doctors in the family?

TR: No, none. I was the first doctor in the family.

I: Right. And what was their response when your parents heard that you wanted to be a doctor?

TR: They were very happy, they thought I was doing the right thing. I must mention that at I was born with a hare lip and a cleft palate and those days there was no plastic surgeon to repair my palate. I still have a cleft in my palate which is closed with a denture. My birth was very traumatic for the entire family. They had not seen anything like that and then I had to go to CMC Vellore many times; even the American surgeon there didn't know how to operate on the palate, and I had to go for speech therapy. My maternal grandmother had offered bells in many temples to pray that her granddaughter should be able to speak well. This was one of the factors that made me feel I should not be dependent on anybody. I did not want to get married. Even then, I started thinking of people who were disabled in many ways and how they would cope with their disabilities.

I: At what point did you decide that you wanted to do psychiatry?

TR: Well, after medical school.

I: What attracted you to psychiatry?

TR: I wasn't sure if I really wanted to do it. I just thought I would try it out and so I applied for a senior residency which was an honorary position in the psychiatric department in General Hospital (attached to the Madras Medical College) with Dr Rajkumar. After three months, I found myself liking it and I continued. I found that I was getting increasingly absorbed and so I decided to go on and applied for my post-graduation.

I: You've been really terrific and amazing in what you have achieved, and building SCARF and making it an internationally known organization, both for research and but, more importantly, for service delivery. You also expanded the work to dementia and child youth mental health. What kind of obstacles did you face?

TR: When we started SCARF in 1984, people didn't know much about schizophrenia. I'm talking of the general public; they wondered what the organization was and many couldn't even pronounce the word schizophrenia. In fact, our friends from the National Institute of Mental Health (NIMH) had suggested that we change the name call it the Mental Health Foundation. But both Dr Menon (founder of SCARF) and I felt that only if we use the word 'schizophrenia' would people really understand it (also see Chapter 12). Therefore, raising money for it was also difficult because people had no idea what it meant. We were able to get initial funding purely because people trusted us. There was always the question of what we should do. Should we deliver care only or also do research?

I was very passionate about research but there were some members of the Board who felt that service delivery was more important. I decided to raise funds for research as an independent stream. The biggest challenge those days was that people around the world thought that research in India was of poor quality and all data were fudged. One of my main tasks was to convince people that we can do credible and ethical research at SCARF. At the World Health Organization (WHO), I spoke to John Orley and convinced him to accept my ongoing work on the outcomes of schizophrenia as part of the WHO's ISOS. I had to do this with other organizations like the NIMH, Johns Hopkins, etc. It took many years but eventually this happened and now we are in a position where people seek us out for collaboration. I think we have reached a stage where we have built a lot of credibility; people know we deliver and carry out high-quality research. It was a long battle hard won.

I: What drives you?

TR: It's largely from inside. I am 68 now. I don't need the money, I don't need to travel, I don't need to go to meetings, I don't even need publications to further my career. So, it's not so much external factors. I don't discount them totally; it's nice to go and meet people, to publish papers. Even today when I was listening to Robin Murray talking about his work, I said to myself 'Oh my goodness! Why didn't we do this kind of research?' I immediately went to my junior colleagues in the hall and said, 'Can't you guys think of doing work like this?' So, I think it is something deep within me which drives it all.

I: Being the first woman in an orthodox Brahmin household going into a profession and having to overcome the disability, do you get the feeling that somehow you have to prove yourself much more than others?

TR: Maybe initially it was like, that although not at a conscious level. It's not like I was saying I had to prove myself in any way. I don't mean to blow my own trumpet but I was top in my school, I was second in my university, I was a gold medallist, I was a good table tennis player. I excelled in most things I did fairly naturally without too much effort. I'm fiercely independent. This did not mean I broke rules; it's just that I need my space, I need my thought processes.

I: Do you have any regrets choosing psychiatry?

TR: Not at all. I think I did the right thing. I mean I'm certainly enjoying it; I just couldn't have been an obstetrician or a paediatrician. In those days you know, a woman doctor had to be either an obstetrician or a paediatrician, And I cannot stand kids who shout and cry all the time, I just can't. I just don't have it in me, and I hated obstetrics because I hated the way some obstetricians were so rude to their patients. I could never have worked in such an environment.

I: You have chosen to stay away from leadership at a national level in the sense of getting involved in Indian Psychiatric Society or getting into obstetrics and challenging obstetricians from the inside, so what was your hesitation?

TR: If I get into something, I have to contribute and the contribution has to be substantial, not just for one or two years. You really have to make an impact; you need to change something, and I knew that was difficult in a Society with a leadership tenure of a year. It's not that I don't respect the Society. I know a lot of good things are happening, but I don't think I will fit in there.

I: When you were going into psychiatry, who were your role models and heroes and heroines?

TR: Definitely Dr Sarada Menon, who selected me for the postgraduate course. She was such a strict disciplinarian and very particular that we wrote good case notes of our patients. Her dedication and commitment were very inspiring; she is the role model for many of us (also see Chapter 12). However, my interest in research was fuelled by Dr Rajkumar who was Professor of psychiatry at the Madras Medical College and gave me my first job in the ICMR study SOFACOS. Then, I've also met along the way people like Dr NN Wig who inspired me in his own way, but I did not have the chance to work with him.

I: In your experience, how has psychiatry changed in your time?

TR: It has changed quite a bit because when we first started, the stigma of seeking help was much greater but now people have much less hesitation in seeing psychiatrists. Young people working in the software industry seek help for sleep, marriage, and sexual problems. This would have been unheard of even 10 years ago. Now people don't mind seeking help for depression and anxiety, although psychosis is still not well understood.

I: What do you think of the current state of psychiatry?

TR: Where? In India?

I: Yes, you can talk about India or internationally or both.

TR: A lot is happening internationally including at the WHO. Much more funding is available for research, although it is still limited in India. But we still have a long way to go in terms of service delivery in the low and middle income countries (LAMIC). Even in the state of Tamil Nadu, which is one of the better states for healthcare, we still have many untreated patients in rural areas with the Duration of Psychosis (or illness) (DUP) of 10 years, 12 years.

I: You've been doing some fascinating work in terms of telehealth. How did that come about? How did you decide that you wanted to send a van around the villages and offer healthcare on the Web or via Skype?

TR: The first tele-psychiatry initiative happened soon after the tsunami in 2004, which affected the two southern districts of Nagapattinam and Cuddalore. Oxfam came to us and requested us to do tele-counselling to the people there. The government of Tamil Nadu was also very encouraging. After the tsunami, we were left with a group of untreated patients with psychosis for whom we gave some support for a few years. I had seen some tele-mobile initiatives of an eye care foundation, Sankara Netralaya, and a few others. I decided we too should have a mobile facility—I'd never heard of one anywhere in the world. That's how it came about. The TATA trusts supported us and Ashok Leyland designed the bus.

I: What do you see as the problems with psychiatry at present?

TR: I don't think the profession works together; I think we don't speak with one voice in many places. There are too many dissenting notes within the profession and now we also have the family groups, carers' groups, the users of services. We should be consistent in the messages we send out to the general public and not confuse them—about medication and its safety, the need to continue treatment, the services available, etc. Then there is the fact that we are still not able to improve the lives of our patients. Even if you take major psychosis, we know that only 30–40% are really functionally improved. And more importantly we don't know what causes schizophrenia. We know that tuberculosis and malaria are caused by organisms/

mosquitoes. With mental illness, we give patients a cocktail of factors which may have caused the disorder. This is not convincing enough.

I: You think psychiatry is brainless or mindless?

TR: No, I won't say it is either. I think there are very bright people in psychiatry now. Around the world I see some really intelligent and bright people in psychiatry but I think we don't work together, we have our own agendas. So, this not coming together and not speaking with one voice is the problem. That is what is going to make a difference at the society level.

I: What do you see, apart from the fact of us not speaking with one voice, are the other characteristics of a good psychiatrist?

TR: I think the first thing is empathy. I mean you really need to understand your patient. You need to understand his problems in life as much as his symptoms; it's his life situation which is so critical, I think that's what we fail to do. We focus on the symptoms and we act more as clinicians, but I think we should really focus more on the patient's family life, on his social life. Or get the case managers to attend to this aspect. When you actually ask the family what causes the burden for them, they don't always talk about the hallucinations or the delusions. They say, 'He's not doing anything; he's not earning or not able to support his family.' But these are not generally addressed by most mental health professionals.

I: Do you think one of the problems may be that in psychiatry, like in most of medicine, we focus too much on symptom reduction rather than social functioning?

TR: Absolutely. One reason is our teaching and curriculum which focuses only on medications.

I: Is it still two weeks of psychiatry training at undergraduate level in India?

TR: Yes, undergraduate training in psychiatry is still only two weeks in most places and everybody goes on leave during those two weeks. I'm even talking of postgraduates' psychiatric curriculum, say in MD psychiatry or a DNB, we don't teach enough of all these social measures or recovery and rehabilitation. I think again the focus is on medications.

I: One of the things that intrigues me is the lack of training or teaching on ethics and probity. Is that a universal phenomenon in India? I don't see it in postgraduate courses.

TR: Nothing. Well, I was not taught any ethics at all. My standard of ethics was partly derived from my family and partly being taught by people like Drs Menon and Rajkumar. It was imbibed, but we didn't have formal teaching in it.

I: I know people who are seeing 100 patients a day; how will they make social contact with their patients?

TR: They have time only to make a diagnosis and prescribe medicines. I also think the onus is on the government to do such things at a macro level. We should have community teams like you have in the United Kingdom. Unless that is done, I can't blame the individual psychiatrist. I think the responsibility largely rests with the government. We should have community outreach teams, trained to deliver psychosocial interventions. We certainly have a manpower crunch but what our community work has clearly shown is that we do not always need highly trained professionals. We need an empathetic brand of volunteers from the community who can be sufficiently trained and who can deliver good treatment of the mentally ill. I would really love to see the day when we have a lot of community teams in rural areas going out and reporting back to the psychiatrist if something is required. Considering that we have so many people who are looking for jobs in rural areas, we can easily use them, but where's the money? Where is the political will? People argue that it is top priority to have psychiatric drugs available from primary health centres, or from district headquarter hospitals. For example, we are now collaborating with a study on antenatal women in Bihar in north India. When we go there we find there are very few psychiatrists. If you want to counsel women on perinatal issues or antenatal issues, who is going to do that?

I: If you were looking back and talking to your younger self, what would you say?

TR: I'll say what you did was great. I have no regrets either personally or professionally. I mean, there are always things you could have done better, but I think under the circumstances I'm very happy with what I have done.

I: What would you have done differently?

TR: I am not sure now, but not many things, I guess.

I: And what are the achievements you are most proud of? What do you want to be remembered for?

TR: When I was just over 30 years of age, we started the non-governmental organization (NGO) Schizophrenia Research Foundation (SCARF), I wrote its constitution and its by-laws, with very little knowledge at that point in time. For 23 years I was the Director—stabilizing the organization, making it financially secure, innovating in terms of starting the international conference ICONS and tele-psychiatry, and building a wonderful team to take it all forward. Now, as you know, SCARF is well known nationally and internationally.

I: What would your advice be to the trainees of today?

TR: I think they first have to be sure of what they really want to do and then pursue it relentlessly.

I: What if you are to redesign the undergraduate curriculum. What would you do?

TR: I would give them at least three or four months in psychiatry and I would definitely expose them not just to the state mental hospital but to other NGOs, good NGOs if there are any in the area. They should learn about community outreach and the social psychological aspects of illnesses. I would tell them how research is really exciting because I don't think at undergraduate level anybody talks to students about research.

I: Have there been any memorable occasions that you can think of either in a clinical setting or in research that you look back and say it had been one of those Eureka moments?

TR: No, no Eureka moments as such. I think my work and my achievements have all been very gradual. No, I really can't think of anything.

I: You touched upon problems in psychiatry, the way it's too medicalized and some so-called anti-psychiatrists would agree with you What would your response be to them? They think that medications should never be given; everything is society's fault, and this is a very Laingian way of thinking.

TR: In some international meetings over 10 years ago, I had a chance to interact with some who felt this way. I gave them case illustrations of how a strong 23-year-old with paranoid symptoms has beaten up his elderly parents to the extent that they had to be hospitalized. Of course, the patient did not think he was ill and he refused treatment. We need to strike a balance.

I: I believe in the bio-psycho-social and anthropo- and spiritual model but it goes back to what you were saying earlier about lack of unified voice. How do we change that? What can a leader do to try and bring about that unified vision?

TR: I think we have to start with the younger cohort of doctors and psychiatrists who may be open-minded and not fixed in their views. If we are able to bring in all these elements starting from ethical factors to social, family, and community factors apart from the genetic and biological, then I think at least the next crop of doctors and psychiatrists will have a much better overall understanding and vision.

I: Thanks very much for your time.

24
Pichet Udomratn

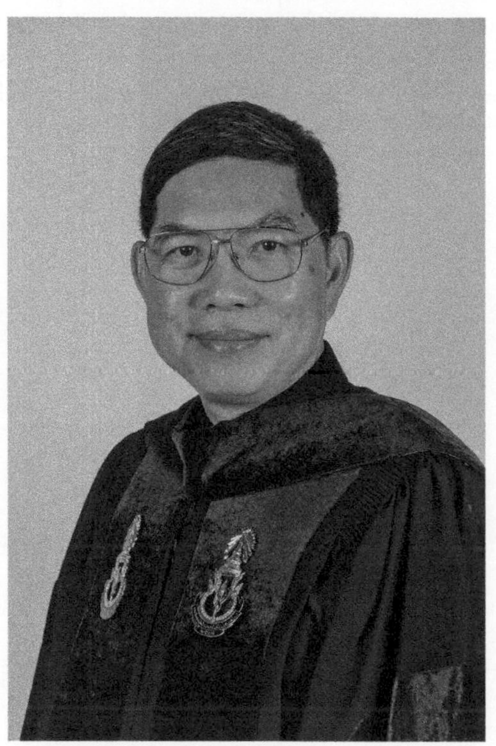

Biography

Prof. Pichet Udomratn received his MD (Hons) in 1980 from Prince of Songkla University, Songkhla, Thailand. During 1988–1989 he received a World Health Organization (WHO) fellowship to work as a research fellow and visiting psychiatrist at the Department of Psychiatry, Royal Edinburgh Hospital, and at the Division of International Medical Education, University of Edinburgh. He also was awarded a British Council Fellowship twice; in 1988 to attend the British Council course on Psychogeriatrics at the University of Nottingham and in 1992 to attend the British Council course on recent developments in psychiatry at the University of Cambridge. In 1994 he was funded by the Exchange Fellow Program of the Thai Ministry of University Affairs and the Federal Ministry of Science and Research of Austria to work as a visiting researcher at the Division of Pharmacopsychiatry and Sleep Research,

Department of Psychiatry, University of Vienna. In 2001, he was awarded a Fellowship to attend the University of Melbourne–Harvard Medical School Leadership Program in International Mental Health at the University of Melbourne.

He was elected by Thai psychiatrists to be President of the Psychiatric Association of Thailand (PAT) for two consecutive terms (2006–2007 and 2008–2009). Later, during 2010–2019 he was elected to be the Founding President of Thai Society for Geriatric Psychiatry and Neuropsychiatry (TSGN).

He is now an Emeritus Professor of Psychiatry of Prince of Songkla University in southern Thailand and presently has been appointed by Thai Medical Council to be the first Chairman of the National Board Examination on Geriatric Psychiatry.

His role in international psychiatry is highlighted by involvement with various professional organizations. He is currently working as follows:

- Vice-President, World Association for Psychosocial Rehabilitation (WAPR)
- Board Member and Zonal Representative of the World Psychiatric Association (WPA) for Zone 16
- WPA Standing Committee on Education
- Working Group for WPA on Public Mental Health
- International Advisory Committee of Japanese Society of Psychiatry and Neurology (JSPN)

In the past he served for many international organizations, including:

- International Advisory Group for WHO on the revision of ICD-10 Mental and Behavioral Disorders
- Working Group for WHO on Psychotic Disorders in ICD-11
- President, Pacific Rim College of Psychiatrists (PRCP)
- President, Asian College of Schizophrenia Research (ACSR)
- President, Asian Federation of Psychiatric Associations (AFPA)
- President, ASEAN Federation of Psychiatry and Mental Health (AFPMH)
- Vice President for Outreach, International Society for Bipolar Disorders (ISBD)
- Chairman and Founding Member, Asian Network of Bipolar Disorder (ANBD)
- Vice-Chair of the WPA Working Group for the Revision of Curriculum on Psychiatric Education
- Member of the WPA-Lancet Psychiatry Commission on the Future of Psychiatry

Professor Udomratn has received many awards from both national and international Organizations, including:

- Kupfer-Frank Distinctive Contribution Award for making a great impact upon the ISBD and its mission (2021)
- WPA Honorary Membership for excellence in service to the World Psychiatric Association (2017)
- ISBD Scholar Award as the Asian Regional Leader for his initiative idea to propose the World Bipolar Day (WBD) to be celebrated on 30 March every year (2015)

- Outstanding Thai Psychiatrist who Devoted Himself for the Benefit of the Professional Community (2013)
- Outstanding Research Psychiatrist from the Psychiatric Association of Thailand (2001)

He has worked with many leaders in psychiatric field by involvement in many international congresses, including:

- Chair of the Scientific Committee of the WPA Regional Congress (India, 2023)
- Member of the Organizing Committee of the WPA Thematic Congress (UAE, 2023)
- Member of the Scientific Committee of the 20th, 21th, 22th WPA World Congress of Psychiatry (Thailand, 2020, Colombia 2021, Thailand 2022)
- Congress President of the 18th International Congress of PRCP (Myanmar, 2018)
- Congress President of the 5th World Congress of Asian Psychiatry (Japan, 2015)

Professor Udomratn is now a member of the Editorial Boards of many international journals such as *Psychiatry and Clinical Neuroscience*, the *Asia Pacific Psychiatry Journal*, the *Asian Journal of Psychiatry*, *Taiwanese Journal of Psychiatry*, and the *International Journal of Social Psychiatry*. He also serves as a peer reviewer for many international journals as well as the *Journal of the Psychiatric Association of Thailand*, of which he is a former editor.

He has authored more than 150 publications including books, research papers, reviews, and special articles. His major fields of interest and research are broad. These fields include psychotic disorders, mood and anxiety disorders, psychopharmacology, geriatric psychiatry, and psychosocial rehabilitation. Recently he joined with other co-authors to write the chapter 'Psychiatric Rehabilitation in the 21st Century' in the WPA book, *Advances in Psychiatry*.

Interview

PU: Thank you for inviting me to join this interesting project and let me be part of your excellent book.

I: Thank you. I mean it's such a great pleasure for me because the book is about interviewing psychiatrists around the world and you know, what got them to where they are, they have achieved and so you have seen the questions.

PU: It looks like a very interesting book.

I: Can you tell me about your childhood and growing up and how you ended up in medicine?

PU: Yes. I was born in 1957 in Hat Yai city, Songkhla province, in southern Thailand, which was nearly 1,000 kilometres from Bangkok. My primary school was not far from my home. When I was young, my father gave me a ride to school but when I was growing up, I walked to school from home by myself. I was lucky, there was an examination in which I ranked number 1 of the class, so at the time it was a tradition in my family that all my brothers and sisters would continue their higher education in famous schools in Bangkok. So I had followed their footsteps. However, life in Bangkok during the years 1972 to 1974 was not easy, especially regarding transportation. Public buses were crowded, there were always traffic jams, bad air pollution, and so on. These are the reasons which later helped me make the decision not to pursue my higher education at the university in Bangkok and come back to my home town. At that time, it was a norm and value that bright and clever students who studied in the science track would choose either medicine or engineering. My oldest brother chose medicine and became a doctor, my other brother chose engineering, so I had no choice; I was left between medicine and engineering. So I chose medicine but the place where I chose to study was not a medical school in Bangkok but I chose to come back and study at Prince of Songkla University (PSU) which was the first new medical school in the southern part of Thailand, located in Hat Yai. At that time, the government thought that there should be more medical schools outside Bangkok, so they built one in the north, one in the north-east, and one in the south. I'm from the second batch of the medical student list at this university and at that time, we didn't have enough facilities. There was no university hospital as it was under construction, and even medical teachers were young people who had just finished their training in Bangkok and they had trouble adjusting to life in a city that was quite a long way from Bangkok. Returning to Bangkok took 20 hours by overnight train, so there was a real brain drain of new medical teachers. When I was a medical student, one of the very sad topics that was being discussed among the medical students was who would be the next of our medical teachers that resigned. In the third year, I made up my minds to try to stay on at Hat Yai and become one of the staff of medical teachers here. I didn't want this situation to get worse. I then had to decide which department I wanted to work for and found that I wanted to attempt psychiatry because my teacher told me that I did a wonderful job. He said, 'You don't only interview the patient to search for diagnosis but you also offer her empathetic understanding and support via some kind of supportive psychotherapy.' When you hear your teacher tell you that you're good at something, your self-esteem increases. The more I learn psychiatry, the more I love it which brings me to my final decision to become a psychiatrist.

I: Did you stay on in Hat Yai to do psychiatry training, or did you go elsewhere for that?

PU: Because our medical school was a new one, they didn't have any course for postgraduate training. So I had to choose a training institute in Bangkok, and the training institute that I chose was the oldest and the first training institute of psychiatry in Thailand. It was called the Somdet Chaopraya Hospital but now it is the Somdet Chaopraya Institute of Psychiatry.

I: Do you ever regret choosing psychiatry?

PU: No, not at all. If I had the chance to choose again, I would still choose psychiatry as my career.

I: Who has been your role model?

PU: My teachers. My first teacher demonstrated to me how to give positive feedback to medical students, and the other teachers taught me how to show empathetic understanding, how to listen to the patients, how to establish therapeutic relationships with the patients, and also how to behave with colleagues. I think many of my teachers were my role models.

I: And over the years, have there been any particular clinical or research points which have remained in your memory?

PU: When I was a resident, the American Psychiatric Association (APA) introduced a new classification called DSM III and it was the first time that the panic disorder appeared as a separate disorder, but during that period of training in Thailand, we also used the WHO classification ICD-9. This was confusing as when we wrote up cases, it seemed to me that some were definitely panic disorder but because we didn't use DSM we had to offer the diagnosis of anxiety states based on ICD-9, which was different from DSM III. After passing the board examination, I had returned to PSU where I met a Thai psychiatrist who had trained in the United States where DSM was used. His advice gave me more confidence in diagnosing panic disorder. So, finally I reported the first case report of panic disorder in Thailand in the local journal of psychiatry.

I: Over the 45 years or so you have been in psychiatry, how has psychiatry changed in Thailand?

PU: Oh, it has changed a lot! The number of psychiatrists has increased, stigmatization has decreased, and the attitude of public towards psychiatry has changed in a positive way. We now also have training in other subspecialties which we didn't have before such as geriatric psychiatry, and sleep psychiatry. So, that has changed a lot during the years.

I: What are your views on the current state of psychiatry?

PU: I think psychiatry is in an era of developing new knowledge, especially in neuroscience and how to understand the brain and behaviour. The role of AI (Artificial Intelligence) is being discussed a lot these days, how it has been used in other subspecialties and how it will come to be used in part of the clinical practice of psychiatry. I don't think AI can replace psychiatrists; we can use it to give us some guidelines or some knowledge but in terms of catching the emotion, feeling, and supporting the patients, AI cannot replace the psychiatrists. But it is great to have technology that we can use to have more contact with patients and with each other, exchange ideas through tele-psychiatry or tele-medicine; it has been especially helpful during the COVID 19 situation.

I: Over the years, what do you see as problems with psychiatry?

PU: Although we say that the stigmatization has decreased in my country I feel that stigma continues to be a problem, stigma not just against psychiatry but against persons with mental disorders. It will take time to overcome this.

I: What's the recruitment into psychiatry like in Thailand? Do you have any problems?

PU: Yes, at the beginning it was due to stigma. Few medical students chose psychiatry but then the situation has changed, we now have more applicants to be trainees than we can accept them perhaps due to what they call 'pull' factors and 'push' factors. I think it's important to begin from medical students. They should learn psychiatry, not only as pure mental disorders but to learn about psychiatry in a broader way. If I had a chance to build a new medical school, I think that the new curriculum of psychiatry would have psychiatrists working together with internal medicine, obstetrics and gynaecology, and in other parts of the hospital, the surgical ward, in the internal medicine ward, in the OB GYN ward. In these, you would have two specialists working together, doing outpatients together, doing the ward rounds on patients together. Then as a psychiatrist you can pick up the mental health problems or mental disorders or comorbidity that are associated with physical disorders which have been neglected or overlooked by other specialists. This would encourage medical students to become interested in psychiatry. In fact, in our medical school, we have a new curriculum, put in place at the time I was the Assistant Dean of Academic Affairs. The new curriculum integrated psychiatry into various blocks, we call it rotation, and medical students would rotate from one block to another, such as health and disease of the elderly, health and disease for women. They also have to learn psychiatry in a specific block in clinical years. We found that students who learned using the new curriculum had a more positive attitude, measured by using Attitudes to Psychiatry-30 (ATP 30), towards the field. The questionnaire had an item that stated 'I would like to be a psychiatrist. The number of medical students who agreed to this item was higher after the last day of rotation compared to the first day, although this number was not statistically significant.

I: Obviously one of the big challenges is how you integrate psychiatry. I like that idea that it should be integrated and part of looking at every condition, but the difficulty is that quite often medical colleges do not wish to change.

PU: Yes, and it's a problem also because the number of the staff rises if you do things this way, but I think we can manage that. We do not need one psychiatrist dedicated to one ward but they can rotate around wards. For example, on Monday they may be at internal medicine, Tuesday at palliative care, so they spend at least one or two hours in the morning on rounds with the other specialists.

I: What do you see as the characteristics of a good psychiatrist?

PU: It seems to me that a good psychiatrist should be a good listener, should be someone who has empathetic understanding, should have a non-judgmental attitude, who is able to support patients. I found that when they interview patients, many new young trainees try to seek information solely for diagnostic purposes; they don't see how to support the patients at the same time. I usually demonstrate that to them and I also tell them that the interview is not only for diagnosis; it also to be for therapeutic intervention.

I: Where do you see are the gaps in training of psychiatrists?

PU: In Thailand?

I: Yes, and globally.

PU: In Thailand, we have psychiatrists who work in mental hospitals where they do not have any medical facilities, so when psychiatrists in general hospitals want to refer cases to mental hospitals, they are uncomfortable accepting those referrals perhaps because these psychiatrists in mental hospitals lack confidence that patients who may have comorbidity with physical or medical conditions will be cared for or looked after with less medical facilities in their hospitals. It seems to me that there should be a gap in the curriculum of postgraduate training which may need to emphasize groups of patients who have comorbidities.

I: And in medical school in Thailand, you said that now you got blocks of training. Is there any specific period of training in psychiatry there?

PU: Yes. In my medical school even though we had blocks these were for the first three years. In the clinical years, students have clerkships, going from one ward to another, and at my university they have to come to the psychiatric ward for two weeks in the fourth and in the last year before they graduate. So, at the same time as the blocks you have to take care of some of the mental patients who have been admitted to the ward. Also, students have exposure not only in the ward but also visiting patients in the family, in the community, in home healthcare projects, and also at outpatient psychiatric clinics.

I: In India, for example, it is a similar thing that you do two weeks of psychiatry in the fourth year so there isn't a kind of integrated model to try and integrate medicine or surgery or obstetrics with psychiatry so you see a very limited number of cases. You probably get to see a very severely ill psychotic patient, which can add to the stigma.

PU: Not all medical schools in Thailand use the new curriculum as the problem-based learning that was divided into various blocks. Some of them still teach using the conventional curriculum and in general, students have to rotate to psychiatry about four weeks in the fourth or fifth year. Some medical schools add an extra two weeks in their last year, and this means that they have to rotate through psychiatry twice. Moreover, the curriculum of psychiatry varies from medical school to medical school, but all medical students have to rotate to both psychiatric wards and psychiatric outpatient departments.

I: What do you think about people with mental illness or with drug addiction? Do they have been treated appropriately?

PU: We have a problem because the number of drug-addicted prisoners in Thailand is increasing. The government has deemed these prisoners now to be classified as patients and they want to send these prisoners for treatment as drug-addicted patients until the doctor says that they have recovered, then will be released or discharged. This decreases the number of prisoners. However, the allocated budget does not permit us to do the job they want us to do. It's less than we expect.

I: This is not dissimilar to the situation in the United States where it's argued that a large number of people with mental illness are in prisons because there are limited number of asylums and there are often limited mental health services to look after them so they end up in prisons, so they are basically in asylum but without treatment.

PU: I see.

I: You have been very involved with Asian psychiatry and you also led the Asian Federation of Psychiatric Associations (AFPA). What was that like?

PU: I think that it is a very good idea to bring all the associations in Asia together to become closer under one roof of AFPA. However, the process sometimes has problems. When I had the chance to become the President of the AFPA, I tried very hard to unify the associations. Finally, we had the Bangkok Resolution in 2013. This Resolution was agreed unanimously by Presidents and Representatives of psychiatric societies in Asia that the unity and collaboration among societies is a major asset in the promotion of mental health and the betterment of psychiatry in Asia. You can find details of the Resolution from the AFPA website (www.afpa.asia/resolution.html.)

I: What were the lessons you learned? You did a very good job during the term. It was a three-year term, wasn't it?

PU: No, it was a two-year term. I was the President from 2013 to 2015 and I learned a lot between this period. During my term, I put all of my efforts to strengthen the relationship between associations and AFPA which later became stronger than before. I initiated many activities such as the *AFPA Bulletin*, the congress in the year between World Congress of Asian Psychiatry (WCAP), initially called Regional Congress of Asian Psychiatry (RCAP) and later changed to be the International Congress of AFPA. I proposed the AFPA Lifetime Achievement Award; you were the only recipient of this award in 2015. We were very proud to have given this distinguished award to you. I also started the relationship between AFPA and European Psychiatric Association (EPA). We agreed to have AFPA-EPA symposium at WCAP and the annual meeting of the EPA. Speakers in the symposium comprised one senior and one junior Asian psychiatrist, together with one senior and one junior European counterpart. This special symposium was first held in the 5th WCAP in Fukuoka 2015, and two weeks later at the 23rd European Congress of Psychiatry in Vienna the same year. However, this collaborative activity between AFPA and EPA has not been continued since my Presidency was ended,

I: Which of your achievements are you most proud of?

PU: I think I have many achievements which I had never thought of before. In Thailand, I have been widely known as the psychiatrist who was the pioneer in ensuring that geriatric psychiatry was recognized because before that, it had not been part of the curriculum in general psychiatry. Later on, with the help of Royal College, when you were the President and we had Memorandum of Understanding between your college and the Thai college, I suggested that we should write the curriculum for this subspecialty and you proposed Yong Lock Ong from Singapore to help us. I would like to inform you that now geriatric psychiatry has been accepted by the Thai Medical Council as a subspecialty of psychiatry and I have been appointed by the Thai Medical council to be the first chairman of the National Board Examination of Geriatric Psychiatry.

I: Congratulations, well done.

PU: Thank you. But the thing that I feel very proud of is my idea about the World Bipolar Day. In the year 2013, I was chairman of the Asian Network of Bipolar Disorder and we held a council meeting in Bangkok. We were lucky because at that time, the President of the ISBD (International Society of Bipolar Disorders), Professor Wilhelm Nolen, wanted to attend to promote the annual meeting of the ISBD which occurred in Seoul in 2014. I invited him to join our council meeting as an observer and in that meeting I voiced the idea that as now we have so many World Days, even World Sleep Day proposed by the World Association of Sleep Medicine, we should have more than just World Mental Health Day and World

Suicide Prevention Day. We all know that bipolar disorder is a serious illness that is treatable so why don't we have World Bipolar Day? Everyone in the meeting room agreed. Then we asked which day should be world bipolar day? As we think that Van Gogh suffered from bipolar disorder we chose his birthday, 30 March. Professor Wilhelm Nolen, President of the ISBD, loved the idea. He thought that this will help the ISBD meeting in Seoul in March 2014 to be really important, the ISBD took this idea and informed the International Bipolar Foundation (IBPF) to support it. Finally, three organizations were involved (including my organization, the Asian Network of Bipolar Disorder (ANBD), but the funding and the big support came from the ISBD and the IBPF. My initial thought was just to celebrate World Bipolar Day with the objectives to increase public awareness about bipolar disorder and to erase the stigmatization of the disorder. We first celebrated this day in March 2014 at the annual meeting of the ISBD. Professor Wilhelm Nolen gave me very short notice for giving an address (after his opening address) in the form of a brief talk about the origin of World Bipolar Day. Then, at the break, Professor Mohan Isaac came to check hands with me and said, 'Oh! I didn't know that you were the father of World Bipolar Day.' It is now well known and has been celebrated worldwide, so I am very proud of this.

I: Looking back, what would you tell your younger self?

PU: I would suggest to my younger self that I should do a PhD in epidemiology because epidemiology is important. Learning medicine is hard, and on top of that we have to learn subspecialties in psychiatry. I wanted my final boards to be my last exams so when the last day of the National Board Examination on Psychiatry came around I felt enormous relief. I had my first daughter that same year. Later, I realized that I wanted to go abroad but just for a short time for a postgraduate fellowship, a short period of time, six months or nine months, but I didn't think of studying for a PhD. If I had the chance to go back, I may have to ask my wife if she would mind if I took leave to study for a PhD in epidemiology for at least three or four years (laughs).

I: What would you advise trainees of today?

PU: In continuing psychiatric education, usually I tell my trainees that you finish, you have the board examination, you pass the board examination, but that doesn't mean that you don't have to learn anything new; this is just the beginning. If you look at panic disorder as an example, it's quite strange that early on, most of the articles published in the journals on panic disorder said that panic disorder cannot be treated by benzodiazepines. The only benzodiazepine that works is alprazolam: why? It took at least 20 years until Sadock and Kaplan published their Textbook with a list of medications that work for panic disorder, including benzodiazepines such as diazepam, clonazepam, and so on. At that time, I discussed this with some researchers in Europe and I told them that colleagues of mine were doing a double-blind trial between diazepam and alprazolam in the treatment of panic disorder. They laughed at me and told me that diazepam doesn't work at all, but finally from our results we found that both drugs are equally effective.

I: Great. Well, I thank we covered almost everything. Thank you.

25
Rutger Jan van der Gaag

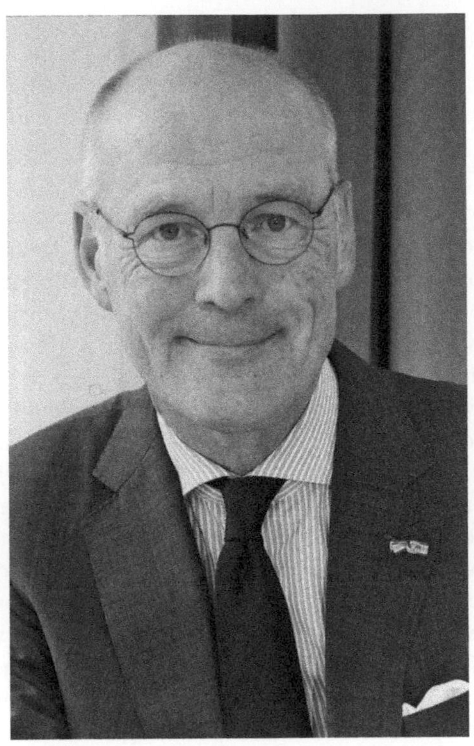

Biography

Professor Rutger Jan van der Gaag MD PhD, Hon. FRCPsych DFAPA ONN (1950) has an international background, having grown up in England and France before moving to Holland in 1968. After his medical studies, he specialized in general practice and moved on to psychiatry in a later phase. He gained international recognition with research in developmental disorders (autism and ADHD) and gender and psychopathology. After a long tenure at the University Medical Centre in Utrecht and experience as director of training in psychiatry (Ermelo), he was appointed as a full professor of psychiatry in Nijmegen (2002). During this period of time, he presided over the Netherlands Psychiatric Association (2008–2012) and the Royal Dutch Medical Association (KNMG, 2012–2016), also serving on the Boards of the European Psychiatric Association, and the Council of the World Medical Association and the

European Medical Doctors (CPME). After becoming emeritus professor in Nijmegen (2016), he was appointed professor of psychosomatics and psychotherapy at the Stradina University in Riga. Currently, among other posts he holds, he is President of the Netherlands Association for Healthcare Executives and he serves on the Executive Board of the University of Paris Cité.

Interview

I: Can we start off by talking about your childhood and your growing up. What was that like?

RJG: I was raised in an atypical family. My parents spent most of the Second World War in hiding. They got married shortly after the war. They adopted two cousins of my mother's whose parents had died in camps. So, I became the fourth child in the family. My father had just completed his studies as an accountant and joined Unilever. We moved to Kent in the early 1950s. At that point, I was an infant on the verge of becoming a toddler. We really lived in very enchanted places. We had a very nice time in England. After the war there was a strong sense of community and incredibly nice schools. I was at St David's College in West Wickham. That all came to an end when my father was moved to France. Dr Shove—an Oxford PhD who was our headmaster said, 'No, worries, lads. English is the universal language.' But obviously he had never been to France. So, when I was eight, on the verge of turning nine, we moved to France. My parents made a mistake in the sense that we were living in a very well-to-do area where there was an international school but at that time it was only for children of diplomats and military. Not being a Catholic, I was sent to a public school, which taught children of people who owned shops or worked at houses as personnel. So, they other children were very hostile towards us as representatives of the upper class. The change in language and circumstances was huge. I can't really tell about my younger brother but I had the feeling that he became very subdued. I became a fighter punching those who were mean to us and aggressive, on the other hand within a year I was the best of the class, and that silenced most of those who had been so harsh and went to secondary school with very good marks. And I must say that from then on, I felt more at home with France even though the French always have something of a touch of xenophobia about them so I never really felt completely accepted as one of them. The circumstances at home changed dramatically too; my parents decided to have two more children. When we were adolescents, my parents were very much engaged and concerned with the two little ones, and we had to look after ourselves. My elder sister and younger brother did it in a very nice way and both were very kind to my parents. I was very rebellious and my rebellious nature brought me into activism in the late 1960s. In 1968, I participated in all kinds of political activities. Eventually I was given notice to leave France for some time. And so, when I was 18 and I had just passed my A levels, I went to Holland where my sister had gone because she did not like the French. My Dutch was poor, my French school did not fit in with what was being taught in the Netherlands so I thought I would be there only for a year. The strange thing was that I was in rather left-wing circles in France but ended up in quite right-wing and more liberal circles in the Netherlands. This was because in my fraternity, most of the people whom I knew were from the nobility, or they were from business families and the diplomatic services who were mostly rather conservative people. I was about to go back to France and had made up my mind that I wouldn't pursue medicine but go into political science. Just before I left I met a very nice girl and she said, 'If you leave, nothing's going to happen'. So I stayed and passed all my exams. We got married on the same day but not to each other. I stayed in Holland and continued my medical studies. I started liking them and I became a very active chair of all kinds of committees. There was a great deal of student participation. Students were heavily involved with changing education programmes, pushing to have more bedside teaching and more mentoring. I was friendly to many of the seniors in the faculty. At that time, I was very interested in gastroenterology. The strange thing is what attracted me to medicine was a very special encounter. I hadn't thought about medicine at all and one day Albert Schweitzer came to play the organ in our church. He would come once in a while to play the organ and there would be a charity gala and people would pay to attend. He would then take that money to Gabon for running hospitals. He asked me what I wanted to do. At that time, I wasn't intending to do much that would make a difference in the world. And then he said, 'That's not going to be a help to your fellow people. Why don't you consider medicine?' I was extremely hesitant about medicine because when I started off in the Netherlands, chemistry and physics seemed important to getting into medicine, and they seemed only remotely linked to what I thought medicine would be about. But one of the senior boys in the fraternity house where I lived in my first year said, 'Well, come to my bedside teaching courses'. So every morning at 7:30 a.m. I would go with him to bedside teaching; neurology, internal medicine, psychiatry. There were really remarkable professors at that time. I remember one of them that I have quoted from for the rest of my life. Professor Jordan always told me to remember that every patient could be your father, your mother, your most dear one; how would you want them to be treated? That really impressed me.

I don't know why I was interested in gastroenterology, maybe because I was doing some research on liver diseases and alcohol and things like that. And then there were two things that really made a huge impression on me: one was when I was reading Martin Buber, who described the idea of building your life in cycles, not doing the same things for more than seven years. The other was one of the things I read at that time, I think it was J.F. Kennedy or Dwight Eisenhower who said, 'Always make sure you have plan B and eventually plan C'. So for the rest of my life there has been a plan B and C.

When I finished my medical studies in 1975 there were two options: either you took your turn of duty in the army for two years or you could go and serve in a peace corps in Africa in a hospital. When I had been training in surgery and gynaecology for only two or three months, my wife Madeleine was given the opportunity to buy a veterinarian practice. In those days, work was scarce for veterinarians, so this was a big opportunity. The other hazard was that she was very concerned that if she stopped working, then she would fall out of the workforce so she was very keen to keep working. I thus had to change gears and that implied that I would have to go into military service, but there was one way of postponing it and that was training as a GP. I did that and it was a revelation, it was so different from having been in the hospital services, meeting people at home and seeing how families work. I liked that very much. There was one practical problem. I still had to do my military service but I could return to the place where I had been training. It was a very nice kind of hybrid village with commuters but also farmers and local businesses, a really interesting place, but I couldn't start a practice there or join the practice that was already there if I didn't live in that community; that was a requirement back then. So, I said to Madeleine that I wouldn't become a GP but would return to internal medicine and gastroenterology. And then she said, 'If you do that, I don't think it would be wise first to have children because you'll never be around. I'm not going to raise them on my own because I'm passionate about working and having my professional independence.' Plan B it was! I remember that on a Saturday, I was reading a newspaper and there was an ad for part-time work for psychiatrists so I decided to go into psychiatry. My wife said, 'If you think that will make you happy, it will work out fine with us, so why not try?' Psychiatry training at that time was for four years. It included one year of neurology, two years of general psychiatry, and then you could specialize. I started with neurology. It was very strange at that time because having been very much involved in the faculty and having completed my study with very good grades, I could just call a professor and ask, 'Could you offer me a position?' and there would be no problem. I loved neurology because it was absolutely precise. I liked the specialty but Madeline said, 'Well, that was not what you were going to do'. The work shifts in neurology were quite long. It was difficult to combine that with the fact that we already had two children. So I turned to psychiatry and I must admit that the two years of training in general psychiatry were a very harsh and challenging experience. I felt somewhat discouraged by the fact that one had the feeling that patients weren't listening. They weren't doing what was advised for them. They were going their own way. Often, they could be rude and aggressive. Things were generally very complicated and at that point in time I was not really sure if this was what I wanted to pursue.

Then, quite by matter of coincidence, I went to a lecture about psychophysiology by Herman van Engeland, a professor in child and adolescent psychiatry. The only thing I can remember from that lecture was that he was talking about development and functioning. He illustrated it by telling what it takes to bake an egg in terms of thinking, anticipating, organizing, planning, etc. What he was telling us was that we now had the means, with electrophysiology, to help us understand what's happening in the brain. I was really hooked and at the end I asked if there were any chance to be enrolled in a child and adolescent psychiatry programme. And there was. So I completed my training in a department where clinical care for children and adolescents with developmental disorders and their families went hand in hand with teaching and research. I realized that I enjoyed working with parents and children a lot and I seemed to be able to connect with them.

In the department where I started there was a very nice mix of things, which I found very interesting. There was clinical work and leadership roles. Thus, at the age of only 31 I was head of the department with about 30 to 40 personnel, and I had to manage them. In the clinic you had to make sure the principles of the clinic were followed. One of the key principles for the personnel was, 'You come here to grow and then you go'. We would attract nurses and say to them that they were going to work with us for five years; they would be trained for two years which would lead to them to work as seniors for two years, and then in the last year they would be supported to look for new professional opportunities to help them move on. I must say I liked that very much because it gave an academic focus: staff were encouraged to develop and change, not stay in that workplace forever. That has been very inspiring, despite the fact that back then I had a very ambivalent relationship with my boss. That had to do with social class. His father repaired bikes and my father was at the top of Unilever. There was a huge social gap between the two of us and he didn't like the fact that I knew many people and moved easily socially. But when it came to being trained in leadership, being trained in clinical work, he was a wonderful role model, and he was very outgoing.

After my first year in the department, my reward was to go to the Maudsley and work with Michael Rutter (see Chapter 18), then go to the Great Ormond Street to work with Philip Graham, and then with Donald Cohen at Yale Child Study Center in New Haven. Cohen was friendly with a rebellious group of French child psychiatrists, under leadership of Prof Gilbert Lelord in Tours. That was the only place in France where no psychoanalyst was in charge of the department, but they were educational and empirical in their approach.

From there I visited the United States regularly. I was often in London at the Maudsley and to see my parents who lived in Wimbledon.

I spent 14 years in that department, seven years of training and doing a PhD, and then seven years as a head of even bigger department within the huge department of child and adolescent psychiatry. After seven years I said, 'Time for a change', and I moved on. I was 45 and became director of training in a community hospital which was quite near the place where Madeleine was working as a teacher then. I worked there for seven years and that was a very rich experience, but also very humbling. I never realized that when you are working in a university hospital, despite the fact that you know nothing, people think you are someone and you have access to all kinds of things. But when you are working a peripheral hospital, you are not very interesting.

I had to broaden my scope as I had only been working with children with autism and ADHD in an academic department. I worked in two places, one was a very traditional Christian place with a huge psychiatric institution so that became my base, the other was in a new town in the polder where everything happened that God had not permitted. There were broken families, drugs, addiction, youngsters with extremely challenging behaviour. My experience as a GP was of great help. I was always very outgoing. I would go to see people at home and that was a really great experience. Moreover I had more time than I had in the university hospital to do research.

Being the director of training has been really one of the most rewarding experiences in my whole professional life. Having residents come for training and having their own struggles, to see them thrive, develop, and then go further was and is very rewarding. At that time, many centres for child and adolescent psychiatry had recruitment problems but I had the embarrassment of choice as everyone wanted to come and train with me. I could even send some trainees to my former boss and other university departments as I was booked completely full. That gave me a very special position within the Netherlands. It was also because I had a very strong position in the autistic society and was given huge credit by parents.

So, despite the fact that I was not in a university position, Donald Cohen from Yale made sure that I kept getting published. And then, in 2002, I was appointed the head of the department of Child and Adolescents Psychiatry in the university hospital of Nijmegen and became professor of psychiatry.

Well, that was a huge challenge because the department was in despair. My predecessor was a paediatrician who had no knowledge of child psychiatry and had never published anything. There were no residents.

My colleague Jan Buitelaar, who became chair of the adult department, and I started off with 25 staff for the child and adolescent department in a beautiful and huge new building. I took quite some effort but we were successful, and after seven years I was running a department with 153 collaborators, 26 residents, and a huge clinical and scientific output. We were running all kinds of programmes and had relationships with all the major institutes in Europe and the United States.

Then I realized that it was time for change again. I wrote a report for my dean saying, 'How can I make myself redundant' (and in the process give opportunities to younger staff with good potential). I began to work part-time there, spending Mondays only in the department but leaving it in good hands for the remainder of the week. My first step outside was a move to the Netherlands Association for Psychiatry. That is where I met you, Dinesh, in our effort to merge the National Psychiatric Associations with the European Psychiatric Association (eventually a successful enterprise).

I remember at that point of the time that one of my big concerns was that my generation was neglecting politics. The generations of my grandfather and my father would engage in politics because their views were that it was something they had to do. Politics was something that was your return on investment to the community. They were mayors, they were representatives in the House of Commons or the Senate, and sometimes Ministers. My generation left it to the clowns. I didn't go into politics because I couldn't find a party I felt I belonged to.

I went into the Psychiatric Association, and I was very fortunate. You may remember Peter Niesink, who was the director and truly remarkable chap. He is more than 20 years younger than I am, but he has an incredible sense of bringing people together and getting things done. We were really very successful, although he did things his way and I did things mine.

We always hosted the annual meeting, attended by 3,000 psychiatrists. I would shake hands with everyone and stand there every morning to welcome the members. One of the nice things was that you had a feeling that people took pride in psychiatry. Early on in my term, we were confronted by the fact that our Liberal Minister of Health decreed that the psychiatric patients had to pay, whereas other patients with 'real' illnesses were exempt.

Within a few days after this stupid idea was launched Peter and I managed to get 10,000 people protesting in The Hague which led to a lot of press exposure. And it forced the Minster to drop her idea.

From then on, we were very successful at lobbying. We were in a position to urge the Ministry of Health to conclude all kinds of arrangements in which healthcare would be self-restricting and professionals wold become more aware of the costs. Those four years as President of the Psychiatric Association were immediately followed by four years as President of the Royal Dutch Medical Association and that was a tough job. I had to do something that was very unpopular, changing things, bringing in young people, but most of the personnel hated me for that. After four years they got a chance to get rid of me. I stepped down a couple of months before my term was over, but I don't regret my time there. I finished that period of seven years on a positive note. My successor, who had not been part of the deconstruction, was able to implement the changes that were necessary. Lesson learned. You cannot be both the bad guy that comes in to overturn the status quo and then expect the personnel to accept you as the good guy and help you reorganize.

Now I have reached the next seven-year period in my life story, one in which returning to society is centre stage. So I tried to pick out things that I think are relevant to something. Dear friends and venerated colleagues such as Dinesh Bhugra, who taught me social justice for vulnerable people, and Sir Michael Marmot, who pointed my attention towards social determinants of (mental) health, have given me guidance in this process. And that's what I'm doing now.

I: Over the years, how do you think psychiatry has changed?

RJG: I think from my perspective, psychiatry has moved out of its comfort zone. When I started in 1977, I did part of my training in an institute where every morning all the patients would walk into their workplaces and they returned to their pavilions at noon and had their meals. That was a very patronizing way of doing psychiatry and yet at the same time, the psychiatrists then knew what they were there to do. They were the ones who were taking care of these institutions and they were the ones offering asylum to people that nowadays roam homeless in the streets. There was tremendous change in the 1990s. Child and adolescent psychiatry was far less prominent than general psychiatry.

In our country from the 1990s there was a complete shift of paradigm. Everyone was supposed to be responsible for his own behaviour. If you were not motivated, you were dismissed. Under the 'flag of auto-determination', psychiatrists and society choose to neglect vulnerable people. In those days, people were kicked out of institutions. All the work and activities that were done in the institutions and that gave patients structure and meaning were abolished. They were not being taken care of. It was probably because there was a kind of paradigm according to which people are responsible for their own behaviour, you shouldn't force anybody to do anything. A complete change of gears from over-patronizing to utter neglect. I met a patient recently whom I knew from my first training and he lived on the premises of the psychiatric hospital. He worked in a bank in town and once in a while he would develop psychosis or something like that. When he was out of work he was in the hospital and when he had recovered, he would go back and he said, 'In the old days, you had more opportunities than now because people were much more inclined to employ you because they knew that these hospitals would take care of you and that you would return. If things were going badly, the employer would get a phone call saying "So-and-so is not coming for the next two to three weeks but that they would be back in due course." Now if you are not stable and run into a crisis once in a while, your employer gets fed up with you and doesn't want you to come back at all.'

I: You said that over the years, psychiatry has moved out of its comfort zone. What do you see as the problems with modern psychiatry?

RJG: One of the problems with modern psychiatry is that the psychiatrist is uncertain about his or her role. In many instances, psychiatrists still have a huge responsibility but the services are all run by psychologists. Psychiatrists are responsible for hundreds of patients that they don't really know but they are not involved in running the department. There is a generation gap between older psychiatrists who are very nostalgic for times when they were considered authorities and young psychiatrists who are far more flexible and are engaged in community care. From my point of view, the younger psychiatrists are idealistic but not really committed to engaging with patients on the longer run. And goodness knows many psychiatric conditions are chronic but still many patients have recurrent relapses. The other day I called a psychiatrist because I needed her help. I said,' I have known this patient since 1981 and I think he needs your help'. Well, it was a phone call so I couldn't see what happened at the other end of the line but I thought that she must have fallen from her chair because of the idea that you could have a relationship for more than 30 years with a patient. She was mostly worried about getting her work remunerated for more than a couple of sessions. Many mental health professionals nowadays work part-time and are not easily accessible When I speak to patients, I have the feeling that they miss someone they can really rely on, and simply having their phone numbers is not enough.

I: What do you see as the characteristics of a good psychiatrist?

RJG: I think that the good psychiatrists are the ones that care for their patients. Those that have real empathy, keeping appropriate distance and showing respect. They dare to have a long-running relationship in which they don't patronize but empower their patients and are highly available through modern media such as secured chats and videocalls or the phone. I think that the ones that are really doing what must be done are the ones that are beating the system and that are not afraid of standing up to their managers. This nice generation of rebellious psychiatrists that care more about patients than about the system, but it takes courage to so.

I: In your opinion, how do you see that psychiatry's social contract can be achieved? Don't you think in some ways rebellion can cause problems in servicing that contract?

RJG: It could be. But I see that compliant psychiatrists are being marginalized. So maybe I am using the word rebellious in the wrong way, but audacity is needed as well as the courage to think. One of the interesting things about my youth is that the culture in France was very different as compared to that in the Netherlands. In the Netherlands, you abide by the rules and then you are a good citizen. In France, you try to beat the rules. So, if you want to apply for something in the Netherlands, just fill in the form and send it in and rely on the system that the form will be duly addressed and that you will get a response. I call someone and say, 'I understand that I have to fill in the form. Can I bring it to you? Can we discuss it?' Or I just do it my way and wait for the system to respond. When it comes to doing things for your patients, I think you should be thinking out of the box. I once had a huge clash with my boss in the academic centre because at noon I had left, so he said, 'Where were you?' and I said, 'I went to a car shop because I thought that would be someone who would be willing to employ one of my autistic patients'. And that happened. I went to see that guy. I described the person who was admitted to the hospital and then I went to the social security service, and I said, 'You are paying this person an invalidity pension. Can I arrange that if my patient's employer says he is doing well and the employer pays, you don't have to pay? If he isn't get well, we will reverse this arrangement.' That is not in the rules but it works. In the Netherlands, there is a huge group of psychiatrists who abide by the rules and think that the rules are more important than life. But there is also another group that challenges the rules in order to deliver better patient care, psychiatrist and mental health professionals acting as advocates to their patients.

I: My own experience says that we were never taught to advocate for our patients.

RJG: No, indeed.

I: And I think that should be one of the core skills for doctors.

RJG: It is an explicit task of physicians to advocate for their patients as stated in the World Medical Association Physicians Pledge (2017). But together with that important document from an ethical point of view, it is neither taken into consideration in the medical curriculum nor in the specialization schemes in most countries. Yet medical doctors in general should know and live up to the fact that they are there for the patients, not the reverse. Yet the perversity of the medical remuneration system is that the doctor gets paid for more illness and not for more health! That paradox reminds me of one of the things that I was really ashamed of when I started. The 1970s were times when money seemed to play no role. The economy was doing well in the Netherlands. And in those times, special schools were booming businesses, admitting more pupils every year. So, if someone was disruptive in the class you could send them to a special school. Those special schools now have 17% of all our pupils in the Netherlands. And I contributed greatly to the growth of special schools by saying that it was wonderful that the children were getting the special care they needed instead of challenging the mainstream schools with the question of why they had so many drop-outs. As a result, children who were struggling were discriminated against and stigmatized. But the special school were proud of figures and their directors earned more every year as their salary was dependent on how many pupils they had. At the turn of the century, I realized that I had contributed to the stigmatization these patients suffered. I had contributed to making these schools bigger and bigger whereas these schools should have disappeared and all these children should have been integrated into the mainstream system. And that is what I am advocating for now.

I: Looking back at your life, what would you tell your younger self?

RJG: Don't worry! If plan A doesn't work, there's always a plan B. But also stick to your oath and be a good doctor!

I: Looking back at your career, what would you see has been your biggest achievement?

RJG: Well, my biggest personal achievement for myself was the courage I had when I was 45 to quit the university hospital. More generally, I think that my professorship, my Presidency of the Psychiatric Association, and my Presidency of the Medical Association have all contributed to destigmatizing psychiatry. One of the things that I am committed to is destigmatizing self-stigmatization by most psychiatrists.

I: How do you mean destigmatize psychiatry?

RJG: Well, stigma is an awkward ordeal that sticks to people. Stigma about mental problems is a big deal. People feel uneasy when dealing with individuals with psychiatric illnesses and problems. And that's something that runs in many cultures. I think that psychiatrists themselves have in part contributed to this image by insisting that psychiatric diseases are very different from other diseases. This has alienated them from the medical corps. Most medical doctors are themselves afraid of psychiatric symptoms and patients. We have started self-stigmatizing ourselves and instead of being in the mainstream of healthcare, we are also seen as the odd one out.

When I opened up opportunities for psychiatrists to be reconsidered as medical doctors, they would say, 'Oh no, we are very different'. To give you a very painful example, when I was in the Medical Association, I would get calls nearly every day from a desperate doctor saying 'My wife has depression, my son is becoming schizophrenic, and I cannot get a hold of a psychiatrist'. So we set up a survey. We called 1,000 medical doctors in one morning. We found that the easiest to reach were the surgeons. We even had surgeons that were in the operating theatre and talking into the phone that some nurse was holding, but they were available. On the other hand, when we called psychiatrists, we got answering machines or their personal assistants saying, 'You will be called back'. But that never happened.

I: What would you like to be remembered for?

RJG: I don't need to be remembered. That's a politically correct answer. I would like to be remembered as someone who never gave up. One of the funny things is that I am lecturing quite a lot about Albert Einstein. Einstein said many brilliant things but one of the things that appeals the most to me in this period of my life is that you cannot solve a problem by using the same way of thinking that created it. I see that happening all the time.

In one of my new roles as President of the Association of Hospital Administrators or Governors I go to hospitals and see that they are concerned about the fact that they cannot fill all their beds because most patients can go home much sooner. I respond that their aim should be to make themselves redundant. The future is going to be different. Your hospital has to change from the buildings to caring for patients. You need to deconstruct existing structures. Learn how to deal with well-informed and assertive patients. That is really something. I may not be remembered as the one who found the solutions but as the one who didn't shy away from the problems.

Many of the problems we encounter are self-organized misery because most doctors and managers are very conservative. They tend to want to keep things as they were, instead of opening to new opportunities. So now I hope that on a bigger scale as a psychiatrist, I'll be able to help people overcome their own neurotic management strategies by thinking, 'OK, that's not the way forward, so let's think out of the box'.

I: Out of all of your achievements, what's the achievement that you are most proud of?

RJG: I don't know if it's an achievement but I think I'm most proud of the many residents that I trained.

I: Any other thoughts?

RJG: We can talk about my idols: I already mentioned Einstein. Currently I am looking in awe when I realize how Dwight Eisenhower managed to mobilize 2 million people to prepare the landing in Normandy in 1944, to which we owe our freedom. He did that by valuing people. Not the highly ranked people alone but those involved in nearly invisible activities, and he did so by convincing them that what they were doing, from digging latrines to manufacturing socks, their contribution was essential to the success of the whole operation. That is true leadership. And I could continue with many more examples. But personally I wouldn't have thrived as much if it weren't for my elementary school experiences.

I: What you have illustrated beautifully is the impact on a young mind of immigration, directly or indirectly, and dealing with different languages and different cultures and trying to come out on top. I think that experience gives one flexibility; you can think outside the box and you can ask what may appear to be silly questions.

RJG: One of the things I remember from St David's College in West Wickham was that we would do mainly school work in the morning and sports in the afternoon, every day. In the winter, we played rugby and soccer, and in the summer cricket and tennis. One of the essential things was that we had a different captain every day. As a result, I became aware that any team is as strong as its weakest link. The school was a very integrated school. In my class there was a boy with Down syndrome. Another boy had such a big head and he knew everything about all the kings of England and when they were born, whom they married, when they died. I was caned when I was seven years old, on a Friday afternoon so that I could recover over the weekend. I was caned because I made fun of that boy. Then on Monday morning, Dr Shove said, 'John was caned because he was bullying J who is not stupid! He is just different.' He was different and that was wonderful. He went on to get a PhD from Cambridge and has done very well. He contacted me once saying, 'It's so strange. I really have a touch of eccentricity but my son who has learning difficulties has been diagnosed with Asperger's and is now a learner with special needs and he won't be given the opportunities we had.' That school was a really wonderful place. And although the transitions to France and Holland were tough, I managed because I was well prepared.

I: Thank you, Rutger for sharing your thoughts and memories. It has been a real pleasure listening to you.

26
Lakshmi Vijayakumar

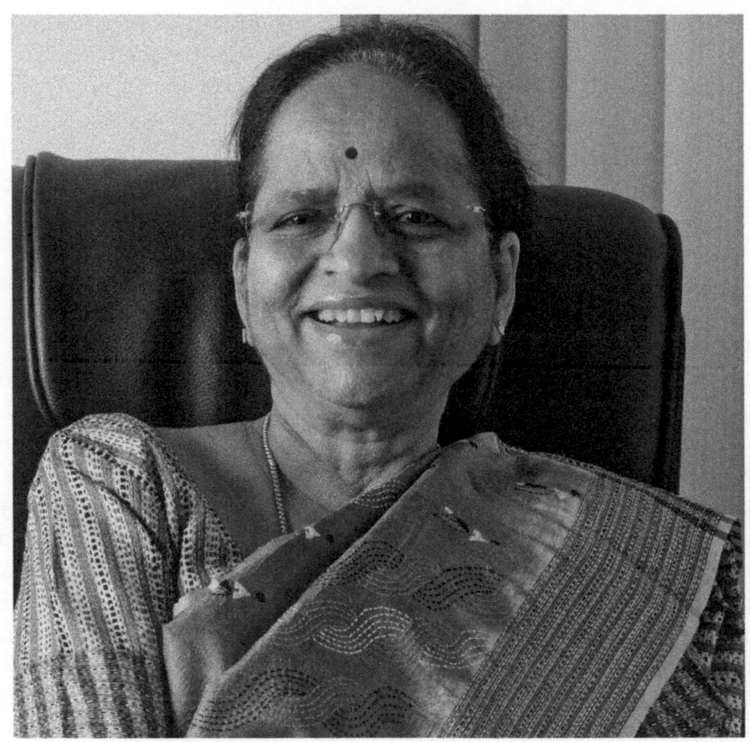

Biography

Dr Lakshmi Vijayakumar is the founder of SNEHA, an NGO in Chennai for the prevention of suicide. She is the Head, Department of Psychiatry, Voluntary Health Services, Adyar, Chennai. She is a member of the World Health Organization's International Network for Suicide Research and Prevention and the only Indian invited to be a member of the International Academy of Suicide Research. She is an Honorary Associate Professor in the University of Melbourne and University of Griffith, Australia.

She was the Vice-President of the International Association for Suicide Prevention (IASP) for four years. She was conferred an Honorary FRCPsych in 2009 for her work in suicide prevention. She was awarded the Ringel Service award by IASP in June 2015. She has been conferred Fellowship of the Royal College of Physicians of Edinburgh.

She was one of the editors of the WHO's report 'Preventing Suicide—A global imperative', published in 2014.

She has published widely in peer-reviewed journals and has authored several chapters. She is a reviewer for numerous journals. She was the editor of the book *Suicide Prevention—Meeting the Challenge Together* and co-editor of *Emergencies in Psychiatry in Low and Middle Income Countries.*

Interview

I: What was it like growing up and how did you end up doing medicine and then psychiatry?

LV: I grew up in small industrial township called Neyveli where they mine lignite. It was a multicultural society and we had good housing, electricity, abundant water, and plenty of open space to play. There was only one school called the Neyveli Boys' High School which had the only section where the language instruction was English. We had about 10 to 12 girls in each class in that boys' school. We were all hugely influenced by our teacher, S. Narayan Swami. He used to make us think and he'd give us projects. Because this teacher was teaching chemistry, I chose chemistry as an elective subject, After SSLC, I moved to Chennai to do PUC and I stayed with my uncle and aunt who were very kind to me, that is my mother's sister and my father's cousin brother were married so I stayed with them. I could have stayed in the hostel but my parents couldn't afford to pay for it. My uncle was doing extremely well at that time. He was one of those people in the 1970s who had a car, a telephone, everything but there was no special treatment, he would drop me in the car in the morning and all of us had to come back on our own. So I did one year of PUC (Pre-University) in Ethiraj College. I had not taken maths as an elective and so I chose physics, chemistry, and biology. Honestly, I was no great shakes in biology at all and I couldn't draw. I had quite a few Malaysian friends and my aunt is a very good cook, so they wanted to come home and eat home-cooked food, and in return help me with my studies. It was a short, one-year course and I think I got probably one of the top marks in physics and chemistry but I just scraped through biology with about 53% or 54%. There were no entrance exams at that time and medical admission was based on qualifying with the best percentage of marks and on the interview. The interview was held in Thanjavur and everyone said that with biology marks of 53%, compared to above 85% in chemistry and physics, there was really no chance of getting into medicine. I had never been to Thanjavur but I had read about the Thanjavur temple and I wanted to go, so I said to my father, 'I want to go for this interview. I really need to'. So my father took me and since I knew that I was not going to get medicine, I thought I'd let my father treat me so we went to a movie the day before the interview. I still remember the place; it was held in Thanjavur Medical college. There were about 100 of us for the morning session, and two or three people who checked the mark sheets. They looked at mine and said, 'Are you sure you want to attend the interview?' Everybody was asking what my marks were. I said, '53, and they started sniggering because they all got 80s and 70s. In those days nobody got 90s or 100s. So I said, 'What is the harm?

Having come, I have half a mind to leave and spend the rest of the day looking at Thanjavur'. But I decided that as I had come, I might as well go through with the interview. Happily, I was relaxed whereas everybody else was tense, reading and preparing. I went in. There were three people on the interview panel and every person got only three minutes or so. There was one guy who was sitting in the corner who asked me, 'Do you really want to do medicine? You have good scores in physics and chemistry and you got just 53% in biology. Do you really want to do medicine?' I said, 'Yes, I do.' If he had asked me in a different way, maybe I might have answered differently but he was very sarcastic and that put my back. I said, 'Yes, because I think what you are taught in PUC is pulling the legs from cockroaches and things like that, which is not medicine'. That is not how you assess a person, whether the person is fit for medicine or not, if you are able to pull a leg from a cockroach it means you may not be suitable for medicine, if you are doing that happily. So I didn't do it happily, I didn't do all these plucking things. There was a person in the middle who was bald and when I saw him, he was like one of those P.G. Wodehouse characters. He started laughing and that put the other guy out, and he obviously liked me. I was not sweaty, I was cool and I was answering like that, I said 'Yeah, that's a good point actually.' He said, 'I'm going to ask you something different' and then he said, 'There is a power plant near where you come from. Are you aware of other nuclear power plants? do you know where they are?' I said, 'Of course I know. There are three.' I gave him the three names (Kalapakkam, Bombay, and Rana Pratap Sagar) and he said, 'that's good! I asked this question to everybody; did you know that? That's great, that's wonderful' and then he asked me questions like this, very general knowledge you know, 'Okay, what kind of disease do you get when you get a dog bite?' I said, 'Rabies' he said, 'so what happens, what are the symptoms?' Hydrophobia I said. So, every time if I get stuck with a question, for example: this guy would ask me 'what is the percentage of the urea in the urine or in the blood?' and I would be blinking, this guy would say, Ok, the urea is made in the Plant in your town isn't it? Okay, who is the current chairman?' like that he would ask and then somehow, he asked 'How many baba's you know?' I said, 'I know Satya Sai Baba.' then he said 'Do you know Homi Bhabha and how he died? I said, 'Yeah, I know he died in an air crash in the Alps and the fringe in Mont Blanc' 'where have you heard of Mont Blanc and I said it's a pen so it went on like that. And then he asked me 'What kind of books do you read?' I said, 'I love P G Wodehouse' 'Oh my god! I love that too and say something from that.' I said, 'something from that, like what?' he said, 'just say something.' Then he asked me, 'Say something and let's see if my co-examiners can understand that'. I said 'You remember where the question is who is bigger-Mr Bigger or Mrs Bigger, one person said it was Mrs Bigger because she became Mrs Bigger 'so he was absolutely thrilled and then I carried on with 'who is Bigger, Mr Bigger or Master Bigger? It is Master Bigger because he is a little Bigger' and we carried on about Mr Bigger and Uncle Bigger and then the other man said, 'Sir, all these questions are fine but then this is all for literature but not for medicine' and then he said, 'No, I didn't ask her literature, PG Wodehouse is not literature, Homi Bhabha is not literature. I wanted to know the general knowledge about how the person is aware of what is happening in the world, many a time we are all concentrated on anything you know.' My interview took 25 minutes. I came out and thought that I wouldn't get in because two of my interviewers were completely unsympathetic towards me. I came back and said, 'Where do I study? What do I study?' My father was in Neyveli at the time so there were two options: I could return to Madras to do a BSc and stay at my aunt's place, or I could go to Chidambaram do a BSc there. My father and mother were a little unsure about sending me back to Madras because my cousin who had done engineering had come back and already two of my cousins were there. She was also there, adding pressure to the person, so I took up a BSc Geology in Annamalai University. I joined the local hostel but because the course was supposed to begin a month later I came home. I was chilling out at Neyveli. At that time, medical admissions were announced in the newspapers and roll numbers would appear of all the people who had been selected. My neighbour came running to me in the morning and said, 'What is your number?' and lo and behold, my number was there. I got admitted! Everyone was happy, although some people in the family told my mother that if I were educated then it would be difficult to find someone to marry me.

I: At what stage had you decided that you wanted to do medicine?

LV: To be very honest, I didn't like the Annamalai University hostel. It was very grotty. At that time I had not decided on medicine.

I: So, you went to see the place. So it wasn't that at the age of 11 that you decided that you wanted to be a doctor.

LV: No.

I: Was there some resistance from the family?

LV: Not my immediate family. It was a general concern but I wouldn't call it resistance.

I: Because you are a woman or because being well-educated may have reduced your chances of marrying?

LV: Both financially and as a woman, my parents were very supportive.

I: And did anybody say, what's a good Brahmin doing, cutting up dead bodies? Or were they quite open-minded about that?

LV: No, nothing like that. I went to Thanjavur Medical college. I studied there; I was a decent student. I won't say I was a great student, I never flunked in any of the exams and I did a lot of fun things.

I: Define fun.

LV: That was at medical college. My friend and I joined Himalayan Mountaineering Institute, climbed a peak, and went water-skiing in the Kashmir Nagin Lake. I was the sports secretary for the college.

I: I would have never thought that you were a sports person.

LV: No, but I was.

I: So, you finished medical school?

LV: I isolated myself from other people and probably started studying because I had to occupy my mind with something. So I started studying for the first time in my life in medical school and I got the medal in medicine from Thanjavur Medical College and the Medicine medal from the University of Madras. There was a lot of pressure on me to do medicine because famous professors were there. You don't win a university medal and not do medicine! I came back to Chennai and stayed with my uncle and aunt, and I joined as a senior house officer in the Madras

Medical College. A new ruling came out which said that even freshers can apply without having to do one year of a senior house officer posting.

I: You can apply for psychiatry from your first year?

LV: Apply for any post-graduation

I: OK.

I: Was the senior house officer role separate from the internship or was that the internship?

LV: No, you do internship one year, you finish it, you get your MBBS degree, then there was a requisition that you do one year as a senior house officer before you apply for any postgraduate course. Normally you do one year as a senior house officer in the speciality which you want to practice. So I joined as a senior house officer in medicine at the Madras Medical College. We finished sometime in January or February, so I joined at the end of February as a senior house officer in medicine and Professor KVT was head of department at that time, I don't know whether you have heard of him, he was the doyen of medicine here. He wanted me to join the first unit but Dr S. Balakrishnan, who was from Thanjavur, h said 'No, you must come to my unit' so I went to that second unit. I was working there for two or three months and while I was there, the rule changed, so I applied for MD General Medicine but I also chose to apply for psychiatry. At that time you could apply for general medicine in Chennai or Thanjavur, and you had two choices. So I applied for general medicine in Madras and for psychiatry in Madras (DPM in Madras). So SB asked, 'why do you want to do psychiatry?' I used to work hard (I'll tell you about an incident later which made me feel suicidal) and I was pretty clever, and because we were in Thanjavur, we had to do a lot of things by ourselves like liver biopsies, spinal taps, etc. whereas at the Madras Medical College, students had never done that. I used to be pretty popular among the interns because I used to teach them how to do intravenous injections, lumbar punctures, and all that. When we went on the rounds, SB would ask questions and I used to rattle off responses. I had all the data ready when he used to go on rounds. I was in charge of one ward and I used to do everything there. One day he looked back and asked me where a patient was from. I didn't know. After he had gone I went back round the ward asking every patient where they were from and the like. I was thinking if in three months I could be like this then I'm going to be like this forever, what am I going to do?

I: You would become more interested in disease rather than the person.

LV: Yes, and that's not why I wanted to join medicine. So I applied for psychiatry. When I applied SB asked me why and I said, 'In case I don't get into medicine'. The fact was I got MD General Medicine in Thanjavur and DPM in MMC. I didn't get the MD General Medicine at the Madras Medical College. I had the choice of going back to Thanjavur for MD General Medicine or staying in Chennai and doing DPM and I chose DPM. SB and even KVT were very upset. SB called my uncle and said, 'Is there anything wrong with this woman?' 'Why is she doing DPM when she got into MD General Medicine?' They said I should go to Thanjavur then they would get me transferred back shortly. I said, 'No, no. I want to do psychiatry.' There were two reasons for that; one is I felt I didn't deserve the university medal. I thought there were people who had worked for it for many years and deserved to have won it. So I thought that in psychiatry I'd make a clean start. And I also felt that psychiatry was more humane than anything. So I joined DPM at the Institute of Mental Health and for the first couple of months I was kicking myself because the mental hospital was not the best place to learn psychiatry; I couldn't get a grasp of it. I felt it was too unscientific. Everything was very subjective. I felt very uncomfortable for the first one or two months but it grew on me gradually. When I was able to put all the logic outside and look at patients as people suffering, I was able to connect with it more, but it took a long time.

I: And when did you decide to do PhD?

LV: That was much later.

I: Not during your training?

LV: No, not during my training.

I: Looking back, who have been your heroes or heroines, your role models?

LV: In psychiatry?

I: Medicine, psychiatry, life.

LV: That's a difficult question

I: If you look back, you mentioned professors who can't say where patients are from and well I mean it's obvious he had a very different way of looking at things.

LV: No, he was wanting to find out because somebody from his village had come.

I: OK.

LV: I didn't know who the patient was. It wasn't anything else.

I: When did you go into suicidology?

LV: That was actually partly from my senior house officer days. There was a case of cyanide overdose, a young man who was unlucky in love. He was a goldsmith and he had eaten cyanide in a banana. Everyone thought nobody could do anything to help, but I rushed him to IMCU. The senior house officer was there and he said, 'What do we do for cyanide poisoning?' I remember reading in a novel that they gave sodium thiosulfate to a case of cyanide poisoning. So I said, 'I remember reading that sodium thiosulfate helps but I don't remember anything else.' He said, 'Whatever it is, sign for it and get it from the biochemistry department.' So I got it, we mixed it, and we gave it to him. The fact is he survived. This is the only case of cyanide poisoning in Madras Medical College up until today who survived. Maybe it's because he had taken such a tiny amount, or maybe because he ate it with a banana, or it was thiosulfate that saved him. For the first time in the history of Madras Medical College, as a junior, senior house officer, I was asked to present this case in the clinical meeting. Once he had recovered, the guy was always very friendly towards me, the family was grateful, and he felt ashamed of what he had done. He said that it was a moment, look at all my family, how much they care for me, things like that. I think that incident has always made me think about what decisions people make when they are in despair, and how a life could be saved despite that. That has been at the back of my mind all the time. Another thing was that one of my friends from college who was a very bright student attempted suicide. I could never figure out why. We were all friends, he could have talked to us easily. What made him do that? That has also remained with me for a long time.

I: At what point did you decide to establish 'SNEHA'?

LV: While I was studying psychiatry, I realized that nobody was dealing with mental retardation and at that time we had hardly any medication for schizophrenia, we only had chlorpromazine, haloperidol, and amitriptyline; it was all pretty depressing. I felt that we may not be able to prevent retardation but we can prevent suicide. Why was no-one looking at this? And so I started reading more about suicide and the only cases I read about involved elderly white males living alone, being depressed, who die by suicide whereas what we saw was young people living in families, impulsive, no depression or anything like that. I collected some data. There was an international conference on suicide prevention in Vienna in 1983 or 1985. I sent a paper saying, 'How different it is down here' and they accepted it and I went to present the paper in Vienna. There were a lot of people who were saying 'we are running this; we are running that.' I went with Vijaykumar and we wanted to convert the trip into a kind of a holiday. We had never been to Europe before. So we went to Vienna and stayed with friends and then went to London to meet some of Vijaykumar's friends. In Vienna, during coffee break, there were a lot of meetings in German going on. I was outside and there was a lady having coffee, Vanda Scott. We started talking and she said, 'We really liked your paper very much. I have seen similar things in Hong Kong. I'm now working for the Befrienders International, so why don't you look at some of the other centres? Why don't you visit some of the Samaritan branches in England?' So I went! Vijaykumar grumbled: 'What is this? This is supposed to be a holiday.' We went on to visit the Samaritans branches in Manchester, in London, and at its headquarters in Slough where the secretariat was. I was really thrilled because I felt suicide was also a social issue and unless we have a social objective and get society involved, we are not going to make any headway. I was quite enthused about it and I came back and I said to Vijyakumar that we should start something. He agreed. 'Let's get a group of people together.' Vijyakumar and I were there. We had two clinical psychologists working with us so we called them. Vijyakumar's cousin was interested as well as Nalli (a famous business person and philanthropist in Chennai), so we called them all to the clinic in Santhome and told them that we should start a suicide prevention centre. Everybody agreed. Nalli gave 25,000 rupees as seed funding. I wrote to the Samaritans and Befrienders International and they introduced us to Meena Dadha. I called her. We made Nalli the President, Meena the Secretary, and me as Director. Nobody would give us a place because of the stigma attached to the issue. Then one gentleman suggested a place which belongs to Krishna Premi, one of the Gurus. I went and prostrated myself before him. Fortunately, it was R. Kuppuwami's property and he donated it to us. It was an absolute wreck; it didn't even have a toilet. So the first job I did after fixing the rent at 1,500 rupees a month was to sweep, clean the cobwebs, wipe the floor, get the place ready. That was how we started. After a few months, we didn't have rent for the next month. I still remember when Vinay (her son, now a psychiatrist) was about three or four years old had very high fever but we needed money. I stayed outside a businessman's office for three hours, with my unwell son, before he would see me. Then he told me that he couldn't help because he didn't believe in the cause. Fortunately someone else agreed to help and that's how we started. We had a lot of financial issues.

I: Looking back, what would you have done differently?

LV: There was a lot of opposition to starting SNEHA. People said, 'You can't run an organization with volunteers, you have to have professionals.' I don't know what I would have done differently

I: Did you find being a woman was an asset or problem, or didn't it make any difference?

LV: I don't think it made a difference. Maybe I'm blind to people being not gender sensitive but I think when I'm focused, I don't care what other people think as long as I get the job done.

I: Looking back, how do you think psychiatry has changed in your lifetime?

LV: It has changed. Some degree of stigma has decreased. Earlier, when I started making a living by practising psychiatry, you would ask a patient if there was any mental illness in the family and they would deny it. Now, people are more open about it. The stigma still exists among the faculty, though. And there are definitely more effective treatment options available these days.

I: If you were redesigning the curriculum at undergraduate and postgraduate levels, what would you see as the major issues?

LV: It's high time we stop emphasizing mitral stenosis, mitral incompetence, murmurs, etc. and talk about how to interact with clients, communication styles with the clients, how to deal with family members of the patient. None of these are taught at all. And also, we should make psychiatry an important component of undergraduate training because 25% of people whom they see have psychological issues and patients are badly managed. They just prescribe benzodiazepines for everything, whether it is psychosis or anxiety or personality disorders.

I: One thing that I'm concerned about is that we don't teach ethics. We don't teach probity, and particularly for psychiatry patients there are questions of boundary violations and vulnerability.

LV: Even in comparative positions, the responsibility of the psychiatrists is to be more ethical because you are dealing with people who are much more vulnerable and marginalized than other people. When I started I said, 'There's no science in psychiatry.' And I was very upset for the first few months but now the more I practise psychiatry, I see that science is of no use unless it is coupled with humanity. Science has no meaning unless it is paired with humanity.

I: You mean humanity or humanities?

LV: Humanity, humanities, humaneness.

I: Do you see psychiatry as mindless or brainless?

LV: I think right now we are focusing on the biology of the brain and not thinking about the mind. I think that should change.

I: How would you describe or define a good psychiatrist?

LV: Somebody who is empathetic, has knowledge and skills, and who will be ethical, and who will treat me as if I am his family member, and who would safeguard me.

I: So it's not only as a family member but also about caring and it's also about compassion?

LV: That's what I mean.

I: We have touched on gaps in practices and training. What do you think psychiatry's social contract should be? How can it be delivered?

LV: I feel that every psychiatrist should spare some amount of time away from the clinic and get into the community. Even if you are able to spend just 10% of your time away from the clinic and in the community, you would make a difference in the community.

I: If you were writing a letter to your younger self. What would you write?

LV: That's a tough one. I would say don't waste so much time over what other people say you can and cannot do or what they think of you. If you believe in something, just get on with it, be grateful for what you have. I would probably also say that we are much narrower-minded when we are young, so I wish I had been more inclusive. I think I'm a little bit more inclusive now than I was when I was young. Be open to people, suggestions, ideas. We think young people have a lot of ideas but it's actually not so. They are so much worn by their peers and things like. They need approval from their peers.

I: I find that the training system in India, as in many other countries, is such that you do what your boss tells you. When I talk to younger trainees in India, it appears that it is the boss who decides what project they do, what research they do. There appears to be no innovation in that sense.

LV: True.

I: What would you like to be remembered for?

LV: A decent human being is good enough.

I: And which of your achievements are you most proud of?

LV: I think starting SNEHA, definitely.

I: In your clinical practice as well as policy development, you have had a major influence on national policy in this country in trying to get act of suicide decriminalized. That is a huge achievement by any measure. But if you look back into your career, what were the 'Eureka!' moments which really left a lasting impression on you?

LV: Three things. Apart from the policy of decriminalisation, I was working hard to make a policy change of having a supplementary exam for those who had failed in their board exams. Many students died by suicide due to failure in exams. I worked very hard with a lot of the media. We put pressure on the government by carrying news stories of failing in exams which led to acts of suicide. We did a small research project and found that people who failed in one or two subjects with minimum marks were more likely to carry out suicidal acts. We pushed the government and made a hue and cry and because of the constant media pressure and pressure from us, the Tamil Nadu government was the first government to introduce the supplementary exams for those who had failed in class 10 and 12. These students could retake their exams within the following one or two months so they didn't lose out on an entire year. We showed that exam failure suicide rates dropped significantly and neighbouring states have taken this on as well. *The Economist* reported this as a real success story. I am very happy to have been involved with this, as it has shown direct results in terms of reduction in exam failure suicides.

I: You said there were three things.

LV: SNEHA, these two policy issues. I think also, to a smaller extent, working with Diego de Leo on the formation of World Suicide Prevention Day. The first poster for World Suicide Prevention Day was from Chennai and we printed it and took it to Stockholm.

I: Thanks very much for your time and sharing the story.

Index

For the benefit of digital users, indexed terms that span two pages (e.g., 52–53) may, on occasion, appear on only one of those pages